Risk Factors
and Multiple Cancer

WILEY SERIES ON
NEW HORIZONS IN ONCOLOGY

Series Editor

Basil A. Stoll

(St Thomas' Hospital and Royal Free Hospital, London)

NEW HORIZONS IN ONCOLOGY
VOLUME 3

Risk Factors and

Multiple Cancer

Edited by

BASIL A. STOLL

*Honorary Consulting Physician to Oncology Departments,
St Thomas' Hospital and Royal Free Hospital, London*

A Wiley Medical Publication

JOHN WILEY & SONS
Chichester · New York · Brisbane · Toronto · Singapore

Library of Congress Cataloging in Publication Data:
Main entry under title:

Risk factors and multiple cancer.

   (New horizons in oncology; v. 3) (A Wiley medical
publication)
   Includes index.
   1. Cancer—Addresses, essays, lectures. 2. Multiple
tumors—Addresses, essays, lectures. I. Stoll, Basil
Arnold. II. Series: Wiley series on new horizons in
oncology; v. 3. III. Series: Wiley medical publication.
[DNLM: 1. Neoplasms, Multiple primary—Etiology. 2.
Neoplasms, Multiple primary—Occurrence. W1
WI53R v. 3]
RC265.R57 1984   616.99′4071   83-21585

ISBN 0 471 10513 9

British Library Cataloguing in Publication Data:
Risk factors and multiple cancer.—(New horizons in
   oncology; v.3).—(A Wiley publication)
   1. Cancer—Genetic factors—Addresses, essays, lectures
   I. Stoll, Basil A. II. Berenblum, Isaac III. Series
   616.99′042   RC268.4

   ISBN 0 471 10513 9

Typeset by Photo-Graphics, Honiton, Devon.
Printed by Pitman Press Ltd., Bath, Avon.

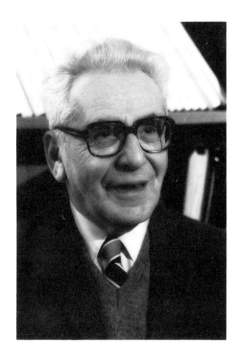

This commemorative volume
is dedicated with affection to

PROFESSOR ISAAC BERENBLUM

on his eightieth birthday.

A tribute to his pioneering research which laid the
foundations for many concepts expressed in this
book.

Contributors

Bruce K. Armstrong, DPhil, FRACP
Director, NH & MRC Research Unit in Epidemiology and Preventive Medicine, University Department of Medicine, Nedlands, Western Australia

J. G. Azzopardi, BSc, MD, FRCPath
Professor of Oncology, Honorary Consultant in Histopathology, Royal Postgraduate Medical School, Hammersmith Hospital, London, UK

Hugh R. K. Barber, MD
Professor and Chairman, Department of Obstetrics and Gynecology, New York Medical College, New York, USA

Isaac Berenblum, MD
Professor, Department of Experimental Biology, Weizmann Institute, Rehovot, Israel

W. H. Butler, MB BS, FRCPath
Assistant Director and Chief Pathologist, British Industrial Biological Research Association, Carshalton, UK

Gerrit DeBoer, BSc, MSc, PhD
Head of Biostatistics Department, Ontario Cancer Institute, Toronto, Ontario, Canada

Jerome J. DeCosse, MD, PhD
Chairman, Department of Surgery, Memorial Sloan-Kettering Cancer Center, New York, USA

H. Elizabeth Driver, BSc, MB BS
Scientific Staff, Toxicology Unit, MRC Laboratories, Carshalton, UK

Peter J. Fitzpatrick, FRCP(C), FRCR
Associate Professor of Radiology, Princess Margaret Hospital, Toronto, Ontario, Canada

Hans W. Grünwald, MD, FACP
Chief, Division of Hematology, Queens Hospital Center, and Associate Professor of Medicine, NY University at Stony Brook, New York, USA

Curtis C. Harris, MD
Chief, Laboratory of Human Carcinogenesis, National Cancer Institute, National Institutes of Health, Bethesda, Maryland, USA

A. R. Harwood, MB, ChB, FRCP(C)
Staff Radiation Oncologist, Princess Margaret Hospital, Toronto, Ontario, Canada

R. J. Heald, FRCS
Consultant Surgeon, Basingstoke District Hospital, Basingstoke, UK

B. Herity, MB, DPH, FFCMI
Lecturer, Department of Community Medicine and Epidemiology, University College, Dublin, Eire

M. J. Hill, PhD, MRCPath
Director, Bacterial Metabolism Research Laboratory, PHLS Centre, Porton Down, Salisbury, UK

T. Krausz, MD, MRCPath
Lecturer, Department of Histopathology, Royal Postgraduate Medical School, Hammersmith Hospital, London, UK

Henry M. Lemon, MD
Professor of Medicine, Section of Oncology/Hematology, Department of Internal Medicine, University of Nebraska Medical Center, Omaha, Nebraska, USA

G. W. Milton, FRCS, FRACS
Professor, Department of Surgery, University of Sydney, Director of Melanoma Unit, Sydney Hospital, NSW, Australia

Paul L. Moots, MD
Department of Neurology, University of Virginia Hospital, Charlottesville, Virginia, USA

Michael P. Osborne, MD, MS, FRCS
Department of Surgery, Memorial Sloan-Kettering Cancer Center, New York, USA

B. A. J. Ponder, PhD, MRCP
CRC Fellow and Honorary Consultant Physician, Institute of Cancer Research and Royal Marsden Hospital, Sutton, UK

James A. Recabaren, MD
Department of Surgery, Memorial Sloan-Kettering Cancer Center, New York, USA

Fred Rosner, MD, FACP
Director of Medicine, Queens Hospital Center and Professor of Medicine, NY University at Stony Brook, New York, USA

Lucien J. Rubinstein, MD
Professor of Pathology, Director, Division of Neuropathology, University of Virginia School of Medicine, Charlottesville, Virginia, USA

A. Scheibner, MBBS
Research Fellow, Sydney Hospital, NSW, Australia

S. M. Sieber, PhD
Office of the Director, Division of Cancer Cause and Prevention, National Cancer Institute, National Institutes of Health, Bethesda, Maryland, USA

Barry S. Tepperman, BSc, MD, FRCP(C)
Department of Radiation Oncology, Princess Margaret Hospital, Toronto, Ontario, Canada

M. H. Thompson, PhD
Deputy Director, Bacterial Metabolism Research Laboratory, PHLS Centre, Porton Down, Salisbury, UK

Robin A. Weiss, PhD
Director, Institute of Cancer Research, Royal Cancer Hospital, Chester Beatty Laboratories, London, UK

J. Whang-Peng, MD
Chief, Cytogenetic Oncology Section, Medical Oncology Branch, Division of Cancer Treatment, National Cancer Institute, NIH, Bethesda, Maryland, USA

James C. Willey, MD
Medical Staff Fellow, National Cancer Institute, National Institutes of Health, Bethesda, Maryland, USA

N. A. Wright, MD, PhD, MRCPath
Professor and Director of Histopathology, Royal Postgraduate Medical School, Hammersmith, London, UK

Contents

Preface to Series

The series is intended to extend the horizons of the very large number of clinicians engaged in the management of the cancer patient. The books will provide a meeting ground between the scientist engaged in research and the practising clinician. The intention is to bridge their divergent philosophy and language so as to provide the clinician with an authoritative and balanced interpretation of new scientific findings and thinking, and to *orientate it specifically to its possible application to the clinical problem.*

Each volume will select a particular aspect of the cancer problem where recent research has suggested a pressing need for new perspectives in the clinical field. It is intended that each volume will be complete in itself.

Preface to Volume 3

In order to recognize those individuals and families at high risk of cancer, the clinician needs to be brought up to date on the multiple environmental and host factors now known to predispose to malignant disease. The rapidly developing knowledge in this field is, however, spread over a wide spectrum of specialized publications, reflecting the diversity of disciplines involved in the study of carcinogenesis, preneoplasia, cytogenetics, cancer epidemiology and aetiology.

For this reason, it was thought appropriate to ask recognized authorities on both sides of the Atlantic to review recent research in their fields, with particular reference to its clinical application. This selective approach is needed because of the highly technical nature of much of the literature on the mechanisms of tumour promotion, markers of carcinogenesis in molecular and cell culture test systems and in mammalian models, and statistical analysis of epidemiological data.

An increasingly common cancer risk in recent years is the manifestation of second primary and multicentric cancers. Recognition of this risk poses important practical questions. Is more effective treatment of a first tumour now resulting in patients surviving long enough to manifest a second primary tumour? Does the presence of the first primary tumour delay development of another, so that removal of the first leads to activation of a second tumour? To what extent could a second tumour be stimulated by the radiation or cytotoxic agent therapy which has been used in treating the first tumour? How often are multiple tumours in the same tissue or organ phenotypically different, and thus likely to respond differently to the same therapeutic agent? Should wide excision be undertaken of suspected precancerous change in contiguous tissue, or can the changes be reversed by newly developing chemopreventive agents?

Evidence is accumulating that some carcinogens are able to switch the same oncogene in more than one organ, thus predisposing to either synchronous or metachronous multiple primary cancers. In addition, various stages in the progression to cancer may be occurring simultaneously in several foci in the same organ or tissue. Further investigation of these new findings in the genesis of multiple cancers, will need close cooperation between clinicians on the one hand, and scientific investigators such as geneticists, epidemiologists, biochemists, and pathologists. It is hoped that this book may encourage such collaboration by setting out some of the problems requiring clarification.

In the interests of clarity, and in order to make each chapter complete in itself, some small points of overlap have been permitted between some of the chapters. I am most grateful to the contributors for the enthusiasm and critical thoughtfulness which they brought to their topics.

London, 1984   BASIL A. STOLL

Part 1

Carcinogenic factors

Risk Factors and Multiple Cancer
Edited by B.A. Stoll
© 1984 John Wiley and Sons Ltd.

Chapter

1   ISAAC BERENBLUM

Two-Stage Carcinogenesis and Multiple Cancers

INTRODUCTION

At the time when human cancer was believed to be a spontaneous, single process of indeterminate nature, the study of multiple primary tumours dealt largely with the question of whether they arose more frequently than could be accounted for by chance. When such multiple tumours were found, they were ascribed to a hereditary predisposition or alternatively to a breakdown of homeostatic mechanisms brought about by the presence of the first tumour. In short, multiple primary tumours were considered a departure from the standard.

This concept has become largely invalid in the light of new knowledge coming mainly from animal experiments, but partly also from epidemiological investigations in humans. Our present view derives from (a) recognition of the various kinds of carcinogens and their different organ specificities; (b) recognition of the initiation–promotion mechanism of carcinogenesis, and its likely impact on human cancer development; (c) recognition that contrary to previous belief, human cancer is predominantly determined by environmental factors. (The term 'environment' is used in its broadest sense, to include not only true carcinogens but also habits, diet, and other precipitating or cocarcinogenic factors.)

Instead of continuing to examine the statistical probability of multiple primary tumours, it is now possible to look at the problem in terms of mechanisms. We can use the evidence derived from basic studies as a guide to the interpretation of the clinical findings.

MECHANISMS IN CARCINOGENESIS

While it is generally assumed that a common mechanism exists for all forms of carcinogenesis – whether by physical, chemical, or viral action – each class of carcinogen (even among the different chemical agents) seems to act in a unique way in reaching the ultimate goal. This apparent paradox is resolved when we consider information derived from animal experiments about the steps involved in the different systems.

The various classes of carcinogens can be distinguished according to (a) their diverse chemical compositions and reactivities; (b) their metabolic fate in the body with respect to activation and/or detoxication; (c) their interactions with cellular constituents; (d) their specificity of action with respect to the different tissues and organs in the body; (e) their slow speed of action or long latent period of carcinogenesis; (f) their somewhat limited effects, taking into account the various kinds of 'permissive' influences as dominant factors in the ultimate development of a tumour. Since the final outcome is a resultant of so many conflicting factors, to regard cancer risk as a single issue is to confuse the problem.

Without going into detail about the chemistry of carcinogenic agents (for reviews, see Arcos *et al.*, 1968, and *IARC Monographs*, 1972–1982), we need to distinguish two major classes of carcinogens with respect to their reactivities with cell constituents: (a) tumour-inducing agents that are relatively non-reactive chemically (better known as 'procarcinogens'), requiring metabolic activation in the body, to convert them into chemically reactive 'ultimate' carcinogens (Miller and Miller, 1981); (b) the highly reactive alkylating agents that do not need prior metabolic or chemical activation (Lawley, 1976).

One might have expected alkylating agents to be the more effective tumour-inducing agents but in fact, they are all very weak carcinogens. This is no doubt due to their capacity to react with so many other constituents in the body, leaving only traces to reach the critical sites in the cell (e.g. the DNA of the nucleus) where the carcinogenic action is to occur. This is in contrast to ultimate metabolites of procarcinogens which are supposedly activated at the sites of the carcinogenic action.

The reason for stressing the metabolic activation of procarcinogens is that they can also undergo metabolic detoxication in the body, so that the effective potency of the majority of carcinogens depends on a balance (varying in degree under different conditions) between activation and detoxication. This is one of the reasons why the potency of a carcinogenic agent cannot be defined in absolute terms.

Another way of classifying chemical carcinogens – this time in functional rather than metabolic terms – is by recognizing three major categories: (a) those, like benzpyrene and other polycyclic aromatic hydrocarbons, which are potentially carcinogenic for all tissues; (b) those, like β-naphthylamine and aflatoxin, which are essentially single-organ carcinogens (for the urinary bladder and liver, respectively); (c) an intermediate group, like the nitrosamines, which are carcinogenic for a strictly limited number of tissues or organs.

Multiple tumours may involve either multiplicity in the same tissue or organ (e.g. multiple tumours of the skin, colon or urinary bladder, bilateral breast cancer, or multiple foci of occult carcinoma in the prostate) or multiplicity affecting several different tissues or organs. The distinction between totipotential, multipotential, and unipotential carcinogens should help to distinguish the different kinds of responses.

Multiplicity of neoplastic response is more common in laboratory animals than in humans for several reasons:

1. Animals used in cancer research are mostly of pure, genetically inbred, strains that respond more uniformly to various stimuli than do random-bred animals. Responsiveness also tends to be very much exaggerated, both positively and negatively, in inbred animals. Thus, some strains of mice have an extremely high incidence of spontaneous tumours, while others have a very low incidence (e.g. close to 100% mammary cancer in C3H mice, in contrast to less than 1% in C57BL mice). The same, though to a lesser degree, applies to responsiveness to extrinsic carcinogenic action, with the likelihood of multiple tumours in the high-responsive strains. The human counterpart to genetically inbred animals is a pair of identical twins, but there is insufficient information about the latter's response to carcinogenic action in comparison with human responses in general (but see Schull and Weiss, 1982).

2. In animals, carcinogens are usually administered under optimal conditions, with consequent high tumour yields and usually more than one tumour per animal. In humans, even under extreme conditions (e.g. in the case of industrial exposure) carcinogenic action is rarely optimal.

3. The conflicting relationship between the long latent period of carcinogenesis and the survival time after appearance of the first tumour. While benign tumours are commonly multiple in humans and animals, in the case of malignant tumours a second tumour is less likely to develop if the survival time after the first tumour is short, because of the long latent period of development of subsequent tumours.

When one considers the separate 'initiating' and 'promoting' components of carcinogenesis, the problem becomes even more complex, though providing a better insight into the intricate mechanism of tumour induction. A short account of the two-stage, initiation–promotion, principle may help to explain the carcinogenic process in basic terms, its precise role in the general scheme of 'cocarcinogenic' influences, and its relevance to human cancer.

Recognition of modifying factors in carcinogenesis, nowadays referred to as 'cocarcinogenic' influences, dates back to the early studies of tar carcinogenesis. For a review of the various modifying influences and the different kinds of cocarcinogenic action, see Berenblum (1969). One form of cocarcinogenic action, known as promoting action, arose from two independent lines of enquiry: one, attempting to verify the neoplastic nature of regressing papillomas in rabbit skin (Rous and Kidd, 1941; Friedewald and Rous, 1944); the other, trying to explain the mechanism of action of the newly discovered cocarcinogen for mouse skin, croton oil (Berenblum, 1941 a,b). Both studies led to the recognition of two separate stages in carcinogenesis: tumour initiation, converting a normal cell into a 'dormant' tumour cell; followed by tumour promotion causing the 'awakening' of the dormant tumour cell and leading to progressive tumour growth.

But more important than the mere recognition of independent components of carcinogenesis is the fact that initiation and promotion differ considerably in their modes of induction, their mechanisms of action, and the way they can be affected by various host factors (age, sex, genetic constitution, hormonal status, and immunological functions) or by extrinsic influences (diet, habits, etc.).

Tumour initiators act very rapidly, a single application being sufficient under experimental conditions to produce the effect. Tumour promoters, on the other hand, act very slowly, covering the greater part of the long latent period of carcinogenesis. Effective tumour induction results only when initiating action *precedes* promoting action, *not in reverse order*. Initiating action is essentially an irreversible process, causing a mutational change in the DNA of the cell. The effect of promoting action becomes irreversible only in its late stages. Its mode of action is not yet properly understood, though a number of possible schemes have been proposed, based on experimental analytical studies (for reviews see Boutwell, 1978; Weinstein *et al.*, 1979). In the case of oncogenic viruses, initiating action would seem to result from incorporation of parts of their nucleic acid components into the DNA of the cell. Thus, unlike the action of chemical or physical initiators which produce a change in the existing cellular DNA, viral initiation represents added genetic information to the cellular DNA.

More detailed information about the two-stage mechanism of carcinogenesis in the more extensively studied systems is outside the scope of this chapter. (See reviews by Berenblum (1982) relating to skin; Pitot (1982) and Farber (1981) for liver; Hicks *et al.* (1978) for urinary bladder; Heidelberger (1980) and Diamond *et al.* (1980) for two-stage transformation in tissue culture.) Information on two-stage carcinogenesis in humans is largely derived from epidemiological studies (Higginson, 1980; Peto, 1982), while recent evidence comes from *in vitro* follow-up studies of 'initiated' dormant tumour cells, in the intestinal mucosa of patients known to be excessively prone to colon cancer (Kopelovich, 1982). The above brief account makes it apparent that factors influencing the development of multiple primary tumours will function very differently in relation to initiation or promotion.

INITIATION, PROMOTION, AND MULTIPLE CANCER

Hypothetically, all mutagens should be effective tumour initiators, and as far as the available evidence goes, this seems to be the case. (The *in vitro* 'Ames test' for carcinogenesis (Ames *et al.*, 1975) is based on the presumption that a mutagenic effect, demonstrable even in a bacterial system, should serve as a reliable indication of tumour initiation, if not actually of total carcinogenesis.) It should nevertheless be stressed that not all somatic cell mutations are necessarily capable of functioning as tumour initiators. Errors in cellular DNA caused by mutagenic action, can be enzymatically repaired (Cleaver, 1973; Trosko and Chu, 1975). Significantly, the disease xeroderma pigmentosum, in which multiple cancers of the skin result from even mild exposures to sunlight, has been shown to be due to absence of the specific enzyme system capable of repairing errors in cellular DNA (Setlow, 1975).

The discrepancy between the postulated frequency of somatic cell mutations and the rarity of multiple tumours in humans could be accounted for in several ways: (a) the proportion of 'tumour' mutations to total mutations might be very small; (b) repair of damaged DNA might operate more commonly than is generally supposed; (c) since promoting action rarely functions to an optimal degree, a majority of dormant tumour cells might remain dormant; (d) other kinds of cocarcinogenic (and anticarcinogenic) influences might affect the outcome of carcinogenic action; (e) homeostatic mechanisms – notably hormonal and immunological – might act as determining factors; (f) survival time after the first appearance of a tumour might be too short to allow subsequent tumours to become clinically apparent.

Before evaluating each of these possibilities, it should be noted that the term 'frequency' whether applied to mutations or tumours, has a different meaning according to whether it is considered in terms of the cells at risk (in which case both are rare phenomena) or in terms of body response (in which case mutations are quite common while tumours are relatively infrequent).

If the infrequency of multiple tumours were due to rarity of tumour mutations, then this should apply to benign as well as to malignant tumours. The fact that multiple benign tumours are not uncommon in humans, renders this explanation of the discrepancy untenable.

That the repair mechanism of damaged DNA might be responsible, is partly borne out by the evidence, already referred to, of multiple skin cancers among those suffering from xeroderma pigmentosum. More information, with respect to other forms of cancer, would be needed before any general conclusion could be reached about the importance of repair mechanisms in relation to multiple primary tumours in humans (Rasmussen, 1980).

The possibility of ineffective promoting or other cocarcinogenic influences (items (c) and (d) above) being responsible for the relative rarity of multiple tumours, calls for deeper consideration. There is ample evidence, from animal experiments, in support of the crucial role of promoting action in carcinogenesis. In mouse skin, for instance, initiating action without subsequent promoting action, is almost totally ineffective in producing tumours; and in the two-stage set-up, many months' delay in the start of promoting action results in a commensurate delay in the appearance of tumours *without significantly affecting the final yield*. Similar results are obtained in other tissues by systemic instead of topical administration of initiators and promoters, though not always so clear-cut in terms of quantitative response.

One of the stumbling blocks in studying *systemic* two-stage carcinogenesis is how to distinguish between true initiation–promotion and other forms of cocarcinogenesis. The difference is important, but while it can be differentiated under experimental conditions, it is likely to cause confusion in human studies. As already mentioned, tumour promotion causes the awakening of dormant tumour cells, after completion of initiating action. Other forms of cocarcinogenesis operate *concurrently* with subeffective carcinogenic action during different stages of the overall process. They may do so in a variety of ways, e.g. by influencing the activation or detoxication of procarcinogens; by facilitating penetration of the ultimate carcinogen into the cell; by changing the sensitivity of the cell; by influencing the potential activity of a causative oncogenic virus; or by influencing normal control mechanisms.

One example of such difficulties in interpretation in human carcinogenesis, is the synergism that exists between inhalation of asbestos dust and cigarette smoking in the development of lung cancer. It is still not certain which of the two is the initiator and which the promoter, or whether the synergism constitutes some other kind of cocarcinogenesis. Similar difficulties in interpretation arise in connection with the low incidence of breast cancer among Japanese women in Japan compared to the second and third generations of Japanese women in the United States who tend to have a high incidence of breast cancer similar to that of other women in the USA. In this case, the high fat diet in Western society is held responsible for the difference, the effect being thought to be an indirect one, by induced changes in the hormonal balance in the body (Carroll, 1975).

HOMEOSTATIC MECHANISMS AND CARCINOGENESIS

This brings us to the issue of homeostatic mechanisms (notably hormonal and immunological) as controlling factors in carcinogenesis, both with respect to tumour incidence and multiple tumour development.

To what extent do hormones influence tumour growth, more particularly the induction process? Whereas most of the experimental findings deal with augmentation of tumour induction in response to artificial hormonal stimulation, clinical information on hormonal influences relates more to inhibitory influences on tumour development, and indirectly, on the chances of such tumours being multiple. The limitations of hormonal influences on tumour induction and development refer to (a) such influences being most pronounced in tissues and organs that are normally under strong hormonal influence; and (b) the fact that tumours that are originally hormone-dependent tend eventually to become hormone-independent, a process known as tumour progression (Foulds, 1954, 1969).

As would be expected, hormonal influences operate very differently during the various stages of carcinogenesis. As far as the *initiating* phase of carcinogenesis is concerned, certain hormones can theoretically exert an influence, by virtue of the fact that mutagenic action is most effective during the mitotic cycle of cell division (Iversen, 1974; Berenblum and Armuth, 1977). When, therefore, proliferative activity is normally under hormonal control (e.g. in mammary tissue), the induction of tumour cells is, to some degree, conditioned by the hormonal balance in the body. Another possible effect of hormones on the initiating phase of carcinogenesis might be in the control of enzymic repair of damaged DNA, though this is purely speculative. That initiating action is not actually dependent on the endocrine system, is evident from the fact that neoplastic transformation of cells is readily brought about *in vitro*.

During the *promoting* stage of carcinogenesis, hormonal influences undoubtedly have greater scope, if only because of the long latent period during which tumour promotion operates. There is, at the same time, a complication here, in so far as hormones may themselves act as tumour promoters, apart from their ability to influence the action of other promoters. It is unfortunately not always possible to distinguish between the two kinds of action, and apart from drawing attention to it, no conclusions can be drawn from the fact that two alternative influences exist. The difference is nevertheless important, both for our understanding of mechanisms of action, and in practice as a guide to cancer prevention.

Indirect evidence of hormonal influence in carcinogenesis is obtained from sex differences in tumour incidence for different organs, and of changes in pattern resulting from gonadectomy. More direct evidence is derived from animal experiments, pointing to influences on the development of cancers of the breast, uterus, ovary, testis, prostate, liver, thyroid, and pituitary; also of the colon, salivary gland, pancreas, and melanoma. (For reviews see Furth, 1982, and Armstrong, 1982.) Though not all the evidence points specifically to the promoting phase as the stage during which the hormonal effects operate, this can be inferred in most cases.

The postulated mechanisms listed by Armstrong (1982) include: (a) facilitation or inhibition of the endogenous production of carcinogens; (b)

effects on the metabolic activation or inactivation of carcinogens; (c) alteration of the susceptibility of tissues to the initiation of cancer; (d) promotion of
the development of clinical cancer from initiated cells; (e) alteration of the
body's capacity to eliminate initiated cells. Only (d) and (e) involve the
promoting phase of carcinogenesis.

There is, in addition, the possibility of a hormonal influence operating
during the post-promotion stage of carcinogenesis, affecting the growth of
hormone-dependent tumours. A particularly striking example of this was the
early report by Foulds (1949) of alternating growth phases during successive
pregnancies, and regression phases between pregnancies, of hormone-
dependent mammary tumours in mice.

A somewhat different picture emerges from the other postulated
homeostatic control of carcinogenesis, known as the immunosurveillance of
tumours (Foley, 1953), postulated that most neoplastically transformed cells
based on the discovery of tumour-specific antigens in chemically induced
tumours (Folwy, 1953), postulated that most neoplastically transformed cells
(initiated dormant tumour cells) were destroyed in the body by circulating
antibodies elicited by the newly acquired tumour antigens, and that only
those tumours that somehow slipped through the immunological barrier,
developed into clinically recognized progressively growing tumours. Its
possible relevance to the control of multiple tumours is obvious.

Unfortunately, this attractive theory did not hold up to subsequent critical
analysis (see Prehn, 1971; Baldwin, 1973; Möller and Möller, 1975; Allison,
1975). Only in the case of virally induced tumours did immunosurveillance
seem to operate to some extent, and this may possibly explain the prevalence
of lymphoid tumours among patients subjected to immunodepression in
connection with tissue transplantation (Penn, 1978).

CONCLUSION

Consideration of the problem of multiple primary tumours has in the past
been prejudiced by the belief that multiplicity was an abnormal phenomenon,
instead of accepting the fact that response to carcinogenic action is generally
conducive to the development of multiple tumours. It is its comparative rarity
in humans which is something abnormal and which calls for explanation.

REFERENCES

Allison, A. C. (1975). Immunological Surveillance Against Tumor Cells. In *Cancer:
A Comprehensive Treatise*, Vol. 4 (ed. F. F. Becker). New York and London:
Plenum Press, p. 237.
Ames, B. N., McCann, J., and Yamasaki, E. (1975). Methods for Detecting
Carcinogens and Mutagens with the Salmonella/Mammalian-Microsome
Mutagenicity Test. *Mutation Research*, **31**, 347.

Arcos, J. C., Argus, M. F., and Wolf, G. (1968). *Chemical Induction of Cancer: Structural Bases and Biological Mechanisms*. New York and London: Academic Press.

Armstrong, B. (1982). Endocrine Factors in Human Carcinogenesis. *IARC Monograph, No. 39. Host Factors in Human Carcinogenesis*. Lyon, France: International Agency for Research on Cancer. p. 193.

Baldwin, R. W. (1973). Immunological Aspects of Chemical Carcinogenesis. *Advances in Cancer Research*, **18**, 1.

Berenblum, I. (1941a). The Cocarcinogenic Action of Croton Resin. *Cancer Research*, **1**, 44.

Berenblum, I. (1941b), The Mechanism of Carcinogenesis: A Study of the Significance of Cocarcinogenic Action and Related Phenomena. *Cancer Research*, **1**, 807.

Berenblum, I. (1969). A Re-evaluation of the Concept of Cocarcinogenesis. *Progress in Experimental Tumor Research*, **11**, 21.

Berenblum, I. (1982). Sequential Aspects of Chemical Carcinogenesis: Skin. In *Cancer: A Comprehensive Treatise*, Vol. 1, 2nd edn. (ed. F. F. Becker). New York and London: Plenum Press, p. 541.

Berenblum, I., and Armuth, V. (1977). The Effect of Colchicine Injection Prior to the Initiating Phase of Two-Stage Skin Carcinogenesis in Mice. *British Journal of Cancer*, **35**, 615.

Boutwell, R. K. (1978). Biochemical Mechanism of Tumor Promotion. In: *Carcinogenesis, A Comprehensive Survey: Mechanisms of Tumor Promotion and Cocarcinogenesis*, Vol. 2. (eds T. J. Slaga, A. Sivak, and R. K. Boutwell). New York: Raven Press, p. 49.

Burnet, F. M. (1967). Immunological Aspects of Malignant Disease. *Lancet*, **1**, 1171.

Carroll, K. K. (1975). Experimental Evidence of Dietary Factors and Hormone-dependent Cancers. *Cancer Research*, **35**, 3374.

Cleaver, J. E. (1973). DNA Repair with Purines and Pyrimidines in Radiation- and Carcinogen-damaged Normal and Xeroderma Pigmentosum Human Cells. *Cancer Research*, **33**, 362.

Diamond, L., O'Brien, T. G., and Baird, W. M. (1980). Tumor Promoters and the Mechanism of Tumor Promotion. *Advances in Cancer Research*, **32**, 1.

Farber, E. (1981). Chemical Carcinogenesis. *New England Journal of Medicine*, **305**, 1379.

Foulds, L. (1949). Mammary Tumours in Hybrid Mice: Growth and Progression of Spontaneous Tumours. *British Journal of Cancer*, **3**, 345.

Foulds, L. (1954). The Experimental Study of Tumor Progression. *Cancer Research*, **14**, 327.

Foulds, L. (1969). *Neoplastic Development*. London and New York: Academic Press.

Foley, E. J. (1953). Antigenic Properties of Methylcholanthrene-induced Tumors in Mice of the Strain of Origin. *Cancer Research*, **13**, 835.

Friedewald, W. F. and Rous, P. (1944). The Initiating and Promoting Elements in Tumor Production: An Analysis of the Effects of Tar, Benzpyrene, and Methylcholanthrene on Rabbit Skin. *Journal of Experimental Medicine*, **80**, 101.

Furth, J. (1982). Hormones as Etiological Agents in Neoplasia. In *Cancer: A Comprehensive Treatise*, Vol. 1, 2nd edn. (ed. F. F. Becker). New York and London: Plenum Press, p. 89.

Good, R. A. and Finstad, J. (1969). Essential Relationship between the Lymphoid System, Immunity, and Malignancy. *National Cancer Institute Monograph*, **31**, 41.

Heidelberger, C. (1980). Cellular Transformation as a Basic Tool for Chemical Carcinogenesis. *Advances in Modern Environmental Toxicology*, **1**, 1.

Hicks, R. M., Chowaniec, J., and Wakefield, J. St. J. (1978). The Experimental

Induction of Bladder Tumours by a Two-Stage System. In *Carcinogenesis, A Comprehensive Survey:Mechanisms of tumor promotion and cocarcinogenesis,* Vol. 2. (eds T. J. Slaga, A. Sivak, and R. K. Boutwell). New York: Raven Press, p. 475.

Higginson, J. (1980). Multiplicity of Factors Involved in Cancer Patterns and Trends. *Journal of Environmental Pathology and Toxicology,* **3,** 113.

IARC Monographs on Evaluation of the Carcinogenic Risk of Chemicals to Humans, (1972–1982) Vols 1–29. Lyon, France: International Agency for Research on Cancer.

Iversen, O. H. (1974). Cell proliferation kinetics and carcinogenesis: A review. *Proceedings Fifth International Symposium on the Biological Characterization of Human Tumours,* (eds W. Davis and C. Maltoni). Amsterdam: Excerpta Medica, p. 21.

Kopelovich, L. (1982). Hereditary Adenomatosis of the Colon and Rectum: Relevance to Cancer Promotion and Cancer Control in Humans. *Cancer Genetics and Cytogenetics,* **5,** 333.

Lawley, P. D. (1976). Carcinogenesis by Alkylating Agents. *ACS Monograph 173: Chemical Carcinogens.* (ed. C. E. Searle). Washington, DC: American Chemical Society, p. 83.

Miller, E. C. and Miller, J. A. (1981). Mechanisms of Chemical Carcinogenesis. *Cancer,* **47,** 1055.

Möller, G. and Möller, E. (1975). Guest Editorial: Considerations of Some Current Concepts in Cancer Research. *Journal of the National Cancer Institute,* **55,** 755.

Penn, I. (1978). Tumors Arising in Organ Transplant Recipients. *Advances in Cancer Research,* **28,** 31.

Peto, R. (1982). Carcinogenesis as a Multistage Process – Evidence from Human Studies. *IARC Monograph 39. Host factors in human carcinogenesis.* Lyon, France: International Agency for Research on Cancer, p. 27.

Pitot, H. C. (1982). The Natural History of Neoplastic Development: The Relation of Experimental Models to Human Cancer. *Cancer,* **49,** 1206.

Prehn, R. T. (1971). Immunosurveillance, Regeneration and Oncogenesis. *Progress in Experimental Tumor Research,* **14,** 1.

Rasmussen, R. E. (1980). Repair of Chemical Carcinogen-induced Lesions. In *Genetic differences in chemical carcinogenesis,* (ed. R. E. Kourl). Florida: CRC Press, p. 67.

Rous, P. and Kidd, J. G. (1941). Conditional Neoplasms and Subthreshold Neoplastic States. *Journal of Experimental Medicine,* **73,** 365.

Schull, W. J. and Weiss, K. M. (1982). Genetic and Familial Factors in Cancer: A Population Perspective. *IARC Monograph 39. Host factors in human carcinogenesis.* Lyon, France: International Agency for Research on Cancer, p. 87.

Setlow, R. B. (1975). Relationships Among Repair, Cancer, and Genetic Deficiency: Overview. In *Molecular mechanisms for repair of DNA,* Part **B** (eds P. C. Hanawait and R. B. Setlow). New York: Plenum Press, p. 711.

Thomas, L. (1959). Reactions to Homologous Tissue Antigens. In *Cellular and humoral aspects of the hypersensitive state,* (ed. H. S. Lawrence). London: Academic Press, p. 529.

Trosko, J. E. and Chu, E. H. Y. (1975). The Role of DNA Repair and Somatic Mutation in Carcinogenesis. *Advances in Cancer Research,* **21,** 391.

Weinstein, I. B., Lee, L.-S., Fisher, P. B., Mufson, A., and Yamasaki, H. (1979). The Mechanism of Action of Tumor Promoters and A Molecular Model of Two Stage Carcinogenesis. In *Environmental carcinogenesis,* (eds P. Emmelot and E. Kriek). Amsterdam: Elsevier/North Holland Biomedical Press, p. 265.

Risk Factors and Multiple Cancer
Edited by B.A. Stoll
© 1984 John Wiley and Sons Ltd.

Chapter

2

JAMES C. WILLEY AND CURTIS C. HARRIS

Interaction Between Host and Environmental Factors

There is convincing epidemiologic evidence that the majority of cancers result from exposure to naturally occurring or man-made environmental carcinogens (Doll, 1977). This conclusion leads us to ask why only some of the people who are exposed to the same risk factors develop cancer, whether a person's susceptibility to a particular environmental cancer risk can be diminished and why some people develop multiple cancers? To answer these and related questions, one must consider the interaction between host and environmental factors (Mulvihill, 1978; Harris, 1983) as studied by laboratory and epidemiologic approaches.

The discussion will be under the following headings:
– Determinants of cancer risk.
– Methods of investigation of host factors.
– Studies of carcinogen metabolism using cultured human tissues.

DETERMINANTS OF CANCER RISK

An individual's risk of developing cancer is determined in part by exposure to carcinogens and cocarcinogens, the quantity and frequency of such exposure, and the interaction of these agents with the target cells (Figure 1). Through epidemiologic methods, it has been established that the likelihood of exposure is dependent on occupation, lifestyle, diet, and personal habits (Fraumeni, 1979). Occupational factors associated with an increased risk of cancer have been recently reviewed (Decoufle, 1982).

Predisposing habits include tobacco use in its many forms (Wynder and Hoffmann, 1982) and consumption of alcoholic beverages (Tuyns, 1982). It

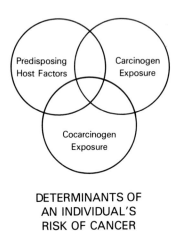

DETERMINANTS OF
AN INDIVIDUAL'S
RISK OF CANCER

Figure 1   Major determinants of cancer risk are shown in this Venn diagram. The size
and contribution of each category of determinant will vary with each individual.

has been estimated that smoking alone accounts for 40% of all cancer (Doll, 1977). Predisposing dietary factors include a high fat and low fiber content (Wynder *et al.*, 1983) and vitamin A deficiency (Bjelke, 1975).

Lifestyle includes such non-specific factors as socio-economic background, place of habitation (e.g. urban or rural), and amount of sun exposure. For example, oesophageal cancer is associated with a poor socio-economic status (Day, 1975), lung cancer with an urban existence (Mulvihill, 1978), and skin cancer with extensive sun exposure (Urbach, 1980). Under the proper conditions, each of the factors mentioned may lead to the development of multiple cancers.

Host factors

Due to the biologically diverse, genetically heterogeneous, human population and the multistep nature of the carcinogenic process, there are differences in susceptibility between individuals to the oncogenic effects of environmental carcinogens.

Genetic factors   Investigation of individuals with multiple tumors has led to the discovery of several hereditary conditions of increased cancer incidence (see Chapter 9). These diseases may be transmitted by single-gene, polygenic, or chromosomal mechanisms. Some hereditary conditions predispose only one type of tissue to neoplasia (e.g. actinic keratosis predisposes to basal cell carcinomas of the skin and familial polyposis coli predisposes to tumors in the gastrointestinal tract) while other hereditary conditions predispose to multiple tumors in different tissues (e.g. hereditary retinoblastoma, Bloom's syndrome, and ataxia telangiectasia).

Most known hereditary causes of multiple tumors were discovered because they manifested as dramatic clinical syndromes with a Mendelian pattern of inheritance. In some of these diseases, host susceptibility to specific environmental agents has been determined, e.g. ultraviolet radiation as a cause of skin cancer in patients with xeroderma pigmentosum. In contrast to these rather rare conditions, most common types of hereditary multiple cancer occur in familial patterns which probably have a polygenetic basis (Fraumeni, 1975).

Experiments using cultured human tissues have established that individuals and tissues differ in their ability to activate and inactivate carcinogens (Harris *et al.*, 1982). Present information suggests that these differences are determined primarily in a polygenetic fashion. Such interindividual differences in carcinogen metabolism may explain why only some individuals in a population exposed to the same carcinogenic influence (e.g. tobacco smoke) will get cancer, and why some smokers are more likely to develop multiple tumors than others.

Age-related factors The direct relationship between aging and carcinogenesis involves metabolic and immunologic changes as well as hormonal changes (see Chapter 10). These conclusions have been drawn from epidemiologic studies (Pitot, 1977) and are supported by experimental animal studies (Nettesheim, 1981; Anisimov, 1982). To explain the age-associated increase in tumor incidence, some interpret available data to mean that it is due to the increasing total dose of carcinogenic agents and that the aging process itself does not influence carcinogenesis (Peto, 1975; Doll, 1978). Other investigators conclude that hormonal, metabolic, and immune shifts increase sensitivity to carcinogens and thus enhance tumor development (Dilman, 1978; Dix *et al.*, 1980).

Effects of aging have been studied in animals by transferring carcinogen-exposed tissues of the same age to mice or rats of different ages (Anisimov, 1982); by observing age-related differences in activation and inactivation of carcinogens, DNA binding of active carcinogen metabolites, and rate of repair of damaged DNA (Anisimov, 1982; Nettesheim, 1981); or by observing the ability of transferred tumors to grow in host mice of different ages (Ebbesen, 1977). So far, these data are conflicting and provide no clear explanation for the correlation of aging with increased risk of cancer.

Immune factors Increasing age is correlated with both an increased risk of cancer and decreased immune competence (Good, 1972). In addition, a number of hereditary and acquired conditions of decreased immune compe-

tence have been shown to be associated with an increased risk of cancer, and
have been summarized recently (Kinlen, 1982).

The relationship between genetically determined immunodeficiency diseases and increased cancer risk is being investigated through an international
registry at the University of Minnesota (Spector *et al.*, 1978). Disorders
included in this registry include ataxia telangiectasia, Wiskott–Aldrich syndrome, severe combined immunodeficiency, and common variable immune
deficiency. Recently, there has been a marked increase in cancer incidence in
patients with disorders included in the Minnesota Registry (Spector and
Kersey, 1979), the most common malignancy in the latest report from the
registry being non-Hodgkin's lymphoma.

Several acquired immune deficiency diseases have been reported to be
associated with increased cancer incidence. An increased incidence of non-
Hodgkin's lymphomas has been reported in patients with Sjogren's syndrome
(Talal and Bunim, 1964), intestinal lymphangiectasia (Waldman *et al.*, 1972),
rheumatoid arthritis (Isomaki *et al.*, 1978), systemic lupus erythematosis
(Green *et al.*, 1978), or pulmonary sarcoidosis (Brinckner and Wilbek, 1974).
People who receive immunosuppressive agents (including transplant recipients) also have an increased incidence of cancer (Hoover, 1977), and here
again, the most marked increase is in non-Hodgkin's lymphoma.

The recognition of acquired immune deficiency syndrome (AIDS)
(Gottlieb *et al.*, 1981) was largely a result of investigation of a high
incidence of Kaposi's sarcoma during 1981 among homosexual men and
intravenous drug addicts (Friedman-Kien *et al.*, 1982). Immunologic investigation of the affected individuals typically demonstrated evidence of
cytomegalovirus and/or hepatitis B virus infection, anergy to a battery of
delayed hypersensitivity recall antigens, poor *in vitro* lymphocyte function
tests, profound depletion of helper T-cells with reversal of the helper/
suppressor (H/S) T-lymphocyte ratio, and normal or high levels of circulating
immunoglobulins with preservation of B-cell function (Gottlieb *et al.*, 1981;
Masur *et al.*, 1981).

Approximately 70% of patients die within two years from either Kaposi's
sarcoma or any of several opportunistic infections. Postulated causes of this
syndrome include the use of 'recreational' drugs (particularly amyl nitrate),
cytomegalovirus infections, or a new biological agent (Durack, 1981). A
recent report of the diagnosis of AIDS in four hemophiliacs (Marx, 1983)
supports the hypothesis that AIDS is caused by an infectious agent since
hemophiliacs receive large amounts of blood products which cannot be
sterilized.

Presently, it appears that immunologic factors are not predominant factors
in the etiology of most cancers in man (Kinlen, 1982). However, it is clear
from the above discussion that immune system incompetence is associated
with tumors such as non-Hodgkin's lymphoma and Kaposi's sarcoma. There

is little to support the idea that immunologic disorders predispose to multiple primary malignant neoplasms except in the case of chronic lymphogenous leukemia (Greene *et al.*, 1978), where it is speculated that the accompanying immune deficiency may account for the increased incidence of malignant melanoma and soft tissue sarcoma seen in these patients.

Host factors relevant to different classes of carcinogens For each class of carcinogenic agent, different host factors are relevant to oncogenic suscepti-bility. Carcinogens may be broadly classified as chemical, physical, or microbial (Table 1). Physical carcinogens include fibers such as asbestos; metals such as nickel compounds; and radiation, non-ionizing as well as ionizing.

The nature of the interaction between host and chemical carcinogen depends on uptake, distribution, and metabolism of the compound within any particular host. In a similar fashion, host interaction with non-ionizing or ionizing radiation depends on the absorptive properties of the skin and the efficiency of DNA-repair enzyme systems. For both of these classes of agents,

Table 1　Environmental determinants of human cancer risk

Class	Example	Primary target site for cancer
Carcinogens		
Chemical		
direct-acting	Mustard gas	Lung
indirect-acting	2-Naphthylamine	Bladder
complex mixture	Tobacco smoke	Lung
Physical		
fiber	Asbestos	Pleura
metal	Nickel compounds	Nasal cavity
radiation	Ultraviolet light	Skin
Viral[a]		
RNA	Human T-cell leukemia– lymphoma virus	Hemopoietic system
DNA	Epstein–Barr virus	Hemopoietic system
	Hepatitis B virus	Liver
Cocarcinogens		
Chemical	Alcoholic beverages[b]	Esophagus
Physical	Asbestos[b]	Bronchus
Viral	Hepatitis[c]	Liver

[a]Although proof of causation is considered to be lacking, these viruses are important contributors to the etiology of specific human cancers.
[b]Interactive effects with carcinogen, tobacco smoke.
[c]Putative interactive effects with chemical carcinogens, e.g. aflatoxin B_1.

it has been possible to describe pathogenetic mechanisms and interindividual variation through experimentation in animal models and human tissues *in vitro*.

There is less known about host factors which allow metals and viruses to be oncogenic. In the Li–Fraumeni syndrome, which involves a familial risk for cancer in several different tissues (Li and Fraumeni, 1969), pathologic studies of 16 tumors revealed variable occurrence of intranuclear cytoplasmic invaginations, intranuclear bodies and acidophilic intracytoplasmic inclusions in eight lesions, suggesting viral damage. Based on pathologic and epidemiologic studies of these findings, it has been suggested that a putative oncogenic virus coupled with hereditary predisposition has led to the production of highly specific histologic varieties of neoplasms (Lynch, 1978).

Factors conferring host susceptibility to inorganic compounds, such as asbestos and glass fibers, and metals such as nickel, chromium and arsenic are currently being investigated intensely (Lechner *et al.*, 1983; Mossman and Craighead, 1980).

Table 2   Cancer sites for which relationships with occupational exposures are well established in human studies

Site	Agent or industrial process
Bladder	Benzidine, β-naphthylamine, 4-aminobiphenyl (xenylamine) Manufacture of certain dyes (e.g. auramine and magenta) Gas retorts Rubber and cable making industries
Blood (leukemia)	Benzene X-radiation
Bone	Radium, mesothorium
Larynx	Ethanol (ethyl alcohol) manufactured by strong acid process (diethyl sulfate?) Isopropyl alcohol manufactured by strong acid process (diisopropyl sulfate?) Mustard gas
Liver (angiosarcoma)	Arsenic (inorganic compounds) Vinyl chloride
Lung, bronchus	Arsenic (inorganic compounds) Asbestos Bis (chloromethyl) ether Chromium compounds Coal carbonization processes (coke ovens, gas retorts, producer gas manufacture)

Environmental factors

Carcinogens

A number of compounds have been evaluated for carcinogenic risk in humans by epidemiologic studies. Such studies will be successful only if there is sufficient variation in levels of human exposure and if the effects of individual agents can be isolated (International Agency for Research on Cancer, 1977). For these reasons, most presently confirmed carcinogens are medications or agents common to certain occupational environments (Table 2). Many agents thus identified can be successfully used to produce cancers in experimental animals. Using laboratory and epidemiologic methods, a number of chemical and physical factors have been recognized as being involved in cancer causation (Table 3).

The list includes natural and synthetic inorganic and organic compounds, and ionizing and non-ionizing radiation. Under certain conditions of exposure and/or hereditary or acquired predisposition, any of these agents can lead to

Table 2 (*Continued*)   Cancer sites for which relationships with occupational exposures are well established in human studies

Site	Agent or industrial process
	Coal tar pitch volatiles (roofing materials, aluminum reduction plants)
	Iron ore (hematite) mining
	Mustard gas
	Nickel refining
	Radiation (radioactive ores)
Nasal cavity, sinuses	Isopropanol (isopropyl alcohol) manufactured by strong acid process (diisopropyl sulfate?)
	Mustard gas
	Nickel refining
	Radium, mesothorium
	Shoe manufacturing (leather dust?)
	Woodworking (wood dust?)
Peritoneum (mesothelioma)	Asbestos
Pharynx	Mustard gas
Pleura (mesothelioma)	Asbestos
Skin (including scrotum) (epitheliomas)	Arsenic (inorganic compounds)
	Coal tar products (mainly coal tar, creosote, pitch, soot)
	Coal hydrogenation
	Mineral oils (from coal, petroleum, shale)
	X-radiation

Table 3   Human chemical carcinogens[a]

Chemical/occupation	Origin/use
4-aminobiphenyl	Rubber antioxidant
Analgesic mixtures containing phenacetin	Medicine
Arsenic and certain arsenic compounds	In ores/preservatives
Asbestos	Natural fibrous silicate, insulation
Manufacture of auramine	Dye intermediate
Azathioprine	Chemotherapeutic agent
Benzene	Solvent, chemical manufacturing
Benzidine	Dye manufacturing
N-N-bis(2-chloroethyl)-2-napthylamine (Chlornaphazine)	Chemotherapeutic agent
Bis(chloromethyl)ether and technical grade chloromethylmethyl ether	Plastics and resins
1,4-butanediol dimethanesulphonate (Myleran)	Chemotherapeutic agents
Certain combined chemotherapies for lymphomas (including MOPP)	
Chlorambucil	Chemotherapeutic agent
Chromium and certain chromium compounds	Protective coating/pigment
Cyclophosphamide	Chemotherapeutic agent
Industries	
Boot and shoe manufacture and repair (certain occupations)	
Furniture manufacture	
Rubber industry (certain occupations)	
Manufacture of isopropyl alcohol (strong acid process)	Chemical manufacturing
Melphalan	Chemotherapeutic agent
Methoxsalen with ultraviolet A therapy (PUVA)	
Mustard gas	Chemical alkylating agent
2-Naphthylamine	Dye and rubber manufacturing
Nickel refining	Steel/alloy manufacturing
Conjugated oestrogens	
Estrogens	Medicine
Diethylstilbestrol	
Soots, tars, and oils	Combustion products
Treosulphan	
Underground hematite mining (with exposure to radon)	
Vinyl chloride	Plastics manufacturing

[a]Adapted from *IARC Monograph*, Supplement 4, 1977.

either single or multiple tumors in humans. Also included in the table are several occupational environments that lead to increased cancer risk. In these cases, it has proved impossible to identify single agents responsible for the observed carcinogenic effect.

Chemical carcinogens are a large group of naturally occurring and synthetic compounds with diverse chemical structures. Most of these chemicals are stable in the environment and require metabolic activation usually within target cells to cause their toxic, mutagenic, teratogenic, and carcinogenic effects (Miller and Miller, 1979) (Figure 2). Competing with the pathways of enzymatic activation are deactivation pathways which generally lead to the formation of polar, water-soluble metabolites. The absorption, activation, and inactivation of carcinogens may be modified by cocarcinogens and anticarcinogens.

The class of physical carcinogens comprises non-ionizing (ultraviolet light) and ionizing radiation, metals, and mineral fibers. Ultraviolet radiation in sunlight is known to be the primary cause of skin cancer. Ionizing radiation can take several forms, including gamma emissions from radioactive materials and X-rays. Metals have also been implicated as causes of cancer (Table 3) and most exposure to these compounds occurs through occupation. Asbestos, a group of naturally occurring mineral fibers, is now recognized as a major health hazard. Because of its unique insulation properties, asbestos has become incorporated into many homes, schools, and office buildings, and is a major component of automobile brake linings.

Cocarcinogens   Cocarcinogens are agents that enhance the effectiveness of carcinogens. These compounds may act by altering the uptake, distribution or metabolism of carcinogens, or the susceptibility of the target cells. Risk of exposure to these compounds is dependent on the same factors as are mentioned above for carcinogens. Many carcinogenic materials, such as tobacco smoke, industrial oils, and petroleum fractions, have potent effects because they contain both carcinogens and cocarcinogens. Examples of cocarcinogens and sources of exposure are given in Table 1.

An example of how exogenous carcinogens and cocarcinogens may interact to cause multiple tumors in contiguous tissues is the synergism between tobacco and alcoholic beverages in causing cancers in the mouth, pharynx, larynx, and esophagus (Schottenfeld *et al.*, 1974). Epidemiologic data reveal an increased risk of these cancers in people who use tobacco (Hammond *et al.*, 1977), and the risk is greatly increased by the heavy use of alcoholic beverages (Rothman and Keller, 1972). Presumably, alcoholic beverages are interacting as cocarcinogens with tobacco. Similarly, lung cancer occurs much more commonly in asbestos workers than in similar populations with no asbestos exposure, and the incidence increases in a multiplicative fashion in

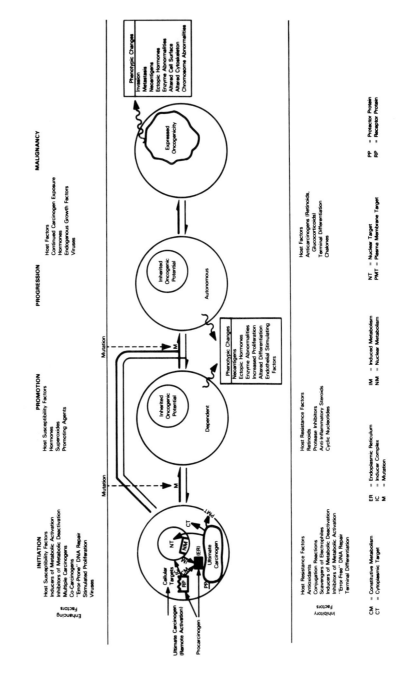

SCHEMATIC REPRESENTATION OF
CHEMICAL CARCINOGENESIS

Figure 2 Schematic representation of chemical carcinogenesis. The circles represent cells at various stages in the process of malignant transformation by chemicals. On the left, a normal cell is exposed to procarcinogens. As the carcinogen enters the cell, it may go directly to cytoplasmic (endoplasmic reticulum, ER) or nuclear (nuclear membrane, NM) sites or constitutive metabolic activity. Alternatively, procarcinogens may complex with a receptor protein (RP), for an inducer complex (IC), and derepress genes controlling enzymatic activity leading to induction of metabolism (IM). Metabolically activated (electrophilic) ultimate carcinogens may complex with other proteins (PP) which prevent immediate degradation or covalent interactions at nearby sites. Ultimate carcinogenic species will interact with a variety of target molecules in the nucleus (NT), in the cytoplasm (CT), or at the plasma membrane (PMT). Carcinogens may also be metabolized in one cell and delivered to other cells in activated form. In both cases, interaction with critical cellular targets, possibly DNA, in a precise way is required for initiation. A number of endogenous and exogenous factors will also influence the probability that the carcinogen–cellular interaction will lead to a permanent state of 'initiation' of carcinogenesis. Similarly, endogenous and exogenous factors determine the level of preneoplastic progression (→) depicted here for schematic purposes as two cells but representing a series of progressive changes. Each preneoplastic change may be stable for long periods and may even revert (←) to a more dependent stage under the proper conditions. As progression toward malignancy continues, the preneoplastic cell becomes more autonomous (perhaps secondary to another mutagenic and/or clastogenic event). A number of phenotypic alterations (→) became apparent during this prolonged process, and the clone size of preneoplastic cells increases. Ultimately, progression results in a malignant clone with clinical expression of cancer. (Adapted from Yuspa and Harris, 1982.)

those who smoke cigarettes (Selikoff *et al.*, 1968). This is presumably due to a synergistic interaction between the effects of the two substances.

METHODS USED FOR INVESTIGATION OF HOST FACTORS

Host factors may be inherited or acquired and the methods used for investigating these factors are clinical (e.g. by epidemiology or pathology) or laboratory (e.g. by animal models or *in vitro* techniques).

Clinical methods

Epidemiologic studies   In order to discern host and environmental factors that are important causes of cancer (and specifically multiple cancers) one can use case reports, evaluation of familial clusters, and descriptive and analytic epidemiologic studies. Descriptive studies may involve evaluating the frequency of a particular cancer (over time, in a particular place and in a particular age cohort) or potential causal factors. Once one has obtained this information, hypotheses concerning the causality of a particular factor with respect to a particular disease can be tested by analytic methods. Such studies may be either of case-control design (retrospective) or cohort design (prospective).

Through retrospective or prospective epidemiologic studies, one can analyse large groups for their risk of developing cancer, and in doing so, develop evidence for the carcinogenicity of specific environmental factors. This evidence can be substantiated by a prospective cohort study which observes the incidence of cancer in a group of people exposed to the same factor. Important additional information derived from such studies is that while the incidence of cancer may be higher than in a non-exposed cohort, not all exposed people develop cancers. Theoretically, the individuals who respond to a carcinogen by developing a tumor may be determined on a purely random basis, but epidemiologic methods have been used to attribute specific host susceptibility factors for many cancers. For example, intercultural epidemiologic studies have demonstrated that colon cancer incidence is higher in the US than in Japan (see Chapter 8). Family case studies have also been useful in attributing specific host susceptibility factors to many cancers, e.g. familial polyposis coli confers increased risk of colon cancer. Familial predisposition to the carcinogenic effects of tobacco smoke has also been reported (Takuhata and Lilienfeld, 1963; Lynch *et al.*, 1982).

Pathologic studies   Assessment of epidemiologic data is dependent on accurate pathologic diagnosis, and determining the tissue of origin and ruling out metastatic disease in instances of suspected multiple cancer is often difficult.

Necropsy studies have also provided valuable clues concerning cancer pathogenesis; for instance, the multistage concept of carcinogenesis is partly based on the identification of preneoplastic lesions (Auerbach *et al.*, 1961; Saccomanno *et al.*, 1971) and the high incidence of occult carcinomas in aged populations (Sugano, 1980).

Experimental methods

Animal models Animal models have been useful for testing the carcinogenicity of compounds, and for studying carcinogen metabolism and cancer pathogenesis. Animal models have been developed for most of the common human malignancies – skin, liver, lung, breast, stomach, colon, pancreas, cervix, endometrium, esophagus, kidney, brain, bladder, and hematologic cancers (Yuspa and Harris, 1982). Furthermore, through inbreeding, one can reduce or eliminate interindividual differences and create strains which have particular characteristics relevant to the study of carcinogenesis. One example of this is the development of strains or stocks of mice with varying susceptibility to tumor promotion, such as Sencar mice, with an enhanced susceptibility to 12-O-tetradecanoyl-13-phorbol ester (TPA), and Recar mice, with a decreased sensitivity (Boutwell, 1964)

Animal studies are reliable as indicators of the qualitative carcinogenicity of a substance in humans, but sensitivity and organ specificity may be different among different animal species. Differences between animal species are pharmacological, temporal, receptor-related, and size-related. The contributions of receptor, time, and size differences are small compared to pharmacological differences between species in response to carcinogens (Thorgeirsson and Nebert, 1977). As an example, 2-acetylaminofluorine, a liver carcinogen in rats, is not carcinogenic in some species, such as the guinea pig, because they have a deficient cytochrome P_{450}-dependent *N*-hydroxylase activity (Thorgeirsson, 1980). Furthermore, using inbred strains of mice, interstrain differences in the carcinogenicity of benzo[α]pyrene or 3-methylcholanthrene are found to be due to differences in the inducibility of aryl hydrocarbon hydroxylase or benzo[α]pyrene hydroxylase (Thorgeirsson and Nebert, 1977).

In vitro *models* Cell and organ cultures have provided a more rapid, quantitative model for carcinogenesis research. One can control the dosage and time of exposure to putative carcinogenic or cocarcinogenic agents, and conduct the experiment in a defined growth medium away from undefined immune and hormonal influences in the host. In explant cultures, the natural organization of various cell types in a tissue remains intact, and this is especially suitable for morphologic and metabolic studies. Again, for more detailed mechanistic studies on the cells of a specific tissue, cell cultures are often preferred. As an example, the great majority of lung cancer originates in the large airways (mainstem and secondary bronchi) and specifically from the epithelial lining of these airways; thus in some metabolic studies, it would be preferable to study the characteristics of the epithelial cells separate from submucosal tissue.

Markers of malignant cell transformation have been determined in cultured animal tissues and cells (Yuspa and Harris, 1982). Such markers include secretion of enzymes that activate plasminogen, altered cytoskeletal structures, changes in surface glycoproteins, heteroploid conversion, and ability to grow in suspension or soft agar. The application of these short-term assays and markers is a major challenge for cancer researchers using cultured human cells.

STUDIES OF CARCINOGEN METABOLISM USING CULTURED HUMAN TISSUES

Cancer research and methodology in cell culture have progressed inter-dependently for over 70 years. There have been successive technological improvements in cell culture techniques, and recently, in the cultures of human epithelial tissues and cells (Harris *et al.*, 1980). A major advance has been the development of defined synthetic media for the growth of normal human epithelial cells (Maciag *et al.*, 1981; Tsao *et al.*, 1982; Lechner *et al.*, 1982).

Carcinogens may interact with DNA by forming DNA–carcinogen adducts, inducing pyrimidine dimer formation, causing DNA strand breaks or affecting the state of deoxycytosine methylation. Most studies examining host–carcinogen interactions have dealt with DNA-adduct or pyrimidine dimer formation, and some of these will be discussed below.

In the past, metabolism of chemical carcinogens by human tissue was studied primarily using subcellular preparations. However, comparison of metabolic capacity between intact tissues and subcellular fractions revealed both qualitative and quantitative differences in enzyme activities, metabolite profile, and carcinogen–DNA adducts formed. For instance, a divergence in the metabolic profile of benzo[α]pyrene (BP) has been shown in human tissues using activation systems of different levels of biological organization (Autrup, 1982). Here, we will describe experiments using human cells and tissues in culture.

Cell specificity

Comparison of BP metabolism in fibroblasts and epithelial cells from the same patient reveals no significant difference in the metabolic profile of BP;

however, the binding level of BP to DNA is three- to fourfold higher in epithelial cells compared to fibroblasts in bronchus (Autrup, 1982), skin (Parkinson and Newbold, 1980) and breast (Bartley *et al.*, 1982). The relatively increased binding in epithelial cells has been demonstrated in intact explants by autoradiographic methods (Harris *et al.*, 1976) and by studying the binding to cellular DNA in separate cultures of epithelial and fibroblast cells initiated from the same bronchus (Lechner *et al.*, 1981). This relative proclivity of epithelial cells to form adducts may explain in part the more frequent occurrence of cancer in these cells relative to fibroblasts.

Organ specificity

It is now well established that certain carcinogens, in particular *N*-nitrosamines, induce tumors with a high degree of organ specificity (Magee *et al.*, 1976). This specificity is determined by a combination of the chemical structure of the carcinogens and as yet poorly understood susceptibility factors of particular organs (Yuspa and Harris, 1982). For example, alkylation of DNA by ethylnitrosourea in susceptible (brain) and resistant (liver) rat organs is qualitatively and quantitatively identical, but the removal from DNA of one particular carcinogen–DNA binding product, O^6-ethylguanine, by DNA repair mechanisms is deficient in the susceptible tissue (Goth and Rajewski, 1974).

Whether host factors cause other carcinogens, such as benzo[α]pyrene (BP) to have organ specificity is unclear. However, using human tissue explant cultures from the same individual it was determined that there are quantitative differences between different organs in the production of the presumed ultimate carcinogen form of BP (Autrup *et al.*, 1982).

Individual differences

The quantity of carcinogen–DNA adducts formed has been shown to vary 50- to 150-fold among cultured tissues from different people (Harris, 1983). These interindividual differences are of the same order of magnitude as those found in pharmacogenetic studies of drug metabolism. Evidence is accumulating that carcinogens and some drugs may be metabolically activated by the same mixed function oxidase. Such drugs may prove to be useful in probing the genetic polymorphism of carcinogen metabolism (Idle and Ritchie, 1983).

We have also measured interindividual variation in activation of carcinogens using human tissue- or cell-mediated mutagenesis assays (Hsu *et al.*, 1978, 1979). A wide variation in human bronchus-mediated frequencies of ouabain-resistant mutations and sister chromatid exchanges in cocultivated Chinese hamster V-79 cells was found. A high degree of correlation between mutation frequency in the V-79 cells and amount of carcinogen–DNA adducts in the bronchial mucosa was observed. These findings further support the contention that carcinogen metabolism and DNA damage have important biological consequences.

Once carcinogen–DNA adducts are formed, DNA repair processes may remove the adduct. The rate of removal of adducts and the interindividual variation in these rates are being investigated. This variation in removal rates of adducts and in activities of DNA repair enzymes may be substantial and biologically significant. Extreme deficiencies in DNA repair are known, with xeroderma pigmentosum being the classic example; although the various complementation groups of xeroderma pigmentosum vary in their deficiencies in DNA repair (Setlow, 1983). The variation in the general population is now being systematically investigated.

Setlow (1983) and co-workers have also observed approximately an eight-fold variation in O^6-methyltransferase activity in lymphocytes from 44 donors. We have observed two to threefold differences in lung or colon tissues from a smaller number of people (Grafstrom *et al.*, 1984). One can predict that studies measuring O^6-methyltransferase and other DNA repair enzymes in larger human populations will uncover even wider variations. The biological significance of variations in rates and fidelity of DNA repair will obviously require further study.

CONCLUSION

Close cooperation between clinicians, epidemiologists, and laboratory investigators has led to progress in several areas of cancer research. Specific carcinogens and cocarcinogens have been identified and refinement of cell and tissue culture techniques have allowed *in vitro* investigations of individual risk. Further valuable information has been obtained by epidemiological and laboratory investigation of families with a high incidence of cancer. For example, the discovery that in xeroderma pigmentosum, family members have a recessively inherited increased risk for developing skin cancer, has led to the discovery of the putative pathogenetic mechanism, i.e. defective DNA repair. Similarly, collaboration between the clinician and laboratory investigator has led to better understanding of the etiology of malignant melanoma, bladder cancer, and lymphoma (Blattner *et al.*, 1983). Physicians and oncologists should interest themselves in etiologic as well as in diagnostic and therapeutic considerations (Mulvihill and McKeen, 1977; Parry *et al.*, 1979; Blattner *et al*, 1983). A checklist of questions has been developed (Mulvihill, 1978) and includes the following: (1) What are the demographic features of the patient? Is the tumor occurring at an unusual site or at a younger or older age than expected? (2) Are there potentially relevant environmental exposures? (3) Are there identifiable host factors such as a positive family history, antecedent disease, or laboratory abnormality? (4) Does the patient have multiple synchronous or metachronous tumours? Patients who are found to be at increased risk should have a careful family evaluation, their tissue cells should be evaluated *in vitro* (and preferably stored frozen) and serum samples should be taken for possible future assay.

Individual differences in host suceptibility show the urgent need for rapid, inexpensive tests to measure individual risk. The ever-expanding list of possible carcinogens underlines the need to develop rapid *in vitro* tests of human carcinogenicity and intensify research into anticarcinogenic compounds.

REFERENCES

Anisimov, V. N. (1982). Carcinogenesis and aging. *Experimental Pathology*, **22**, 131.

Auerbach, O., Stout, A., and Hammond, E. (1961). Changes in bronchial epithelium in relation to cigarette smoking and in relation to lung cancer. *New England Journal of Medicine*, **265**, 253.

Autrup, H. (1982). Carcinogen metabolism in human tissues and cells. *Drug Metabolism Reviews*, **13**, 603.

Autrup, H., Grafstrom, R. C., Brugh, M. *et al.* (1982). Comparison of benzo(a)pyrene metabolism in bronchus, esophagus, colon, and duodenum from the same individual. *Cancer Research*, **42**, 934.

Bartley, J., Bartholomew, R., and Stampfer, M. R. (1982). Benzo(a)pyrene in human mammary epithelial and fibroblastic cells. *Journal of Supramolecular Structure and Cellular Biochemistry Supplements*, **5**, 165.

Bjelke, E. (1975). Dietary vitamin A and human lung cancer. *International Journal of Cancer*, **15**, 561.

Blattner, W. A., Greene, M. H., Goedert, J. J., Mann, D. L. (1983). In *Human carcinogenesis* (eds C. C. Harris and H. Autrup). New York: Academic Press (in press).

Boutwell, R. K. (1964). In *Progress in experimental tumor research*, Vol. 4 (ed. F. Homberg). Basel/New York: Karger, p. 207.

Brinckner, H. and Wilbek, E. (1974). The incidence of malignant tumors in patients with respiratory sarcoidosis. *British Journal of Cancer*, **29**, 247.

Day, N. E. (1975). Some aspects of the epidemiology of esophageal cancer. *Cancer Research*, **35**, 3304.

Decoufle, P. (1982). In *Cancer epidemiology and prevention* (eds D. Schottenfeld and J. F. Fraumeni). New York: W. B. Saunders, p. 318.

Dilman, V. M. (1978). Aging, metabolic immunodepression and carcinogenesis. *Mechanisms of Aging and Development*, **8**, 153.

Dix, D., Cohen, P., and Flannery, J. (1980). On the role of aging in cancer incidence. *Journal of Theoretical Biology*, **7**, 163.

Doll, R. (1977). The prevention of cancer. *Journal of the Royal College of Physicians London*, **11**, 125.

Doll, R. (1978). An epidemiological perspective of the biology of cancer. *Cancer Research*, **38**, 3573.

Durack, D. T. (1981). Opportunistic infections and Kaposi's sarcoma in homosexual men. *New England Journal of Medicine*, **305**, 1465.

Ebbesen, P. (1977). Effect of age of non-skin tissues on susceptibility of skin grafts to 7,12-dimethylbenz(a)anthracene (DMBA) carcinogenesis in BALB/c mice and affect of age of skin graft on susceptibility of surrounding recipient skin to DMBA. *Journal of the National Cancer Institute*, **58**, 1057.

Fraumeni, J. F. (1975). *Persons at high risk of cancer: An approach to cancer etiology and control.* New York: Academic Press.

Fraumeni, J. F. (1979). In *Carcinogens: Identification and mechanisms of activation* (eds A. C. Griffin and C. R. Shaw). New York: Raven Press, p. 51.

Friedman-Kien, A. E., Laubenstein, L. J., Marmor, M. *et al.* (1982). Disseminated Kaposi's sarcoma in homosexual men. *Morbidity and Mortality Weekly Reports,* **30,** 305.

Good, R. A. (1972). Relations between immunity and malignancy. *Proceedings of the National Academy of Sciences,* **69,** 11026.

Goth, R. and Rajewsky, M. F. (1974). Persistence of O^6-ethyl guanine in rat brain DNA: correlation with nervous system-specific carcinogenesis by ethylnitrosourea. *Proceedings of the National Academy of Sciences,* **71,** 639.

Gottlieb, M. S., Schroff, R., Schauker, H. M. *et al.* (1981). Pneumocystis carinii pneumonia and mucosal candidiasis in previously healthy homosexual men: evidence of a new acquired cellular immunodeficiency. *New England Journal of Medicine,* **305,** 1425.

Grafstrom, R.C., Pegg, A.E., Trump, B.F. and Harris, C.C. (1984). O^6-Alkylguanine-DNA transalkylase activity in normal human tissues and cells. *Cancer Research,* in press.

Green, J. A., Dawson, A. A., and Walker, W. (1978). Systemic lupus erythematosis and lymphoma. *Lancet,* **2,** 753.

Greene, M. H., Hoover, R. N., Fraumeni Jr, J. F. (1978). Subsequent cancer in patients with chronic lymphocytic leukemia – a possible immunologic mechanism. *Journal of the National Cancer Institute,* **61,** 3378.

Hammond, E. C., Garfinkel, L., and Seidman, H. (1977). In *Origins of human cancer,* Vol. A (eds H. H. Hiatt, J. D. Watson, and J. A. Winsten). Cold Spring Harbor: Cold Spring Harbor Laboratory, p. 101.

Harris, C. C. (1980). Individual differences in cancer susceptibility. *Annals of Internal Medicine,* **92,** 809.

Harris, C. C. (1983). In *Human carcinogenesis* (eds C. C. Harris and H. Autrup). New York: Academic Press (in press).

Harris, C. C., Genta, V., Frank, A. *et al.* (1976). Binding of [^{3}H]-benzo(a)pyrene to DNA in cultured human bronchus. *Cancer Research,* **36,** 1011.

Harris, C. C., Trump, B. F., Grafstrom, R., and Autrup, H. (1982). In *Mechanisms of chemical carcinogenesis* (eds C. C. Harris and Cerutti). New York: A. R. Liss, p. 289.

Harris, C. C., Trump, B. F., and Stoner, G. D. (eds) (1980). *Methods in cell biology,* Vol. 2, parts A and B. New York: Academic Press.

Hoover, R. (1977). In *Origins of human cancer* (eds H. H. Hiatt, J. D. Watson, and J. A. Winsten). Cold Spring Harbor: Cold Spring Harbor Laboratory, p. 369.

Hsu, I.-C., Autrup, H., Stoner, G. D. *et al.* (1978). Human bronchus-mediated mutagenesis of mammalian cells by carcinogenic polynuclear aromatic hydrocarbons. *Proceedings of the National Academy of Sciences,* **75,** 2003.

Hsu, I.-C., Harris, C. C., Trump, B. F. *et al.* (1979). Induction of ouabain-resistant mutation and sister chromatid exchanges in Chinese hamster cells with chemical carcinogens mediated by human pulmonary macrophages. *Journal of Clinical Investigation* **64,** 1245.

Idle, J. R., and Ritchie, J. C. (1983). In *Human carcinogenesis* (eds C. C. Harris and H. Autrup). New York: Academic Press (in press).

Isomaki, H. A., Hokulinen, T., and Joutsenlahti, U. (1978). Excess risk of lymphomas, leukemia and myeloma in patients with rheumatoid arthritis. *Journal of Chronic Diseases,* **31,** 691.

International Agency for Research on Cancer (1977). Monograph: *Evaluation of carcinogenic risk of chemicals to man*, p. 15.

Kinlen, L. J. (1982). In *Cancer epidemiology and prevention* (eds D. Schottenfeld and J. Fraumeni). New York: W. B. Saunders, p. 494.

Lechner, J. F., Haugen, A., Autrup, H. *et al.* (1981). Clonal growth of epithelial cells from normal adult human bronchus. *Cancer Research*, **41**, 2294.

Lechner, J. F., Haugen, A., McClendon, I. A., and Pettis, E. W. (1982). Clonal growth of normal adult human bronchial epithelial cells in a serum-free medium. *In Vitro*, **18**, 633.

Lechner, J. F., Haugen, A., Tokiwa, T., Trump, B. F., and Harris, C. C. (1983). In *Human carcinogenesis* (eds C. C. Harris and H. Autrup). New York: Academic Press (in press).

Li, F. and Fraumeni, J. F. (1969). Soft tissue sarcomas, breast cancer and other neoplasms. *Annals of Internal Medicine*, **71**, 747.

Lynch, H. T. (1978). Genetic and pathologic findings in a kindred with hereditary sarcoma, breast cancer, brain tumors, leukemia, lung, laryngeal, and adrenal corticoid carcinoma. *Cancer*, **41**, 2055.

Lynch, H. T., Fain, P. R., Albano, W. A. *et al.* (1982). Genetic/epidemiological findings in a study of smoking-associated tumors. *Cancer Genetics and Cytogenetics*, **6**, 163.

Maciag, T., Nemore, R. E., Weinstein, R., and Gilchrest, R. A. (1981). An endocrine approach to the control of epidermal growth: serum-free cultivation of human keratinocytes. *Science*, **211**, 1452.

Magee, P. N., Montesano, R., and Preussmann, R. (1976). In *Chemical carcinogens* (ed. C. E. Searle). Washington, DC: American Chemical Society, p. 491.

Marx, J. (1983). Spread of AIDS sparks new health concerns. *Science*, **219**, 42.

Masur, H., Michelis, M. A. Greene, J. B. *et al.* (1981). An outbreak of community-acquired pneumocytis carinii pneumonia. *New England Journal of Medicine*, **305**, 1431.

Miller, E. C. and Miller, J. A. (1979). Milestones in chemical carcinogenesis. *Seminars in Oncology*, **6**, 445.

Mossman, B. T. and Craighead, J. E. (1980). Asbestos-induced epithelial changes in organ cultures of hamster trachea: inhibition by retinyl methyl ether. *Science*, **207**, 311.

Mulvihill, J. J., and McKeen, E. A. (1977). Discussion of multiple primary tumors. *Cancer*, **40**, 1867.

Mulvihill, J. J. (1978). In *Pathogenesis and therapy of lung cancer* (ed. C. C. Harris). New York: Marcel Dekker, p. 53.

Nettesheim, P. (1981). Host and environmental factors enhancing carcinogenesis in the respiratory tract. *Annual Review of Pharmacology and Toxicology*, **21**, 133.

Parkinson, E. K., and Newbold, R. F. (1980). Benzo(a)pyrene metabolism and DNA adduct formation in serially cultivated strains of human epidermal keratinocytes. *International Journal of Cancer*, **26, 289.**

Parry, D.M., Mulvihill, J.J., Miller, R.W., and Spregel, R.J. (1979). Sarcomas in a child and her father, *American Journal of Diseases of Children*, **133**, 130.

Peto, R. (1975). Cancer and aging in mice and men. *British Journal of Cancer*, **32**, 411.

Pitot, H. C. (1977). Carcinogenesis and aging – two related phenomena. A review. *American Journal of Pathology*, **87**, 444.

Rothman, K. J., and Keller, A. Z. (1972). The effect of joint exposure to alcohol and tobacco on risk of cancer of the mouth and pharynx. *Journal of Chronic Diseases*, **25**, 711.

Saccomanno, G., Archer, V. E., Auerbach, O., Kuschner, M., Saunders, R. P., and

Klein, M. G. (1971). Histologic types of lung cancer among uranium miners. *Cancer*, **27**, 515

Schottenfeld, D., Gantt, R. C., and Wynder, E. L. (1974). The role of alcohol and tobacco in multiple primary cancers of the upper digestive system, larynx, and lung: a prospective study. *Preventive Medicine*, **3**, 277.

Selikoff, I. J., Hammond, E. C., and Chung, J. (1968). Asbestos exposure, smoking and neoplasia. *Journal of the American Medical Association*, **204**, 106.

Setlow, R. B. (1983). In *Human carcinogenesis* (eds C. C. Harris and H. Autrup). New York: Academic Press (in press).

Spector, B. D., and Kersey, J. H. (1979). Lymphoreticular malignancies in patients with genetically determined immunodeficiencies: Evaluation by surface markers and/or histology. *Proceedings of the American Association for Cancer Research and the American Society of Clinical Oncology*, Vol. 20, p. 374.

Spector, B., Perry III, G. S., and Kersey, J. H. (1978). Genetically determined immunodeficiency disease and malignancy: report from the immunodeficiency-cancer registry. *Clinics in Immunology and Immunopathology*, **11**, 12.

Sugano, H. (1980). Natural history of human cancer. *Transactiones Societatis Pathologicae Japanicae*, **69**, 27.

Talal, N., and Bunim, J. J. (1964). The development of malignant lymphoma in the course of Sjogren's syndrome. *American Journal of Medicine*, **36**, 529.

Thorgeirsson, S. S. (1980). Carcinogenesis studies in experimental animals. *Annals of Internal Medicine*, **92**, 809.

Thorgeirsson, S. S. and Nebert, D. W. (1977). The Ah locus and the metabolism of chemical carcinogens and other foreign compounds. *Advances in Cancer Research*, **25**, 149.

Tokuhata, G. K. and Lilienfeld, A. M. (1963). Familial aggregation of lung cancer in humans. *Journal of the National Cancer Institute*, **30**, 289.

Tsao, M. C., Walthall, B. J., and Ham, R. G. (1982). Clonal growth of normal human epidermal keratinocytes in a defined medium. *Journal of Cellular Physiology*, **110**, 219. 219.

Tuyns, A. J. (1982). In *Cancer epidemiology and prevention* (eds D. Schottenfeld and J. F. Fraumeni). New York: W. B. Saunders, p. 293.

Urbach, F. (1980). Ultraviolet radiation induced skin cancer in man. *Preventive Medicine*, **9**, 227.

Waldmann, T. A., Strober, W., and Blaese, R. M. (1972). Immunodeficiency disease and malignancy. *Annals of Internal Medicine*, **77**, 605.

Wynder, E. L., and Hoffmann, D. (1982). In *Cancer epidemiology and prevention* (eds D. Schottenfeld and J. F. Fraumeni). New York: W. B. Saunders, p. 277.

Wynder, E. L., Kay, R. M., Reddy, B. S. *et al.* (1983). In *Human carcinogenesis* (eds C. C. Harris and H. Autrup). New York: Academic Press, (in press).

Yuspa, S. H., and Harris, C. C. (1982). In *Cancer epidemiology and prevention* (eds D. Schottenfeld and J. F. Fraumeni). New York: W. B. Saunders, p. 23.

Yuspa, S. H., Ben, T. B., Hennings, H. and Lichti, U. (1980). Phorbol ester tumor promoters induce epidermal transglutaminase activity. *Biochemical Biophysical Research Communications*, **97**, 700.

Risk Factors and Multiple Cancer
Edited by B.A. Stoll
© 1984 John Wiley and Sons Ltd.

Chapter

3   ROBIN A. WEISS

Role of Oncogenic Viruses

Several kinds of virus can cause cancer in man and animals. These viruses probably induce malignancy by different mechanisms, and interact with different environmental and host cofactors. Malignant disease is a rare result of infection and may occur many years after initial infection. In many cases the viral genome, or a part of it, persists in the tumour cell and may, therefore, contribute directly to its malignant properties; in other malignancies, the virus may no longer be present when the tumour appears.

Much of our knowledge of oncogenic viruses comes from animal and cell culture studies, although the role played by viruses in multifactorial cancer is better understood in the epidemiology of human disease. The literature on tumour viruses is extensive and the reader is referred to Klein (1980), Essex *et al.* (1980), Tooze (1980), Weiss *et al.* (1982) for discussion of the natural history, epidemiology, and pathogenesis of the better known tumour viruses. In this chapter, references will be cited only for more recent studies and hypotheses.

HUMAN ONCOGENIC VIRUSES

Table 1 lists seven human malignancies in which viruses appear to play an aetiological role. Epstein–Barr virus (EBV) (Epstein and Achong, 1979) is the cause of infectious mononucleosis, as well as being associated with three kinds of malignancy, Burkitt's lymphoma, immunoblastic lymphoma in immunodeficient patients, and nasopharyngeal carcinoma.

EBV is an example of an ubiquitous human herpes virus which usually infects infants with subclinical effects. Some B-cells, and also probably some epithelial cells in the throat, remain chronically but latently infected throughout life, with sporadic activation. It is those few individuals not infected as infants who are at risk of developing infectious mononucleosis as adolescents

Table 1   Human malignancies probably caused by viruses

Type of cancer	Associated virus
Burkitt's lymphoma	Epstein–Barr virus
Immunoblastic lymphoma in renal transplant patients	Epstein–Barr virus
Nasopharyngeal carcinoma	Epstein–Barr virus
Hepatocellular caricinoma	Hepatitis Barr virus
Squamous carcinoma (especially uterine cervix)	Herpes simplex virus type II Papilloma virus types 6 & 11
Kaposi's sarcoma	Cytomegalovirus
Adult T-Cell lymphoma–leukaemia	Human T-cell leukaemia retrovirus

or young adults when infected with high virus doses in the saliva of their partners.

The virus was first discovered in Burkitt's lymphoma cells grown in culture, and almost all African cases of Burkitt's lymphoma harbour the virus and express its nuclear antigen (EBNA) in the tumour cells. Similarly, the EBV genome and EBNA are found in the cells of nasopharyngeal carcinoma prevalent in southern Chinese. Most infected individuals have persistent EBV-infected B-cells which are potentially immortal when grown in culture.

EBV appears to induce an early 'transformation' step in the oncogenesis of B-cells which may require further changes such as specific chromosome translocations for fully malignant expression (Nilsson, 1982; Klein, 1983). EBV-transformed cells are continuously monitored by the immune system, and, as discussed below, immunodeficient patients have a higher risk of developing EBV-induced lymphoma.

The case for viral involvement in the development of hepatocellular carcinoma is similar to that for EBV-associated tumours (Szmuness, 1978; Zuckerman, 1982). Epidemiologically, primary liver cancer is most prevalent in those parts of the world and those communities where hepatitis B virus (HepBV) is most common (Beasley, 1982). Longitudinal studies of Alaskan Eskimos (Heywood *et al.*, 1982) indicate that seroconversion in HepBV infection may occur 10 years or more before tumour presentation, and infection is frequent in infancy. Like EBV, the HepBV genome can be demonstrated in the carcinoma cells (Shafritz *et al.*, 1981). Related hepatitis viruses of ducks and of woodchucks induce liver cancer in infected animals. Although primary liver cancer is relatively rare in the Western countries, it is one of the most frequent carcinomas world-wide, and we may, therefore, consider HepBV as a major environmental carcinogen.

The evidence for viral aetiology in squamous carcinomas is not as compelling as in EBV-associated malignancies and liver cancer. Epidemiological studies strongly indicate that a transmissible, probably infectious, agent is a factor in cancer of the uterine cervix, but a virus has not been consistently identified. The incidence of cervical cancer is correlated with promiscuity of the patient, or more likely of her sexual partner (Skegg *et al.*, 1982), and is also known to be associated with penile cancer in sexual partners.

For many years, most emphasis has been placed on herpes simplex type II (HSV-II), but more recently, human papilloma viruses (HPV types 6 and 11) have attracted increasing attention. Evidence for HSV-II infection is frequently found in cervical cancer patients and is more closely associated with the malignancy than with evidence of other venereal infections. Furthermore, HSV-I and HSV-II genome fragments are able, at very low efficiency, to transform fibroblastic cells in culture. However, the HSV genome is not invariably found in the carcinoma cells and this has led Galloway and McDougall (1983) to support a 'hit-and-run' mechanism for HSV oncogenesis which does not require persistence of viral DNA in the carcinoma cells.

Zur Hausen (1982) has postulated that HSV may act synergistically with HPV in causing cervical cancer. Dysplastic cells infected with HPV may progress to fully malignant variants on exposure to HSV or other factors such as heavy smoking. HPV types 6 or 11 have been found in several cervical cancers (Gissmann *et al.*, 1983), and there may be further HPV serotypes not yet characterized which are associated with this disease. HPV may also be involved in squamous carcinoma of other sites, including the skin (Ostrow *et al.*, 1982; Spradbrow *et al.*, 1983).

Kaposi's sarcoma is a rare malignancy in the Western world, occurring mainy in patients of Jewish or Mediterranean origin, but the tumour is relatively common in parts of Africa. Boldogh *et al.* (1981) have detected antigens, RNA and DNA of cytomegalovirus (CMV) in African Kaposi's sarcoma tissues, and it is generally believed that CMV is aetiologically associated with this tumour.

A highly malignant form of Kaposi's sarcoma has recently become evident as a frequent consequence of acquired immunodeficiency syndrome (AIDS) now becoming prevalent among promiscuous male homosexuals (Drew *et al.*, 1982; Waterson, 1983). The agent causing AIDS remains to be identified and is probably not CMV itself, but AIDS patients may be especially susceptible to certain CMV-infected cells emerging as Kaposi's sarcomas (see discussion of immunodeficiency below).

Adult T-cell leukaemia-lymphoma (ATL) was first identified in southwestern Japan (Uchiyama *et al.*, 1977; Hanaoka *et al.*, 1982) as a malignancy of mature T-cells distinguishable from classical mycoses fungoides/Sezary's syndrome by the aggressive course of the disease, visceral involvement, and hypercalcaemia. More recently further endemic areas have been discovered, notably the Caribbean basin (Blattner *et al.*, 1982).

A retrovirus known as human adult T-cell lymphoma virus (HTLV or ATLV) is now known to be causally associated with this disease. The virus was first isolated by Poiesz *et al.* (1980) in a lymphoma cell line derived from an American patient and subsequently in Japan (Yoshida *et al.*, 1982). The US, Japanese, and Caribbean isolates appear to be members of the same virus family (Popovic *et al.*, 1982). The mode of transmission of the virus is not yet known, although it is not an inherited, endogenous genome (Reitz *et al.*, 1981) and, therefore, must be infectious. As with the other human tumour viruses, malignancy is a late and rare consequence of infection.

In Japan, the incidence of infection judged by sero-positive individuals increases with age throughout life, and infection becomes more frequent in wives than husbands, suggesting male to female sexual transmission (Tajima *et al.*, 1982). Clinical presentation with the malignancy is more prevalent in the summer, suggesting some seasonal cofactor such as mosquito-borne microfilariasis (Tajima *et al.*, 1981). In contrast to Burkitt's lymphoma, however, the geographical clustering of this lymphoma appears to result from the incidence of primary virus infection rather than from a secondary cofactor.

Lastly, mention should be made of two ubiquitous groups of human viruses which can be shown to have oncogenic properties under experimental conditions, but are not linked epidemiologically with human malignancies. Human adenoviruses are common respiratory tract viruses, of which types 5 and 12 readily cause malignant tumours in hamsters and rats and can transform cells in culture. Similarly, the human polyoma viruses, BK and JC, are high oncogenic in rodents but are apparently non-malignant in man. JC has been associated with progressive multifocal leucoencephalopathy and BK frequently becomes an active urinary tract infection in transplant patients. It remains to be seen whether these potentially oncogenic viruses will one day be causally related to human malignancies.

RISK FACTORS IN HUMAN VIRAL ONCOGENESIS

In the foregoing discussion, human malignancies have been described for which virus infection appears to be a necessary component of oncogenesis. Clearly, then, exposure to the virus is the primary risk factor. Because infection with some of the viruses, e.g. EBV, HSV and CMV, affects a substantial proportion of the human population, whereas the associated cancers are relatively rare, secondary risk factors may play a determining role in the incidence of the disease. This is exemplified by a secondary environmental factor, namely holoendemic malarial infestation, for Burkitt's lymphoma in tropical Africa and New Guinea, and a secondary host genetic factor, namely HLA subgroups and dietary or environmental factors in ethnic southern Chinese, predisposed to nasopharyngeal carcinoma (Henderson *et al.*, 1976; Epstein and Achong, 1979; Yu *et al.*, 1981).

Virus-induced cancers are not unusual in having a multifactorial evolution but it is often difficult to apportion quantitative risks to individual factors, especially when they act synergistically. Thus, it will be difficult to determine accurately the respective roles of HSV and HPV in cervical carcinoma, as proposed by Zur Hausen (1982), or the role of dietary carcinogens, such as aflatoxins or alcohol, in HepBV-associated hepatocellular carcinoma (Larouze *et al.*, 1976).

Squamous skin cancer might be attributable to papilloma viruses (Spradbrow *et al.*, 1983) with exposure to ultraviolet light as the best documented environmental factor, inherited defects in enzymatic repair of UV-damaged DNA (*xeroderma pigmentosum*) and susceptibility to papillomavirus infection (*epidermodysplasia verruciformis*) as well delineated genetic factors, and immunosuppression (see below) as a recognized predisposing pathophysiological factor.

IMMUNODEFICIENCY AND CANCER

The notion that malignant cell clones continuously arise in the body but are quickly eliminated by immune surveillance mechanisms has been discredited because immunodeficient mice and men do not show a markedly higher incidence of most types of cancers. However, those cancers which are known to have a viral aetiology do present at a significantly higher rate in immunodeficient hosts. Thus a major risk factor in viral carcinogenesis is impairment of the immune system (Penn, 1982).

Renal and other organ transplant patients have an increased incidence of non-Hodgkin's lymphomas, Kaposi's sarcoma, liver cancer, and skin cancers. Kinlen (1982) and Purtilo (1982) have, therefore, proposed that the increase in squamous carcinoma of the skin and in melanoma among transplant patients implies a viral factor, possibly HPV, though this remains to be firmly established. Squamous skin cancer is also elevated in non-transplant patients treated with immunosuppressive drugs.

Immunoblastic lymphomas (reticulum cell sarcomas) in patients with iatrogenic immunosuppression (Purtilo and Klein, 1981) and in genetic X-linked immunodeficiency (Purtilo, 1982) contain EBV DNA and antigens. A clonal tumour emerges following polyclonal lymphoid hyperplasia in these patients (Hanto *et al.*, 1982) and in persistent infectious mononucleosis (Abo *et al.*, 1982).

In AIDS, Kaposi's sarcoma and lymphoma are the most frequent tumours observed (Waterson, 1983). One may surmise that late steps in the oncogenesis of CMV-infected cells are normally suppressed by a competent T-cell system. AIDS patients, however, being deficient in T-cells, may be considered as the human equivalent of nude mice, and it is possible that the Kaposi's sarcoma results from the transfer of occult malignant cells from donor to immunodeficient recipient. The development of tumours of donor origin following organ transplantation is now well documented (Kinlen, 1982), and Kaposi's sarcoma in AIDS might conceivably represent an analogous cellular transmission between sexual partners.

PROSPECTS FOR PREVENTING VIRAL MALIGNANCIES

Wherever viruses prove to be the primary cause of cancer, prevention by immunization against viral infection must be seriously entertained. None of the viruses implicated in human cancer is endogenous in the sense of being genetically transmitted (Weiss, 1982), although CMV (Stagno et al., 1982) and possibly HTLV may sometimes be congenitally transmitted. Immunization against postnatal infection should be feasible with oncogenic viruses such as EBV (North et al., 1982), especially with the prospects of chemically synthesized antigenic peptides and of recombinant DNA methods for economically producing viral antigens free of live virus in bacterial systems. Immunization against HepBV will be a specially important task in view of the overall morbidity including liver cancer caused by this virus (Blumberg and London, 1981; WHO Scientific Group, 1983).

Where primary immunization is not practical, intervention at the level of a rate-limiting cofactor could effectively prevent the great majority of viral cancers developing to a clinical presentation. For example, prevention of malarial infection, which is so desirable owing to the direct morbidity of the *Plasmodium* parasite itself, would incidentally eliminate all but a small number of sporadic cases of Burkitt's lymphoma.

Prevention of iatrogenic infection is an important matter. The necessity for HepBV detection in donated blood is well recognized. There is evidence that both the AIDS agent (Ragni et al., 1983) and HTLV (Miyoshi et al., 1982; Saxinger and Gallo, 1982) are transmitted by the transfer of blood or blood products. It is of great importance to devise rapid screening methods if the risk of blood transfusion is to be eliminated.

MOLECULAR MECHANISMS OF VIRAL ONCOGENESIS

How viruses transform cells into a neoplastic state is not yet understood clearly, although remarkable advances have recently been made in probing the molecular genetics of animal tumour viruses. With the DNA tumour viruses, such as herpes, hepatitis or papovaviruses, full replication of the virus is cytopathic so that the infected cell is destined to die rather than transform to malignancy. However, replication is frequently incomplete, either because the infected cell is of a type that does not support the complete viral life cycle or because the virus has lost genetic information essential for later stages of replication.

With the RNA retroviruses, full replication is not usually cytocidal, so the infected cell may support virus production as well as becoming neoplastic. Nevertheless, many retrovirus infections are non-productive, and the most highly oncogenic retroviruses are defective for viral replication owing to the substitution of oncogenes in place of genes essential for virus production.

Tumour viruses could induce neoplasia by a variety of mechanisms:

1. Non-specific tissue damage inducing proliferation

The chronic cytopathic effects of virus infection may stimulate regeneration or hyperplasia in neighbouring uninfected cells that eventually become neoplastic. One could envisage such events, for example, in liver tissue infected with hepatitis B virus. There is evidence, however, that viral transformation is more specific, as only a small number of cytopathic viruses are oncogenic. Furthermore, in many cases the viral genome, or part of it, can be found in each of the tumour cells, implying that specific viral genetic information is important in viral oncogenesis.

2. 'Hit-and-run' mutagens

In cases where the viral genome cannot be found in the cancer cells, it is thought that precancerous cells ancestral to the tumour have been infected by the virus and that the virus has caused mutations – just as physical and chemical carcinogens do – without persisting in the malignant clone. Such a model has recently been proposed for cervical carcinogenesis by herpes simplex virus (Galloway and McDougall, 1983). Some lymphomas in cats and cattle, while strongly linked epidemiologically with retroviruses, are virus-negative.

3. Tumour viruses as insertional mutagens

The DNA of retroviruses and some papovaviruses integrates into host chromosomal DNA. Integration itself is a recombinational event that causes changes in the organization of host genetic information. The site of viral integration into host DNA has been studied extensively for these viruses, and in most cases it appears to be largely random, that is, the viral genome integrates at a different site, and often in a different chromosome for each infected cell. Some of these integration events will be mutagenic, and in rare cases could lead to neoplasia, analogous to mutagenesis by chemical carcinogens. Polyoma viruses, for example, are mutagenic and also induce chromosome breaks and rearrangements.

In the case of avian retroviruses causing bursal lymphomatosis, there is evidence that integration of the viral genome can alter the expression of neighbouring host genes, in particular by activating their expression ectopically. Of the many millions of bursal cells infected with the avian retrovirus, a clonal lymphoma is derived from one cell in which the virus has integrated in a suitable position to enhance the expression of a particular cellular gene, knows as *c-myc*. The human *c-myc* gene is amplified in some myeloid leukaemias and solid tumours, and it is translocated from chromosome 8 to active immunoglobulin gene sites on other chromosomes in Burkitt's lymphoma (Klein, 1983; Rowley, 1983).

Whereas activation of *c-myc* in avian bursal lymphomagenesis is probably an early step in viral oncogenesis, the translocation of *c-myc* in human Burkitt's lymphoma is a late step apparently unrelated to the earlier 'immortalization' of the lymphoblast by EBV but closely related to its final emergence as a malignant clone. Cellular genes like *c-myc*, which are thought to exert oncogenic properties, are collectively called *c-onc*, for cellular oncogenes. Most *c-onc* genes have been identified by their close resemblance to viral oncogenes (*v-onc*).

4. Viral oncogenes

Some acutely oncogenic retroviruses carry transforming genes in place of the virus's normal replication genes. These genes are not required for viral replication; indeed, they render the virus defective but can induce cell transformation (Bishop, 1982). They are collectively known as *v-onc* genes and the best studied is the *src* gene of Rous sarcoma virus. The *src* gene codes for a 60,000 dalton protein which exhibits a protein kinase activity, phosphorylating tyrosine residues.

Mutants of Rous sarcoma virus which are temperature-sensitive for the maintenance of the neoplastic state of the infected cell are temperature-sensitive for the kinase reaction, indicating that this enzyme activity is important for the oncogenic effect of the virus. Several other *v-onc* genes also code for protein kinases. The target proteins in the host cell, which become phosphorylated by these oncogene products, are currently under intensive study. Other *v-onc* genes code for different products. The *v-myc* gene encodes a DNA-binding protein and *v-ras* encodes a GTP-binding protein. Thus there is no common function to the products of oncogenes.

Molecular hybridization studies show that *v-onc* genes have been derived from cellular genes. By incorporation into the viral genome they come under viral control signals and may also be packaged and transmitted infectiously when viral replication is complemented by a related non-defective 'helper' virus. The *v-onc* genes of defective, transforming retroviruses represent the converse situation to the *c-onc* genes activated by non-defective retroviruses. Instead of the virus causing ectopic gene expression by inserting itself next to the cellular gene, it picks up that gene and carries it as part of the virus. The result is that all the cells that the virus infects are likely to become neoplastic.

Such transducing oncogenic viruses occur only very rarely outside the laboratory, perhaps because they are so pathogenic that they will not be maintained in natural host populations, as they do not play a role in virus replication. However, they are proving to be immensely powerful tools for investigating the molecular biology of cancer. Because *v-onc* genes are derived from cell genes that are well conserved in evolution, it is proving possible to use *v-onc* genes of chicken or mouse retroviruses as probes for the molecular rearrangement and ectopic expression of homologous genes in human malignancies, even when a virus is not involved in its causation.

A number of *c-onc* genes have been isolated from non-viral human carcinomas, sarcomas, and leukaemias (Marshall, 1983). Using DNA transfer and manipulation techniques, the human *c-onc* genes can be identified by transformation of preneoplastic cells in culture. In at least two cases, an altered gene product rather than changed control of gene expression determines the oncogenic property of the allele found in malignant cells. However, the functions of the normal alleles of *c-onc* genes remain to be elucidated.

In contrast to retroviruses, DNA tumour viruses code for viral proteins essential for early phases of viral replication which also play a role in cellular transformation. For instance, the large T antigen of SV40 is required for initiating replication of viral DNA, but also stimulates cellular DNA synthesis. Viral T antigen forms complexes with a cellular protein, called p53, and it is probably the complex that activates cell division (Lane and Harlow, 1982). The p53 protein is also synthesized in normal cells, but it is rapidly degraded. When complexed to T antigen it becomes stabilized and may trigger uncontrolled cell proliferation. An adenovirus protein similarly binds to p53, and an analogous complex between viral and cellular proteins is found in EBV-transformed cells. Several non-viral tumours also express high levels of unusually stable p53 protein.

Thus, transiently expressed cellular proteins which are probably involved in the normal activation of DNA synthesis may induce neoplasia if they persist unnaturally in the cell, either because they form complexes with viral proteins, or due to some other alteration in non-viral tumours.

CONCLUSION

The elucidation of molecular events in oncogenesis caused by viruses is helping us to understand neoplasia generally. Nevertheless, as Logan and Cairns (1982) have noted:

We need to keep in mind that natural human carcinogenesis is a multistep process. We do not know what the rate-limiting steps are, nor which of them are most sensitive to environmental influences and therefore a proper object for preventative strategies. But we can at least feel that the technology for studying genes and their patterns of expression are now advancing so fast that the molecular biologist will soon be telling the epidemiologist what to look for.

It may become feasible in the not too distant future to exploit our knowledge of oncogenes and their products for the diagnosis and treatment of human cancer.

REFERENCES

Abo, W., Takada, K., Kamada, M. *et al.* (1982). Evolution of infectious mononucleosis into Epstein–Barr virus carrying monoclonal malignant lymphoma. *Lancet,* **1,** 1272.

Beasley, R. P. (1982). Hepatitis B virus as the etiologic agent in hepatocellular carcinoma. Epidemiologic considerations. *Hepatology,* **2,** 215.

Bishop, J. M. (1982). Retroviruses and cancer genes. *Advances in Cancer Research,* **37,** 1.

Blattner, W. A., Kalyanaraman, V. S., Robert-Guroff, M. *et al.* (1982). The human type-C retrovirus, HTLV, in Blacks from the Caribbean, and relationship to adult T-cell leukemia/lymphoma. *International Journal of Cancer,* **30,** 257.

Blumberg, B. S., and London, W. T. (1981). Hepatitis B virus and the prevention of primary hepatocellular carcinoma. *New England Journal of Medicine,* **304,** 782.

Boldogh, I., Beth, E., Huang, E.-S. *et al.* (1981). Kaposi's sarcoma. IV. Detection of CMV DNA, CMV RNA and CMNA in tumor biopsies. *International Journal of Cancer,* **28,** 469.

Drew, W. L., Conant, M. A., Miner, R. C. *et al.* (1982). Cytomegalovirus and Kaposi's sarcoma in young homosexual men. *Lancet,* **2,** 125.

Epstein, M. A., and Achong, B. G. (eds) (1979). *The Epstein–Barr virus.* New York: Springer-Verlag.

Essex, M., Todaro, G. J., and zur Hausen, H. (eds) (1980). *Viruses in naturally occurring cancers.* Cold Spring Harbor Laboratory.

Galloway, D. A., and McDougall, J. K. (1983). The oncogenic potential of herpes simplex viruses: evidence for a 'hit-and-run' mechanism. *Nature,* **302,** 21.

Gissmann, L., Wolnik, L., Ikenberg, H. *et al.* (1983). Human papillomavirus types 6 and 11 DNA sequences in genital and laryngeal papillomas and in some cervical cancer biopsies. *Proceedings of the National Academy of Science, USA,* **80,** 560.

Hanaoka, M., Takatsuki, K., and Shimoyama, M. (eds) (1982). Adult T-cell leukemia and related diseases. *Gann Monograph on Cancer Research,* **28,** 1.

Hanto, D. W., Frizzera, G., Gajl-Peczalska, K. J. *et al.* (1982). Epstein–Barr virus-induced B-cell lymphoma after renal transplantation. Acyclovir therapy and transition from polyclonal to monoclonal B-cell proliferation. *New England Journal of Medicine,* **306,** 913.

Henderson, B. E., Louie, E., Jing, J. S. *et al.* (1976). Risk factors associated with nasopharyngeal carcinoma. *New England Journal of Medicine,* **295,** 1101.

Heyward, W., Bender, T. R., Lanier, A. P. *et al.* (1982). Serological markers of hepatitis B virus and alpha-fetoprotein levels preceding primary hepatocellular carcinoma in Alaskan Eskimos. *Lancet,* **2,** 889.

Kinlen, L. (1982). Immunosuppressive therapy and cancer. *Cancer Surveys*, **1**, 565.

Klein, G. (ed) (1980). *Viral oncology*. New York: Raven Press.

Klein, G. (1983). Specific chromosomal translocations and the genesis of B-cell-derived tumors in mice and men. *Cell*, **32**, 311.

Lane, D., and Harlow, E. (1982). Two different viral transforming proteins bind the same host tumour antigen. *Nature*, **298**, 5874.

Larouze, B., London, W. T., Saimot, G., Werner, B. G., Lustbader, E. D., Payet, M., and Blumberg, B. S. (1976). Host responses to hepatitis B infection in patients with primary hepatic carcinoma and their families. *Lancet*, **2**, 534.

Logan, J., and Cairns, J. (1982). The secrets of cancer. *Nature*, **300**, 104.

Marshall, C.J. (1983). Oncogenes. *Cancer Topics*, **4**, 102.

Miyoshi, I., Fujishita, M., Taguchi, H. *et al.* (1982). Caution against blood transfusion from donors seropositive to adult T-cell leukemia-associated antigens. *Lancet*, **1**, 683.

Nilsson, K. (1982). Phenotypic and cytogenetic characteristics of human B-lymphoid cell lines and their relevance for the etiology of Burkitt's lymphoma. *Advances in Cancer Research*, **37**, 319.

North, J. R., Morgan, A. J., Thompson, J. L., and Epstein, M. A. (1982). Purified Epstein–Barr virus mr 340,000 glycoprotein induces potent virus-neutralizing antibodies when incorporated in liposomes. *Proceedings of the National Academy of Science, USA*, **79**, 7504.

Ostrow, R. S., Bender, M., Niimura, M. *et al.* (1982). Human papillomavirus DNA in cutaneous primary and metastasized squamous carcinomas from patients with epidermodysplasia verruciformis. *Proceedings of the National Academy of Science, USA*, **79**, 1634.

Penn, I. (1982). The occurrence of cancer in immune deficiencies. *Current Problems in Cancer*, **6**, 2.

Poiesz, B. J., Ruscetti, F. W., Gazdar, A. F. *et al.* (1980). Detection and isolation of type C retrovirus particles from fresh and cultured lymphocytes of a patient with cutaneous T-cell lymphoma. *Proceedings of the National Academy of Science, USA*, **77**, 7415.

Popovic, M., Kalyanaraman, V. S., Sarngadharan, M. G. *et al.* (1982). The virus of Japanese adult T-cell leukemia is a member of the human T-cell leukemia virus group. *Nature*, **300**, 63.

Purtilo, D. T. (1981). Immune deficiency predisposing to Epstein–Barr virus-induced lymphoproliferative diseases: The X-linked lymphoproliferative syndrome as a model. *Advances in Cancer Research*, **34**, 279.

Purtilo, D. T. (1982). Viruses, tumours, and immune deficiency. *Lancet*, **1**, 684.

Purtilo, D. T., and Klein, G. (1981). Introduction to Epstein–Barr virus and lymphoproliferative diseases in immunodeficient individuals. *Cancer Research*, **41**, 4209.

Ragni, M. V., Lewis, J. H., Spero, J. A., and Bontempo, F. A. (1983). Acquired immunodeficiency-like syndrome in two haemophiliacs. *Lancet*, **1**, 213.

Reitz, M. S., Poiesz, B. J., Ruscetti, F. W., and Gallo, R. C. (1981). Characterization and distribution of nucleic acid sequences of a novel type C retrovirus isolated from neoplastic lymphocytes. *Proceedings of the National Academy of Science, USA*, **78**, 1887.

Rowley, J. D. (1983). Human oncogene locations and chromosome aberrations. *Nature*, **301**, 290.

Saxinger, W. C., and Gallo, R. C. (1982). Possible risk to recipients of blood from donors carrying serum markers of human T-cell virus. *Lancet*, **1**, 1074.

Shafritz, D. A., Shouval, D., Sherman, H. I. *et al.* (1981). Integration of hepatitis B virus DNA into the genome of liver cells in chronic liver disease and hepatocellular carcinoma. *New England Journal of Medicine*, **305**, 1067.

Skegg, D. C. G., Corwin, P. A., Paul, C., and Doll, R. (1982). Importance of the male factor in cancer of the cervix. *Lancet*, **2**, 581.

Spradbarrow, P. B., Beardmore, G. L., and Francis, J. L. (1983). Virions resembling papillomaviruses in hyperkaryotic lesions from sun-damaged skin. *Lancet*, **1**, 189.

Stagno, S., Pass, R. F., Meyer, E. D. *et al.* (1982). Congenital cytomegalovirus infection. The relative importance of primary and recurrent maternal infection. *New England Journal of Medicine*, **306**, 945.

Szmuness, W. (1978). Hepatocellular carcinoma and hepatitis B virus. Evidence for a causal association. *Progress in Medical Virology*, **24**, 40.

Tajima, K., Tominaga, S., Shimizu, H., and Suchi, T. (1981). A hypothesis on the etiology of adult T-cell leukemia/lymphoma. *Gann*, **72**, 684.

Tajima, K., Tominaga, S., Suchi, T. *et al.* (1982). Epidemiological analysis of the distribution of antibody to adult T-cell leukemia-virus-associated antigen: possible horizontal transmission of adult T-cell leukemia virus. *Gann*, **73**, 893.

Tooze, J. (ed.) (1980). *Molecular biology of tumor viruses*, 2nd edn, Part 2. *DNA tumor viruses*. Cold Spring Harbor Laboratory.

Uchiyama, T., Yodoi, J., Sagawa, K. *et al.* (1977). Adult T-cell leukemia in Japan. Clinical and hematological features of 16 cases. *Blood*, **50**, 481.

Waterson, A. P. (1983). Acquired immune deficiency syndrome. *British Medical Journal*, **286**, 743.

Weiss, R. A. (1982). The persistence of retroviruses. In *Virus Persistence* (eds B. W. J. Mahy, A. C. Minson, and G. K. Darby). *Symposium 33, Society for General Microbiology*. Cambridge: Cambridge University Press, p. 267.

Weiss, R. A., Teich, N. M., Varmus, H. E., and Coffin, J. M. (eds) (1982). *Molecular biology of tumor viruses*, 2nd edn, Part 3. *RNA tumor viruses*. Cold Spring Harbor Laboratory.

WHO Scientific Group (1983). Prevention of primary liver cancer. *Lancet*, **1**, 463.

Yoshida, M., Myoshi, I., and Hinuma, Y. (1982). Isolation and characterization of retrovirus from cell lines of human adult T-cell leukemia and its implication in the disease. *Proceedings of the National Academy of Science, USA*, **79**, 2031.

Yu, M.C., Ho, J.H.C., Ross, R.K. and Henderson, B.E. (1981). Nasopharyngeal carcinomas in Chinese—salted fish or inhaled smoke? *Preventive Medicine*, **10**, 15.

Zuckerman, A. J. (1982). Primary hepatocellular carcinoma and hepatitis B virus. *Transactions of the Royal Society of Tropical Medicine and Hygiene*, **76**, 711.

Zur Hausen, H. (1982). Human genital cancer: synergism between two virus infections or synergism between a virus infection and initiating events? *Lancet*, **2**, 1370.

Risk Factors and Multiple Cancer
Edited by B.A. Stoll
© 1984 John Wiley and Sons Ltd.

Chapter

4

J. WHANG-PENG and S. M. SIEBER

Chromosomal Damage by Radiation and Antitumor Agents

INTRODUCTION

Radiation and antitumor agents are capable of damaging DNA and producing chromosome aberrations. Some individuals are more susceptible to DNA-damaging agents than others; these individuals include those with chromosome breakage syndromes such as ataxia telangiectasia, xeroderma pigmentosum, Fanconi's anemia, Bloom's syndrome, Cockayne syndrome, and Down's syndrome. Susceptibility also differs with age, decreasing with age in early life and increasing in later life. It is becoming increasingly clear that those who are more susceptible to DNA-damaging agents are also at increased risk of cancer (Setlow, 1978; Cohen et al., 1982).

With improvements in cytogenetic techniques, many specific chromosomal abnormalities have now been associated with certain malignancies. Acquired chromosomal abnormalities include: the Ph^1 chromosome in chronic myelocytic leukemia (Nowell and Hungerford, 1960); t(15;17) in acute promyelocytic leukemia (Rowley et al., 1977a); t(8;14) in Burkitt's lymphoma (Manolov et al., 1971); and del 3p(14–23) in small cell lung cancer (Whang-Peng et al., 1982). Congenital chromosomal abnormalities include del 13q14 in retinoblastoma (Yunis and Ramsay, 1978) and del 11p13 in patients with aniridia–Wilms's tumor (Riccardi et al., 1978). However, the relationship between the origin of these abnormal chromosomes and neoplasia is still unclear.

Mitelman et al. (1981) in a retrospective study of patients with acute non-lymphocytic leukemia (ANLL), found that clonal chromosomal aberrations were significantly more common in patients occupationally exposed to potentially mutagenic/carcinogenic agents (chemical solvents, insecticides,

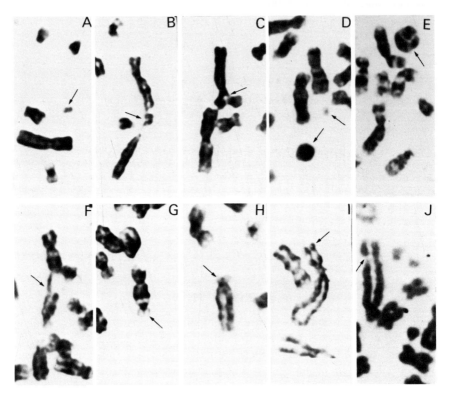

Figure 1   Representative chromosome aberrations induced by X-irradiation. Human peripheral lymphocytes were exposed to 50–100 r of X-irradiation, and 48–72 hours later metaphase spreads were prepared. (A) and (B) chromosome fragments; (C) single chromatid break; (D) micronucleus and chromosome fragment; (E) ring chromosome; (F) decondensation of one chromatid; (G) dicentric chromosome; (H), (I), and (J) giant marker chromosomes. Arrow in J indicates single chromatid break.

and petrol products) than in patients with no history of occupational exposure to such agents.

Chromosomal damage by radiation and anti-tumor agents would not be detectable without an adequate demonstration of chromosome morphology subsequent to production of mitotic figures. The development of banding techniques (Caspersson *et al.*, 1970) opened a promising new avenue in the area of cytogenetics. Chromosomal aberrations can be divided into the following categories (Figure 1):

1. A simple deletion, which results from a single break in a chromosome, producing a gap, a break, or an acentric fragment and a deletion.

2. An exchange, which can produce either stable or unstable chromosome aberrations. It involves at least two breaks and an exchange of broken parts, either:
    (a) between different chromosomes resulting either in dicentric chromosomes (unstable) or reciprocal translocations (stable);
    (b) between different parts of the same chromosome, producing rings (unstable) or paracentric or pericentric inversions (stable). Unstable chromosomes (ring, dicentric or acentric chromosomes) are so termed because they will be eliminated during subsequent cell divisions. Stable chromosomes are usually marker chromosomes, and they usually remain in cells for generation after generation.
3. Micronuclei, which arise from chromosome fragments that are not incorporated into daughter nuclei; their presence can be used as a rapid assay for chromosomal damage.
4. Polyploidy, is an aberration readily shown immediately after exposure to toxic agents *in vivo* or *in vitro*. Polyploidism is usually dose-related within the range of exposure; hence the number of these aberrations can be used as an indicator of exposure in humans.

The introduction of the sister chromatid exchange (SCE) technique has also provided a useful method of assessing chromosome effects induced by chemicals and radiation (Figure 2). The growth conditions for SCE studies require special modifications from regular PHA (phytohemoagglutinin)-stimulated lymphocyte cultures.

RADIATION

The chromosomal aberrations caused by radiation are categorized as stable or unstable abnormalities (Buckton *et al.*, 1962), and include chromosomal intrachanges and interchanges. Intrachanges represent events that occur within a chromosome, including breaks (terminal deletions and interstitial deletions), breaks and reunions (centric rings and fragments, acentric fragments with marker chromosomes), and inversions (pericentric or paracentric). Interchanges represent interactions of two or more chromosomes, such as formation of a dicentric chromosome and a fragment, or formation of two marker chromosomes. These two types of interchanges occur with approximately equal frequency.

Although irradiation causes chromosomal changes in Hela cells (Nias and Ockey, 1965), a progressive reduction in chromosome number has not been associated with exposure to radiation or to changes in radiosensitivity, regardless of whether cells are exposed to single doses or to continuous irradiation (30 r/day). An increase in the proportion of polyploid cells has been noted in irradiated subjects (Tough *et al.*, 1960; Buckton *et al.*, 1962),

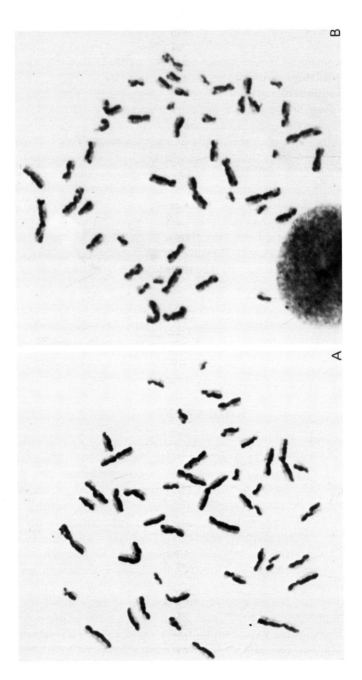

Figure 2   Sister chromatid exchange assay in human lymphocytes: (A) normal control cells; (B) lymphocytes incubated with *m*-AMSA (0.01 µg/mℓ) for 48 hours. Numerous sister chromatid exchanges are apparent in the metaphase chromosomes.

and a high incidence of polyploid cells has also been produced by irradiating leukocyte cultures *in vitro* (Ohnuki *et al.*, 1961; Bell and Baker, 1965).

Several types of chromosome aberrations are useful for the study of radiation exposure, including dicentric chromosomes, polyploidism, and micronuclei. Not only do these tests provide a rapid assay for radiation exposure but they also can provide a rough estimate of the level of exposure or radiation dose.

1. *Dicentric chromosomes* Dicentric chromosomes are easy to recognize and score. Many published data indicate that the frequency of dicentric chromosomes correlates linearly with the dose within 200 r (Evans, 1972).
2. *Polyploidy* An increased incidence of polyploid cells occurs in irradiated individuals (Tough *et al.*, 1960; Buckton *et al.*, 1962). Polyploid cells also occur at a high incidence in leukocyte cultures irradiated *in vitro* (Ohnuki *et al.*, 1961), Ishihara and Kumatori (1966) studied cells irradiated under either *in vivo* or *in vitro* conditions. They found that the incidence of polyploidy was 0.05% in control (unexposed) cells; the incidence of polyploidy in irradiated cells was 0.2% (50 r), 0.3% (100 r), 0.5% (200 r) and 2.7% (350 r).

   In comparison, the incidence of polyploidy in individuals exposed to Thorotrast was 0.26% and in individuals irradiated at Bikini was 0.3%. The majority of the polyploid cells contained abnormal chromosomes, such as dicentrics, tricentrics, rings, and acentric fragments. Dicentrics were the most frequently observed chromosome abnormalities. The frequency of polyploid cells showing structural chromosome abnormalities increased with the dose of radiation and the abnormal chromosomes were apparently able to duplicate since they frequently were present in pairs.
3. *Micronuclei* Micronuclei arise from chromosome fragments that are not incorporated into daughter nuclei at mitoses because they lack a centromere. Countryman and Heddle (1976) noted that the increase in micronucleus frequency begins at the time of the first mitosis after irradiation and found a quantitative relationship between the incidence of chromosome aberrations and incidence of micronuclei. Therefore, the authors suggested using the micronuclei count as a rapid assay for chromosomal damage induced by X-rays.

Reddy *et al.* (1980) studied 15 healthy age-matched individuals as controls, 10 adults aged 23–43 who received 200–768 r between the ages of 22 to 559 days for alleged thymic enlargement, and 7 cancer patients who received therapeutic irradiation at doses ranging between 4000 and 6000 r. The frequency of micronuclei in controls was 2.43±0.24 (mean±SE) micronuclei per 1000 cells; it was 3.54±0.34 in individuals irradiated for thymic enlargement, and 8.21±1.78 for cancer patients. The incidence of micronuclei in cells from non-irradiated cancer patients was 4.17±0.91.

INTERNAL IRRADIATION

Some radioactive contrast media, Thorotrast in particular, not only cause significant chromosomal aberrations but are also associated with an increased incidence of neoplasms as well, Isotopes such as ^{131}I, ^{32}p, ^{198}Au and ^{19}Y have been used as clinical therapeutic agents for both benign and malignant diseases. In addition, some environmental or occupational contaminants such as ^{226}Ra, ^{228}Ra, ^{222}Ra and ^{220}Ra are considered to present a cytogenetic hazard.

Radiocontrast media and radiation

Adams *et al.* (1977) measured chromosome aberrations and micronuclei in lymphocytes from seven patients in which angiocardiography using Renografin was used. Their results indicated that the chromosome damage observed in patients was due not only to an increased absorption of X-rays, but also to breakage of chromosomes even in the absence of X-rays. Norman *et al.* (1978) confirmed their results, also suggesting that the contrast medium was largely responsible for the observed cytogenetic damage.

Thorotrast was extensively used as a radiographic contrast medium between 1930 and 1947. In a study of 1689 individuals given thorium dioxide in West Germany between 1935 and 1951, Van Kaick *et al.* (1978) found a high incidence of hemangioendothelioma of the liver; other malignancies which developed in these patients included osteosarcomas, two of which occurred in persons given thorium dioxide at 13 and 16 years of age. In addition to malignancies arising at the sites of thorium deposition, there is an increased incidence of leukemia and aplastic anemia in individuals exposed to Thorotrast (da Silva Horta *et al.*, 1965; Bastrup-Madsen *et al.*, 1971).

A Danish series of 1005 patients receiving Thorotrast was described by Faber (1973). A total of 312 patients had died, and 11 of these had developed leukemia. The time interval between Thorotrast administration and the development of leukemia was variable, averaging about six years. Myeloid, lymphoid, and erythroid leukemias have all been reported following Thorotrast exposure (Trübestein and Citoler, 1973). A cytogenetic study was performed on 36 patients who had received Thorotrast by intra-arterial injection from 11 to 31 years previously (Buckton *et al.*, 1967). The incidence of unstable chromosomal aberrations (rings, dicentrics or acentric fragments) was 9.2%. Many cells contained more than one aberration and a 3.8% frequency of tricentrics was also noted. There was no correlation between the incidence of chromosome aberrations and dose of Thorotrast given, nor were any sex differences apparent. Stable chromosome rearrangements were present in only 5.7% of cells.

Radioactive iodine (^{131}I)

Iodine-131 enters the iodine pool, and some is concentrated in the thyroid gland while the remainder is excreted in urine. The iodine pool in adults ranges from 20 to 30 liters and corresponds to extracellular fluid. ^{131}I in the iodine pool will irradiate most body tissues uniformly with both beta- and gamma-radiation. When the thyroid gland is destroyed by an ablative dose of radioiodine, the mean half-line of radioiodine in the gland is about five days. It is probable that most of the body lymphocytes will be irradiated while they circulate through the gland.

Lloyd *et al.* (1976) studied 11 patients receiving large ablative doses of ^{131}I (6 received 80 mCi) for the treatment of thyroid carcinoma. Forty-five patients received an additional 200 mCi for metastatic lesions. The authors used the number of dicentrics induced to estimate the approximate radiation dose. The number of dicentrics per cell ranged from 0 to 0.094 with a mean of 0.04. The biological effects of radiation in patients treated with ^{131}I are also manifested as chromosomal breakage in peripheral blood lymphocytes (Nofal and Beierwaltes, 1964; Cantolino *et al.*, 1966). A statistically significant increased incidence of structural and numerical chromosomal abnormalities was observed acutely and to a lesser extent chronically in such patients. These abnormalities were detected as early as 30 minutes after therapy and persisted for at least 14 years (Nofal and Beierwaltes, 1964).

Malignancy arising as a complication of therapy in patients who received treatment for hyperthyroidism or thyroid carcinoma was not noted in over 10,000 cases treated with radioiodine for thyrotoxicosis (Pochin, 1960). However, hypothyroidism in infants whose mothers were treated during pregnancy with ^{131}I has been described (Goh, 1981).

Radioactive phosphorus (^{32}p)

Phosphorus-32 is used extensively to treat polycythemia vera (PV). In a review of published data on 239 untreated patients with PV, aneuploidy was seen in 53 (22.2%). In contrast, aneuploidy was seen in 42 (67.7%) of 62 PV patients receiving ^{32}p and/or chemotherapy (Whang-Peng and Young, 1978). A small F chromosome (20q12-) is the only common chromosome abnormality found with regularity in this disease. Lawler *et al.* (1970) showed a deleted F-group chromosome in 10 of the 79 (12.6%) cases they described; 9 of these 10 patients had received ^{32}p and one had been treated with busulfan.

In a review by Modan and Lilienfeld (1965), a marked predisposition to leukemia was identified in patients with polycythemia vera. Approximately one in six patients developed leukemia after an interval of 10–15 years, and abnormal clones are found in a large proportion of ^{32}p-treated patients. These clones are thought to be radiation-induced and sometimes involve 100% of the metaphases examined during the terminal stages of the disease. The leukemia is usually of the acute or subacute myeloid variety.

Radioactive gold (^{198}Au); radioactive yttrium (^{19}Y)

Intra-articular injection of radioactive gold of yttrium has been used for the treatment of rheumatoid arthritis. The half-life of ^{198}Au is 65 hours. Examination of blood samples obtained one day to eight years following treatment with ^{198}Au showed increased chromosomal aberrations (Stevenson *et al.*, 1973). The authors account for the chromosome changes by hypothesizing that aberrations were induced in lymphocytes because of the irradiation they received as they passed through the lymph nodes. The risk following intra-articular irradiation would appear to be less for ^{90}Y than for ^{198}Au.

Radium

The accumulation in the body over a short period of time of large amounts of radium or mesothorium leads to the early production of bone damage, to septic necrosis, and to the development of bone tumors. Severe anemia and leukopenia are also noted. One chromosome study showed that watch dial painters using paint containing radium (with radioactivity ranging from non-measurable to 0.56 μCi of radium-226) had an increased incidence of structural chromosome abnormalities. The incidence of unstable aberrations was 2.36% versus 1.64% in controls. The frequency of stable aberrations was 10% versus 1.17% in controls. The authors found a consistent gradient of increasing structural abnormalities with increasing body burden of radium (Boyd *et al.*, 1966).

Fischer *et al.* (1971) described the results of cytogenetic studies performed on the peripheral lymphocytes of 6500 individuals residing in Bad Gastein, Austria. This population was examined because they were exposed to an elevated level of naturally occurring radioactivity, mostly from ^{222}Ra and ^{220}Ra present in spring water. These individuals exhibited a significant increase in the incidence of chromosome aberrations.

Uranium mine workers have a high incidence of lung cancer, especially small cell lung cancer. Many small cell lung cancers have a specific chromosome abnormality such as del 3p(14–23) (Whang-Peng *et al.*, 1982). Whether the tumors developing in uranium miners carry the same marker remains to be determined.

EXTERNAL RADIATION

External radiation includes that from diagnostic X-rays, household appliances, cosmetic exposure (ultraviolet light), X-ray treatment for benign conditions, irradiation for malignant conditions, and radiation exposure related to accidents and military activities.

Diagnostic X-irradiation

Peripheral lymphocyte chromosome studies were performed on 11 patients exposed only to diagnostic X-ray procedures (Bloom and Tjio, 1964). Each patient served as his own pre-irradiation control. Although no chromosome aberrations were found in six patients exposed to 20–80 milli r during X-ray examination of the chest, definite evidence of X-ray-induced aberrations was apparent within 72 hours after irradiation. Fluoroscopy was performed on the remaining five patients. In three of these patients an upper gastrointestinal series was performed, and barium enema studies were carried out in the other two. The skin doses ranged between 12 and 35 r, as determined by a Victorine Chamber.

The authors found dicentrics, fragments or ring chromosomes in 1–4% of metaphase cells in post-irradiation cultures. In three of the five patients, the aberrations appeared in peripheral lymphocytes within 30 minutes after irradiation; in the other two patients, the aberrations appeared at 72 hours after irradiation. The aberrations had disappeared from the lymphocytes of four patients by two weeks after irradiation, whereas in the fifth patient the aberrations persisted for at least 2½ months after irradiation.

Therapuetic irradiation

Ankylosing spondylitis

Buckton *et al.* (1962) examined peripheral blood cultures from 58 patients with anklylosing spondylitis, none of whom had had more than one course of X-ray therapy to the spinal axis. Cultures were studied immediately before X-ray therapy to periods of up to 20 years after therapy. The authors categorized the chromosomal aberrations noted as either unstable or stable. The incidence of unstable abnormalities rose to a peak value at two to three weeks after the end of treatment, and then declined. A small number of abnormal cells persisted for five years. The incidence of stable abnormalities did not change over the years from the level reached shortly after the end of treatment; dicentrics were present for up to five years and small fragments from 5 to 19 years. X-irradiation also caused a striking increase in number of polyploid cells in blood cultures from these patients.

The risk of leukaemia developing in spondylitic patients is related not only to the X-ray dose but also to the age at exposure, the risk being greater in older than in younger subjects. Of the 11 patients with acute leukemia whom the authors studied, two showed a remarkable degree of polyploidy in blood and in the marrow. Both patients had an acute erythroleukemia and both had had extensive X-ray therapy for ankylosing spondylitis.

Mastitis

Seventy-two patients ranging in age from 18 to 40 years had received 75–1400 r for acute mastitis 12–33 years prior to evaluation. No significant differences between controls and irradiated patients were noted with regard to incidence of chromosome aberrations or in proportions and absolute numbers of T, B, and null lymphocytes. There is high incidence of breast neoplasms in irradiated mastitis patients, which the authors suggested is due to an increased mutation rate in breast tissue caused by irradiation (Reddy *et al.*, 1977).

Irradiation after mastectomy

Kucerova (1970) performed cytogenetic studies on a patient who had received a total of 16,000 r of fractionated radiation after resection of a mammary tumor. A gradual but significant rise in the number of lymphocytes with chromosomal aberrations was found, which persisted from 35 to 69 weeks after termination of treatment. During radiotherapy the number of polyploid mitoses rose significantly, but by 35 weeks after radiotherapy was discontinued had returned to normal.

In another study, six female patients were treated for mammary carcinoma with neutron radiation (telecobalt). The mean incidence of dicentrics and ring chromosomes increased from 1% in controls to 4%, 9.4%, and 17.8% in patients who had received 6 Gy, 16 Gy, and 22 Gy, respectively (Antoine *et al.*, 1981). Schmid *et al.* (1980) studied 17 patients with various tumors before, during and after 14 MeV (DT) neutron therapy. They noted that the total damage to chromosomes (dicentrics, centric rings, and excess acentrics) showed a positive correlation with the dose to skin.

Irradiation of the thymus

Goh *et al.* (1976) reported a significant increase in chromosome breaks in adults whose thymus had been irradiated 28–41 years previously.

Ultraviolet radiation

Chu (1965) studied a clonal line of Chinese hamster ovary cells and noted that the aberration frequency was wavelength-dependent and reached a broad maximum between 2400 and 2800 Å. The effects of psoralen plus ultraviolet light were evaluated in Chinese hamster ovary cells *in vitro* and it was found that a radiation dose of 1.34×10^2 J/m^2 produced micronuclei in 6.5% of exposed cells, and that the incidence of micronuclei rose sharply to 45.2% when the radiation dose was increased approximately threefold (Ashwood-Smith and Grant, 1976).

Non-medical irradiation

Accidental irradiation

The wind shifted unpredictably after detonation of a high-yield nuclear device at Bikini, accidentally producing radioactive fallout. Chromosome preparations were made from 51 individuals during an annual review of Marshall islanders in 1964. Thirty of those who had been exposed to 175 r whole body gamma irradiation showed an average chromosome aberration rate of 22%. The incidence of aberrations in 13 individuals who had been exposed to 70 r was 21%, whereas the incidence in unexposed individuals was 9% (Lisco and Conard, 1967).

Eight men were exposed to whole-body irradiation in June of 1958, at the Y-12 Plant in Oak Ridge, Tennessee. They received doses of mixed γ-rays and fission neutrons estimated to have ranged between 22.8 and 365 r. Cytogenic studies were carried out in these individuals at various times (Goh, 1975). At eight years, the incidence of chromosomal aberrations was 12.2% (8.4–16.7%) in the peripheral blood of four patients, and 27% (26–64%) in bone marrow of five patients.

Atomic-bomb exposure

Studies on peripheral blood from exposed individuals have been performed (Sasaki and Miyata, 1968; Bloom *et al.*, 1968) and cytogenetic analysis of these preparations revealed that a dose–response relationship existed for stable-type chromosome aberrations.

Kamada and Uchino (1972) studied five atomic bomb survivors who developed leukemia. They all had had blood disorders such as anemia and/or leukopenia for 5 to 13 years preceding the terminal development of acute leukemia. Of the five cases, three were within 1000 meters of the hypocentre when the explosion occurred. Three of the cases were erythroleukemia and two were acute monocytic leukemia. Chromosome aberrations were observed in four of the five cases before their leukemia became overt clinically.

An excess of breast cancer has also been detected in Japanese women exposed to A-bomb radiation (Tokunaga *et al.*, 1982). A study was performed in a group of 24 women who had been exposed to atomic-bomb irradiation when they were less than 10 years of age. The conclusions were that women exposed to more than 50 r Kerma (average breast tissue dose was estimated to be 125 r) showed a breast cancer rate more than 7 times higher than women exposed to less than 10 r. The youngest case was diagnosed with breast cancer at the age of 29.

Exposure to microwaves

The increasing use of microwave generating systems has aroused concern as to potential genetic hazards. Monkey kidney epithelial cell cultures were irradiated with microwaves 10 cm in length at a power density of 5–7 mW/cm^2, applied several times for a few days in 15 minute treatments. Such exposure produced an increase in chromosome aberrations described as chromosome bridges, chromatid gaps, dicentric chromosomes, and chromosome pulverization (Barański *et al.*, 1969). These chromosomal aberrations, as well as hyper- or hypo-ploid mitoses, were also noted in human lymphocytes *in vitro* (Barańska, 1969).

Irradiation of germ cells and the embryo

Most of the information on germ cell irradiation effects is derived from animal studies. After males are exposed to an acute dose of X-irradiation, most spermatogonia are killed. The few suriving ones will repopulate the testes and testicular regeneration is usually complete within three to four months. Some chromosome aberrations are present in surviving spermatogonia; a proportion of these aberrations are selected out and disappear, but others will be carried in the zygote. Translocation configurations involving four chromosomes have been the most frequently occurring type of aberration recorded. The rate of induction of translocations in spermatogonia of mice is related linearly to X-ray doses between 100 and 600 r (Léonard and Deknudt, 1968).

There are relatively few reports on the effects of irradiation of the embryo. Soukup *et al.* (1965) removed embryos from the uterus shortly after irradiation in order to demonstrate early chromosome changes. The frequency of chromosome aberrations correlated linearly with the radiation dose.

To summarize, therefore, external and internal exposure to ionizing radiation will affect both somatic and germinal cells, causing cell death and/or cell damage. Non-visible aberrations, such as point mutations, will not be detected until the mutational effect is expressed. The readily visible aberrations are chromosomal abnormalities. Some of the aberrations are of the unstable type and generally will be eliminated by subsequent cell divisions. Stable-type aberrations are able to survive cell division. If such an aberration confers a selection advantage on a cell, then the formation of a clone of cells with this aberration may develop. There is sufficient evidence that some leukemias and other neoplasms originate as a single cell with a selection advantage.

Ionizing radiation can cause somatic mutations, immunological disorders, neoplasia, and premature ageing (Curtis, 1963). There is no direct evidence to show that there is a particular type of radiation-induced chromosome damage which is specifically involved in development of neoplasia.

ANTITUMOUR AGENTS

Antineoplastic agents include a vast number and variety of substances, from inorganic and organic chemicals, hormones and antibiotics to natural products. All of these drugs have cytostatic or cytotoxic effects, and most, if not all, are capable of causing subtle genetic damage. Some of the damage (e.g. point mutations) is not readily demonstrable even by up-to-date methods, whereas other lesions (e.g. chromosome damage) can be readily demonstrated in chromosome preprations. Improvements in cancer treatment have led to significant increases in survival in some types of neoplasia. However, second primary tumors appear to be developing with increasing frequency in long-term survivors of a first tumor (Sieber and Adamson, 1975a,b; Schmähl *et al.*, 1982). This phenomenon has raised concerns as to the consequence of chromosome damage in normal cells due to exposure to antitumor agents.

ALKYLATING AGENTS

Nitrogen mustard (HN2), the prototype of the alkylating agents, was the first chemotherapeutic agent of proven benefit against human malignancies (Goodman *et al.*, 1946). The major site of attack of compounds of the mustard type is on nucleic acids and it is this action that leads to their cytotoxic and mutagenic activity at the molecular level. Some of the alkylating agents have been called 'radiomimetic' because of the similarity of their clinical spectrum of activity to that of ionizing irradiation.

Nitrogen mustard

The major mechanism of the cytotoxicity of HN2 is thought to be its combination with the negatively charged guanine moieties of DNA (Goldenberg *et al.*, 1971). Fox and Scott (1980) published an extensive review of the literature along with their own results on the genetic toxicology of nitrogen and sulphur mustards. Cytotoxicity in cultured mammalian cells appears largely to result from unrepaired DNA cross-links which constitute a complete block to DNA replication. HN2 is teratogenic and carcinogenic in animals; whether it represents a hazard to man has yet to be determined.

Melphalan

In vitro exposure of peripheral blood lymphocytes to melphalan induces chromosome aberrations, and an increased incidence of SCEs was noted in a study of lymphocytes from cancer patients treated with this drug (Lambert *et al.*, 1978). Patil *et al.* (1980) described two patients receiving melphalan as adjuvant chemotherapy after surgical removal of breast cancer. The patients had received total doses of 680 mg and 735 mg, respectively, and both developed leukemia after approximately one year. Both had aneuploid clones and although multiple chromosomes were affected, all involved rearrangement of chromosomes 11 and 12. Patil also studied patients receiving chemotherapy who had not developed leukemia and eight cancer patients who had not received chemotherapy. Cytogenetic evaluation of bone marrow from these patients revealed no evidence of clonal aneuploid cells.

Busulphan (Myleran)

Chromosome damage has been reported following *in vivo* and *in vitro* exposure to this alkylating agent (Richmond and Kaufman, 1969; Gebhart, 1974). The frequency of gaps induced is dose- and cycle-dependent and it has been shown that the number of gaps and breaks can be reduced by simultaneous treatment with the radio-protector L-cysteine (Gebhart, 1971). A good correlation between *in vitro* and *in vivo* studies was found with respect to the pattern of induced gaps, which were clearly non-randomly distributed. The distribution of breaks was also non-random, but there were some differences between chromosomes.

ANLL developed in 8 out of 553 women following long-term treatment with Treosulfan (dihydroxybusulfan) for ovarian carcinoma. The leukemias developed from 21 to 58 months (median 50 months) after institution of chemotherapy. Cytogenetic studies of bone marrow performed after development of the leukemia showed hypodiploidy and loss of B- and C-group chromosomes in all five of the eight patients examined. No banding data were available (Pedersen-Bjergaard *et al.*, 1980).

Chlorambucil

Chlorambucil is an antitumor agent which is also used as an immunosuppressant in a variety of non-malignant conditions. *In vitro* exposure of normal peripheral lymphocytes to chlorambucil (Reeves and Margoles, 1974) produces primarily chromatid-type damage. The mechanism of chlorambucil-induced chromosome lesions is not clear. Reeves *et al.* (1975) studied peripheral blood cultures from 12 patients who received this drug for various forms of uveitis. The dosage ranged from 65 mg to a total of 2940 mg. The authors were unable to show an increased frequency of chromosome break-age as compared with the normal control group. Similarly Snaith *et al.* (1973) found no chromosome damage attributable to chlorambucil in a group of patients treated with this drug for systemic lupus erythematosis.

Silverstein *et al.* (1979) determined the risk of developing leukemia in a controlled prospective study in which PV patients were randomly assigned to treatment with phlebotomy alone, chlorambucil, or ^{32}p. Acute leukemia developed in 1 of the 134 (0.7%) patients treated with phlebotomy alone, 15 of 141 (10.6%) patients receiving chlorambucil, and 6 of 156 (3.8%) patients being treated with ^{32}p. In this series an increased incidence of solid tumors was not observed.

Thio-TEPA [N,N',N'-(triethylenethiophosphamide)]

Quantitative analysis of chromosomal damage following thio-TEPA treatment of leukocyte cultures showed an exponential dose-dependent increase in the percentage of metaphases with chromosome aberrations. The mean count of breaks per metaphase rose approximately linearly with the applied dose. The dose which causes chromosomal damage in 50% of the metaphases *in vitro* is 5 µg/mℓ of the culture medium (Hampel *et al.*, 1966).

Cyclophosphamide (Cytoxan)

It is known that cyclophosphamide requires metabolic activation prior to exerting cytotoxic, teratogenic or mutagenic effects *in vivo* or *in vitro*. When cyclophosphamide 0.2–0.4 µg/mℓ) was added directly to a culture medium containing lymphocytes, it did not cause chromosomal damage (Hampel *et al.*, 1966). However, plasma taken from rats one hour after they were injected with cyclophosphamide (500–1000 mg/kg) produced numerous chromosomal aberrations in leukocyte cultures. The aberrations were similar to those caused by other alkylating agents.

Tolchin *et al.* (1974) studied patients with rheumatoid arthritis and scleroderma who received cyclophosphamide at a dose of 0.5–2.0 mg/kg day. They found a significantly higher frequency of hypodiploidy and chromosome-type breaks in the cyclophosphamide-treated patients than in a comparable control series.

Nitrosoureas

The chloroethylnitrosoureas are highly lipid-soluble, chemically reactive compounds which have clinical activity against lymphomas, malignant melanoma, brain neoplasms, and gastrointestinal carcinomas. Active drugs in this category are BCNU, CCNU, and methyl-CCNU.

Boice *et al.* (1983) assessed the risk of ANLL, an acute myelodysplastic syndrome and preleukemia in 3633 treated patients with gastrointestinal cancer enrolled in nine randomized clinical trials. The relative risk of leukemic disorders among patients given methyl-CCNU compared to those receiving other forms of therapy was 12.4. Among 2067 patients given methyl-CCNU as adjuvant therapy, 14 developed leukemic disorders. The risk increased significantly with time after treatment. The risk of leukemic disorders did not differ by sex, race, age at treatment, or by initial tumor type, nor was it enhanced by concomitant radiotherapy or immunotherapy. This study provides the first quantitative evidence that nitrosoureas are leukemogenic in man.

Procarbazine (MIH, Matulane, Natulan)

Chromosomal damage has been observed in lymphocytes and bone marrow cells of patients treated with procarbazine for various diseases. A 66-year-old male Peyronie's disease patient developed acute myelofibrosis and bone marrow hypoplasia after being treated for six months with procarbazine. Chromosome preparations from blood of this patient showed 28.8% aneuploid cells and 6.8% of cells with structural abnormalities such as breaks, deletions, translocations, and dicentrics; however, no marker chromosome was found (Pinedo *et al.*, 1974).

Chromosomal damage (chromatid breaks, gaps, isogaps, fragments, and dicentric chromosomes) has also been observed in the lymphocytes and bone marrow cells of patients treated with procarbazine for rheumatoid arthritis (Von Vormittag, 1974). Approximately 60% of the lymphocytes cultured from 67 patients receiving procarbazine had a greater than 1% chromosomal aberration rate and 4% of the cells contained chromatid breaks and exchanges (Schinzel and Schmid, 1976).

In vivo animal studies with procarbazine have indicated that the drug causes marked depression of spermatogenesis and death of spermatogenic cells leading to testicular atrophy (Hilscher and Reichelt, 1968). Lee and Dixon (1972), using both biochemical and serial mating techniques, demonstrated that a maximally effective single dose of procarbazine affected all spermatogenic cell types except late spermatids and mature spermatozoa, and that recovery of affected cells was delayed. In clinical studies, persistent azoospermia and antifertility effects in Hodgkin's disease patients have been associated with combination chemotherapeutic regimens containing procarbazine (Van Thiel *et al.*, 1972).

DTIC (Dacarbazine, dimethyltriazeno-imidazolecarboxamide)

DTIC functions as an alkylating agent, and is active against a broad spectrum of murine solid and ascitic tumors; however, its clinical effectiveness is limited to Hodgkin's disease, malignant melanoma, and soft tissue sarcomas. No cases of second neoplasms have been reported in humans treated with DTIC as a single agent. One case of acute myeloid leukemia was reported to have developed in a patient with mammary carcinoma and an intraabdominal adenocarcinoma 84 months after treatment with BCNU, DTIC, 5-fluorouracil, vincristine, cyclophosphamide, and dibromodulcitol (Portugal *et al.*, 1979).

Cis-Dichlorodiammine platinum(II) (cis-DDP)

The cytogenetic effects of *cis*-DDP on human lymphocyte cultures have been evaluated (Meyne and Lockhart, 1978), and the drug was shown to produce a dose response for both mitotic inhibition and induction of chromosomal aberrations (primarily of chromatid breaks). Although *cis*-DDP has been shown selectively to inhibit DNA synthesis, there does not appear to be a significant degree of cell-cycle phase dependence for the killing effect of the drug (Harder and Rosenberg, 1970).

The non-random distribution of *cis*-DPP-induced break-points between individual chromosomes is of interest. The most obvious non-randomness is the predominance of break-points in light-staining G-bands. DNA-binding studies indicate that *cis*-DDP may preferentially bind guanine–cytosine-rich regions of DNA, and there appears to be a correlation between guanine–cytosine content and lightly staining G-bands (Miller *et al.*, 1973).

ANTIMETABOLITES

Antimetabolites are cycle-active drugs which affect cells by specifically interfering with the enzymatic conversion of essential metabolites. Some drugs in this category are methotrexate, 6-mercaptopurine, Imuran (azathioprine), cytosine arabinoside, hydroxyurea, and 8-azaguanine.

Methotrexate [MTX, 4-amino-N^{10}-methyl-pteroyglutamic acid (amethopterin)]

Jensen (1967) studied bone marrow material of four patients with psoriasis after they had received 25–50 mg of MTX by i.m. injection. He found metaphases with structural abnormalities at a frequency of 0–2% in the control group and at frequencies of 2, 6, 10, and 22% in the bone marrow of the MTX-treated patients. No aberrations were noted in the peripheral blood of these patients, nor were any abnormal clones found.

Several groups have performed cytogenetic studies on psoriatic patients receiving MTX and none found evidence of an increased incidence of chromosomal abnormalities. However, Voorhees *et al.* (1969) observed that *in vitro* exposure of lymphocytes to MTX at 3 and 30 times (1 and 10 μg/mℓ) the peak plasma MTX concentration attained *in vivo* produces chromosome damage. Melnyk *et al.* (1971) found mitotic chromosome damage in bone marrow cells but not in cultured lymphocytes or fibroblasts from a patient receiving MTX for psoriasis. Since no meiotic chromosome damage was detected in a testicular biopsy taken from the same patient, the authors suggested that a comprehensive evaluation of human chromosome damage after MTX exposure may require examination of several different tissues.

6-Mercaptopurine(6-MP)

Wanders *et al.* (1981) described a patient with myasthenia gravis and a thymoma who did not respond to thymectomy. She was treated with 6-MP for 12½ years and subsequently developed Ph^1 positive CML. The authors speculate that the large amounts of 6-MP (more than 400 g) administered over many years might have played a role in the development of CML.

Azathioprine (Imuran)

Azathioprine is a *S*-substituted derivative of 6-mercaptopurine. It is believed that thioglucosidases in the organism split the *S*-linkage of azathioprine and that the cytotoxic and immunosuppressive effects of the drug are, therefore, due, at least in part, to the presence of 6-MP in the tissue (Jensen, 1967). Jensen studied the bone marrow cells for patients treated with azathioprine and showed that there was a significantly increased number of structural chromosome aberrations during treatment as compared to the number present before treatment. The frequency of aberrations ranged between 0 and 4% before treatment to between 4 and 24% during treatment.

Adler *et al.* (1978) described the case of a 22-year-old white man who, after two renal transplants and prolonged immunosuppressive therapy with azathioprine and methylprednisone, developed Ph^1-positive (translocation to chromosome number 7) CML. They also reviewed a population of 25,000 renal transplant recipients and found five cases of CMLs, a five-fold increased incidence of this neoplasm.

Cytosine arabinoside (1-beta-D-arabinofuranylcytosine hydrochloride)

Cytosine arabinoside causes chromatid breakage in S and G_2 phases of the cell cycle. The drug primarily affects the activity of DNA polymerase, and it has been suggested that chromatid breakage induced by ara-C during the G_2 phase is related to inhibition of scheduled DNA synthesis (Karon and Benedict, 1972).

Bell *et al.* (1966) studied 10 patients receiving five-day courses of rapid daily ara-C injections at doses of 150–200 mg/m² body surface area. Within 24

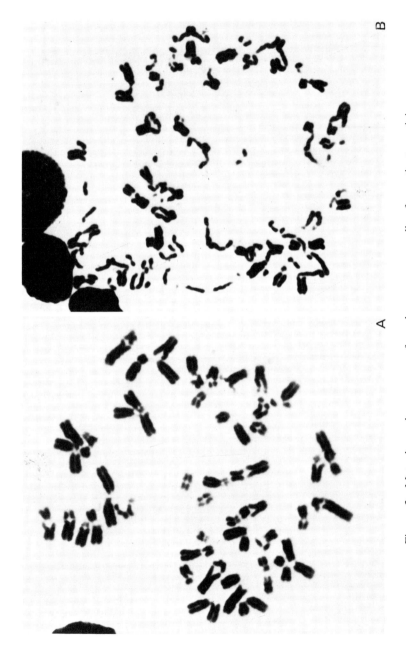

Figure 3 Metaphase chromosomes from bone marrow cells of a patient receiving cytosine arabinoside by intravenous injection. A sample of bone marrow was obtained at the end of a five-day course of cytosine arabinoside given at doses of 150–200 mg/m^2. (A) and (B) show different degrees of precocious separation of chromatids at the centromeric region.

hours after dosing there was a high incidence of chromosomal aberrations in both granulocytic and erythroid marrow cells. These aberrations consisted of chromatid breaks, erosion, despiralization, precocious separation of the chromatid at the centromeric region, and extensive fragmentation involving up to 95% of the cells in the marrow (Figure 3). These abnormalities rapidly disappeared after cessation of therapy.

Hydroxyurea

Hydroxyurea is known to be an inhibitor of ribonucleotide diphosphate reductase. It does not produce chromatid breakage during G_2 phase but does so during S phase (Booth *et al.*, 1971).

8-Azaguanine (5-amino-7-hydroxy-1H-v-triazolo(d)-pyrimidine)

This compound was found to be the most potent purine inhibitor among the triazolopyrimidines, and when injected into the peritoneal cavity of rats bearing the ascitic form of Yoshida sarcoma, 8-azaguanine produced mitotic arrest at metaphse by inactivating the mitotic apparatus. Although an effect on chromosomes of tumor cells was not observed, the drug causes spherical deformation of the chromosomes, leading eventually to the death of the affected tumor cells (Yosida and Hirumi, 1960).

ANTITUMOR ANTIBIOTICS

The antitumor antibiotics considered below are adriamycin, daunomycin, actinomycin D, mitomycin C, bleomycin, and streptonigrin. m-AMSA is also considered in this section. Although it is a synthetic agent, rather than a substance produced by microbes, it is included here because its proposed mechanism of action resembles that of the antitumor antibiotics.

Adriamycin (ADR)

ADR inhibits DNA synthesis by intercalating between adjacent base pairs of the DNA helix (DiMarco *et al.*, 1975). This drug can delay the cell cycle in the G_1 phase, in the S to G_2 phase, and finally irreversibly in G_2, eventually leading to cell death (Barlogie *et al.*, 1976). By using human peripheral blood lymphocytes, Vig (1971) was able to demonstrate that ADR, in as low a concentration as 0.02 μg/mℓ for 24 hours, caused chromosome damage; exposure to higher concentrations (0.05, 0.10 or 0.15 μg/mℓ) for shorter intervals (three to four hours) induced a similar degree of damage. The aberrations ranged from intra- or inter-chromatid and intra- or inter-chromosome to the chromatid–chromosome types, with a high frequency of chromosome-type fragments and asymmetrical exchanges. The distribution of exchange points along the length of chromosomes was nonrandom. Chromosomes 3 and Y appear to be far more resistant to the effect of the drug than other chromosomes.

Daunomycin

This drug is effective in acute leukemia and certain solid tumors in children. *In vitro* studies on normal human lymphocytes indicate that daunomycin affects RNA and DNA synthesis (Theologides *et al.*, 1968), interfering with the cell cycle during the G_2 phase (Whang-Peng *et al.*, 1969). It also appears to have the unique capacity to delay the onset of mitosis in cells which have already synthesized DNA. Cells exposed to daunomycin show fragmentation, chromatid exchanges, and chromatid breaks (Figure 4).

Seven patients with acute lymphocytic or granulocytic leukemia received total doses of daunomycin ranging between 80 and 420 mg/m^2. The highest percentage of major chromosomal aberrations (80–90%) appeared soon after treatment *in vivo*. These aberrations consisted of chromatid breaks, fragments, chromatid exchanges, ring chromosomes, dicentrics and extensive fragmentation. The aberrations disappeared within one to two weeks after cessation of treatment. The aneuploid leukemic cells from two patients showed fewer structural chromosome aberrations than did normal diploid cells from the same patient.

Actinomycin D

It has been shown that actinomycin D is a potent inhibitor of DNA-dependent RNA synthesis. Reich (1964) postulated that this antibiotic is hydrogen-bonded to guanine in the minor groove of the DNA molecule, thus competing with the activity of RNA polymerase which binds to the same site. Arrighi and Hsu (1965) treated Chinese hamster cells *in vitro* with actinomycin D and noted two major chromosomal abnormalities: decondensed chromosomes and chromatid breaks, and eventually inhibition of cell division.

Mitomycin C

This antibiotic is an inhibitor of DNA synthesis, but RNA and protein synthesis are not affected. Peripheral blood from cancer patients receiving treatment with mitomycin C was studied by Ohtsuru *et al.* (1980). Eleven patients received mitomycin C by i.v. injection at a dose of 4 mg, given twice a week for two weeks. Cytogenetic examinations were carried out after the first and second treatments. The frequency of SCEs increased with time after

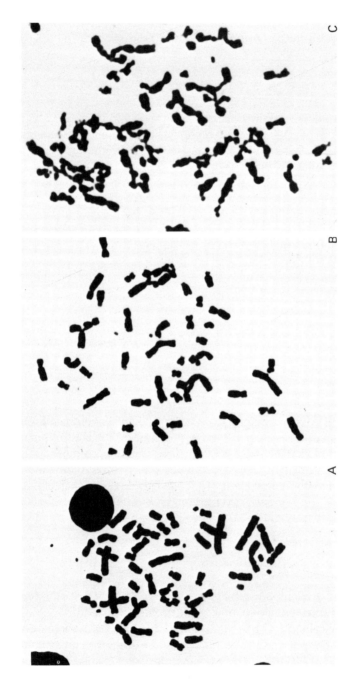

Figure 4   Effect of daunomycin on chromosomes of human peripheral lymphocytes incubated for 48 hours with drug concentrations ranging between 0.03 and 0.3 $\mu g/m\ell$. (A), (B), and (C) show different degrees of chromosomal damage, including fragments and chromatid exchanges.

treatment, reached a peak in about 24 hours (with nearly double the SCE frequency as compared with pretreatment levels), and then returned to the pretreatment level in about 48 hours.

Bleomycin

Bleomycin selectively inhibits incorporation of thymidine into DNA of mammalian cells and causes DNA fragmentation at doses as low as 0.1–1.0 μg/mℓ (Terasima *et al.*, 1970). It also causes single strand scission of DNA and polynuclotides (Umezawa, 1974). The effects of bleomycin on the chromosomes of cultured lymphocytes were investigated by Ohama and Kadotani (1970), who showed that aneuploid cells and chromosome abnormalities increased with the concentration of the drug in the medium. The aberrations observed were mostly gaps, breaks and fragments with a few dicentric and ring chromosomes.

Streptonigrin (SN)

Streptonigrin, a derivative of *S. flocculus*, possesses antitumor and antibiotic properties. Rarely used clinically due to its extreme cytotoxicity, SN is a DNA inhibitor and induces chromosome breaks in cultured lymphocytes.

m-AMSA [4'((9-acridinyl)-amino) methanesulphon-*m*-anisidide]

This is an acridine derivative which has proven to be effective in the treatment of acute myelocytic leukemia. It binds strongly to DNA *in vitro* and intercalates between adjacent base pairs in a manner similar to the parent molecule, 9-aminoacridine (Cain and Atwell, 1974). *In vivo* and *in vitro* studies have been performed by Kao-Shan *et al.* (1983). In the *in vivo* studies, eight patients receiving m-AMSA (30 mg/m^2/day by continuous infusion) were evaluated, and an increased incidence of chromosome aberrations was found; in the treated patients the median aberration incidence was 12% whereas no aberrations occurred in untreated controls.

MISCELLANEOUS AGENTS

Stathmokinetic agents

Stathmokinetic agents are mitotic inhibitors, perhaps because they selectively affect cellular microtubules; thus they interrupt formation of mitotic spindles and cause mitotic arrest and cell death. Drugs in this group are vinblastine (Velban, VLB), vincristine (oncovin, VCR), and colchicine (Malawista, 1971). They are highly specific cycle-active antimitotics.

Prednisone

The results of chromosome studies performed on bone marrow aspirates from patients treated with prendisone alone indicate that this synthetic corticosteroid has no effect on chromosome number or morphology (Jensen, 1967).

Marihuana and Δ-9-tetrahydrocannabinol (Δ9-THC)

This category of drugs was recently approved for use in cancer patients for the relief of pain and for the side effects of chemotherapy. Conflicting results have been reported from studies of their cytogenetic effects *in* human lymphocytes exposed *in vivo* and *in vitro*. Some workers have reported a small increase in chromosome aberrations in healthy marihuana users who were not using other drugs (Matsuyama *et al.*, 1973). Stenchever *et al.* (1974) studied 49 users of marihuana, examining cultures prepared from their peripheral lymphocytes for the presence of chromosome breaks. An average of 3.5% breaks was found in the user group in comparison with a frequency of 1–2% in normal controls.

Diphenylhydantoin (Dilantin)

This drug is often used in conjunction with other chemotherapeutic drugs for control of seizures in brain tumour patients or in patients with brain metastases. Chromosome studies were performed on bone marrow cells and peripheral blood lymphocytes from 10 patients with epilepsy treated with diphenylhydantoin. No increase in chromosomal damage was noted, nor was there an increase in the number of micronuclei compared with control persons (Alving *et al.*, 1977).

COMBINATION CHEMOTHERAPY

Patil *et al.* (1980) carried out cytogenetic studies of four patients receiving a combination of L-PAM with 5-FU, 5-FU and MTX or 5-FU and tamoxifen citrate. No obvious structural chromosome abnormalities could be detected in their bone marrow samples. Kaung and Swartzendruber (1969) performed chromosome studies on peripheral blood leucocytes from 20 patients with lung cancer before and during chemotherapy. The chemotherapeutic agents included Cytoxan, MTX and hydroxyurea or streptonigrin. Peripheral blood studies on the chromosomes revealed a slightly increased incidence of major (fragments, dicentrics, translocations) and minor (breaks) chromosome aberrations during chemotherapy.

Cancer patients receiving combination chemotherapy appear to be at increased risk of developing acute leukemia. (see Chapter 19). Eleven patients with a variety of collagen vascular diseases who developed ANLL were studied by Sheibani *et al.* (1980). All received alkylating agents and 10 of the 11 patients received two or more cytotoxic agents (including nitrogen mustard, cyclophosphamide, chlorambucil, uracil mustard, MTX, azathioprine, and 6-MP). Other drugs administered included prednisone, adrenocorticotropic hormone, and hydroxychloroquinone. Five of these patients had various degrees of aneuploidy, and in all instances abnormalities in C group chromosomes were found.

Kapadia *et al.* (1980) evaluated 20 patients who developed ANLL following chemotherapy for non-Hodgkin's lymphoma, carcinomas, multiple myeloma, CLL and rheumatoid arthritis. Leukemia developed after latent periods from 11 to 132 months (mean 60 months). Cytogenetic studies were performed on 15 patients, and chromosomal abnormalities were found in all but one.

Effects on chromosomes of gestational exposure to chemotherapy or radiation

Cohen *et al.* (1971) studied five women treated for choriocarcinoma and seven children born of these women subsequent to chemotherapy. The drugs were MTX and/or actinomycin D. In almost all cases, similar frequencies of cells with chromosome damage were observed in members of a given mother–child pair. The results suggested no evidence of significant cytogenetic damage to the ova from which the offspring were derived. Similarly, there was no evidence of an increase in fetal wastage, congenital abnormalities or pregnancy complications.

Li *et al.* (1979) assessed the possible adverse genetic effects of cancer in childhood in offspring of patients enrolled in the Sidney Farber Cancer Institute and the Kansas University Medical Center. The patient population included 146 patients (84 women and 62 men) and 293 pregnancies. Of the total pregnancies, 286 went to term, there were 242 live births (1 set of twins), 1 stillbirth, 25 spontaneous abortions, and 19 therapeutic abortions. One female offspring whose mother received radiotherapy for a brain tumor during childhood developed ANLL. Chromosome studies of a few of the offspring did not reveal damage from preconception exposure to cancer chemotherapeutic agents or radiotherapy.

COMBINED RADIATION AND CHEMOTHERAPY

Aggressive therapies employing combinations of chemotherapy and/or radiotherapy have led to an improved cure rate in cancer patients, but there is evidence of a considerably increased incidence of iatrogenic leukemia in this group of patients; leukemia is most frequently ANLL (Whang-Peng *et al.*, 1979; Thiery *et al.*, 1981). Some characteristic cytogenetic findings among leukemic cells from this population include a high incidence of hypodiploidy and complex and extensive structural aberrations. Chromosome numbers 5 and 7 are the most common chromosomes involved in aneuploidy (Whang-Peng *et al.*, 1979; Thiery *et al.*, 1981).

Effects in childhood cancer

Miller *et al.* (1978) studied 66 childhood cancer patients and 4 non-cancer control subjects in an attempt to measure the effects of cancer chemotherapy and chemotherapy plus radiotherapy on chromosomes. The frequencies of aberrant cells were 1/306 in non-cancer controls, 1/377 in cancer patients prior to therapy, 1/15 in cancer patients currently on therapy, and 1/32 in post-therapy patients. The frequency of cells with chromosomal aberrations did not appear to change with time among post-therapy patients. The aberrations noted in on-therapy patients were mostly unbalanced rearrangements and other aberrations of the unstable type; the post-therapy patients had mostly balanced rearrangements.

Fischer *et al.* (1977) studied peripheral blood lymphocytes from a group of children with leukemia after intensive chemotherapy and cranial irradiation. Prolonged intensive chemotherapy resulted in a significant rise in the number of chromatid aberrations when evaluated at 12 months after beginning therapy. After cranial irradiation a sharp increase in chromosome aberrations was present at about three months, but the incidence fell after one year to levels present in cases treated with chemotherapy alone.

Effects in adult cancer

Canellos *et al.* (1975) determined the incidence of second malignancies developing in a series of 452 Hodgkin's disease patients treated with standard chemotherapy or radiotherapy, combination chemotherapy alone, intensive radiotherapy alone, or both intensive radiotherapy and combination chemotherapy administered in sequence. Patients receiving both chemotherapy and radiotherapy were at highest risk of developing a second tumor and those patients who had a complete remission after intensive radiotherapy followed by a relapse of disease prior to receiving combination chemotherapy had the highest risk; in this group the risk for developing a second malignant tumor was 18.5 times greater than expected. Two of the 16 second malignancies developing in this group were leukemias, and in both cases only 45 chromosomes were present with a C-group deletion (no banding studies were performed).

Whang-Peng *et al.* (1979) noted seven cases of ANLL and one patient with a malignant myeloproliferative syndrome among a series of 189 non-Hodgkin's lymphoma and CLL patients. These patients were treated primarily with intensive radiotherapy, although four patients also received chemotherapy. The complex and extensive nature of the chromosomal aberrations seen, and the long interval during which cytogenetic abnormalities were present prior to the diagnosis of leukemia in these patients may be characteristic of leukemia as a second primary tumor in radiation-treated lymphoma, and the presence of such anomalies may predict leukemic transformation.

Rowley *et al.* (1977b) performed cytogenetic studies on a series of 10 patients who developed ANLL after receiving treatment for malignant lymphoma. Seven of the patients had Hodgkin's disease and three had non-Hodgkin's lymphoma, the poorly differentiated lymphocytic variant. Six of the patients were treated with both radiotherapy and chemotherapy, two received radiotherapy only and two were treated with chemotherapy only. Many of the karyotypes were bizarre with marker chromosomes and minute chromosomes; 70% of the patients had fewer than 46 chromosomes and 40% had fewer than 45 chromosomes.

Whang-Peng *et al.* (1979) performed serial cytogenetic analyses in eight patients with ANLL or a malignant myeloproliferative syndrome which developed following radiotherapy for non-Hodgkin's lymphoma or CLL. The authors were unable to correlate directly the appearance of chromosome abnormalities with the development of leukemia.

Zarrabi and Rosner (1979) described 19 patients who developed acute myeloblastic leukemia following treatment for a variety of solid tumors (seminoma, melanoma, ovary, colorectal, bladder, cervix, endometrium, and larynx). The mean interval between the diagnosis of the first tumor and leukemia was 5.8 years, but in two patients the diagnoses of the first tumor and the leukemia were within six months of each other. One patient was treated by surgery only, eight patients received radiotherapy, five patients were treated with chemotherapy, and five received both chemotherapy and radiotherapy. Cytogenetic studies were done on three patients. Two of the patients had hypodiploid karyotypes and the Ph^1 chromosome was present in the third patient.

Marinello *et al.* (1980) have stressed the importance of double minute chromosomes in human leukemia, and Weh *et al.* (1982) have suggested that they may be markers for acute leukemias developing in patients previously treated for other neoplastic diseases.

CYTOGENETIC CONSIDERATIONS

Spontaneous mutations producing a potentially leukemogenic gene have been estimated to occur at a frequency of about one per 10^6/year in mammalian cells (Burch, 1964). Such mutations may render the cell incapable of subsequent cell division, leading to cell death. Repair of DNA may occur so that no remnants of the damage may be visible; alternatively, the DNA damage may alter the gene in such a fashion that the cell continues to live, but in a mutated form which causes somatic and/or genetic effects. Genetic effects can appear in subsequent generations, whereas somatic effects may predispose cells to neoplastic changes. Radiation and antitumor agents are capable of producing chromosome damage, increasing the mutation rates over background levels, and inducing teratogenic and carcinogenic effects.

Most human cancer appears to result from a complex interaction between multiple environmental agents and endogenous host factors. The development of neoplasia proceeds through multiple steps, i.e. initiation, promotion, and progression. It appears that radiation and antitumor agents may act synergistically, since the risk of developing leukemia is greater in patients treated with both modalities than in those receiving chemotherapy alone (Coleman *et al.*, 1977).

Chromosomal abnormalities caused by ionizing radiation and antitumor agents are detectable by cytogenetic analysis. An estimate of the number of unstable and stable aberrations can provide information on the extent of exposure in individual cases. For radiation, there is a linear relationship between dicentrics and dose up to about 200 r; the frequency of marker chromosomes is also correlated with exposure to irradiation. Increases in the incidence of polyploidy is another indicator in irradiated patients, as are abnormal Ag-Nors, inhibition of mitosis, and increases in the frequency of micronuclei. Evaluation of the frequency of SCEs is useful for detecting effects of antitumor agents, since in most instances the incidence of SCEs seems to correlate with chromosome damage induced by these drugs.

There are a number of endogenous (genetic) factors which place an individual at increased risk of developing leukemia and solid tumors. Persons with abnormal sex chromosomes (e.g. XO individuals) or autosomal chromosome abnormalities (e.g. Down's syndrome) are known to be at increased risk for leukemia (Newman and Gross, 1967; Wald *et al.*, 1961). There is also a predisposition to cancer in groups with inherited chromosome instability syndromes (Hecht and McCaw, 1977). Specific chromosome defects are associated with some tumors, such as the 13q14- in patients with neuroblastoma (Yunis and Ramsey, 1978), and 11p13- in patients with aniridia–Wilms's syndrome (Riccardi *et al.*, 1978).

A genetic basis for some types of neoplasia is indicated by the observation that identical twins of children with leukemia are at risk for leukemia (McMahon and Levy, 1964) and the occurrence of family aggregations of leukemia and congenital defects (Fraumeni, 1969). Tissues from patients with some types of genetic disorders appear to be more susceptible to *in vitro* transformation by oncogenic viruses and radiation damage.

Technical improvements have made it possible to study both T and B lymphocytes in isolation. Kamada *et al.* (1979) stimulated the B lymphocytes of two apparently healthy atomic-bomb survivors with Epstein–Barr virus and showed that, 30 years after exposure to ionizing radiation, the incidence of chromosomal aberrations was 50% and 12.5%, respectively. One of the individuals had a karyotypically abnormal clone of B lymphocytes. It will be of importance to elucidate the malignant process underlying acute lymphocytic leukemia, B-cell lymphoma and multiple myeloma in high-risk groups having a history of accidental or therapeutic exposure to radiation or radiomimetic drugs.

In animals, alkylating agents have long been known to be leukemogenic, but in man, the first clear evidence was provided by the accumulation of case reports of ANLL developing in cancer patients receiving chemotherapy (Sieber and Adamson, 1975b). A significant risk of developing ANLL following treatemt with some alkylating agents has now been established. The precise mechanism by which chemotherapy and/or irradiation induces leukemia in man is still not known. Published data show a 10- to 37-fold increased risk for ANLL in patients treated for non-Hodgkin's lymphoma (Zarrabi, 1980; O'Donnell *et al.*, 1979). All the patients had chromosomal abnormalities, as well as hypoplasia or dysplasia of bone marrow. The two chromosomes most frequently involved were chromosome numbers 5 and 7. Deletion, rearrangement or absence of these two chromosomes may allow for the emergence of a clone of cells with growth and selection advantages which ultimately lead to leukemia.

Skinner and Schwartz (1972) suggested that lymphocyte stimulation may allow hidden oncogenic 'virogene' material in lymphocytes to become activated and perhaps to produce tumors. An organ homograft or other antigenic stimulus could initiate persistent unwanted immunological activity (Greenwood *et al.*, 1972; Schwartz, 1972). During a rejection episode, a large number of transformed lymphocytes are present (Hersh *et al.*, 1970).

Antigenic stimuli produce a state of chronic lymphoproliferation which may also be important in the production of neoplasms, particularly those involving the lymphoid system (Schwartz, 1975). Hoover and Fraumeni (1973) reviewed 6297 transplant recipients and found a 350-fold increase in incidence of reticulum cell sarcoma. Factors selectively promoting the growth of lymphoid tumors could include chronic immunological stimulation, expression of an oncogene, or loss of immunological surveillance. One or more of these factors may also be of importance in Kaposi's sarcoma (Warner and O'Loughlin, 1975), a malignancy in which a reaction involving antigenically altered or transformed lymphocytes occurs.

Gange and Jones (1978) reviewed 19 patients (including three of their own) who developed Kaposi's sarcoma after an average of 25.6 months following treatment with immunosuppressive drugs. Eighteen patients received steroids, eight patients received azathioprine, two patients received cyclophosphamide, two patients received antilymphocyte serum and one patient was treated with melphalan. The authors added Kaposi's sarcoma patients to the group of patients with other malignancies (lymphoma and squamous cell epithelioma) prone to develop tumors as a result of immunosuppression. They suggested that factors selectively promoting the growth of lymphoid tumors could include chronic immunological stimulation, expression of viral oncogenes or loss of immunological surveillance. CMV (cytomegalovirus) infection was suggested as an underlying cause of the immunosuppressed state because of the known active shedding of virus in homosexual populations (Drew *et al.*, 1981); hepatitis B virus was also commonly encountered in this group of individuals (Haverkos and Curran, 1982). The impairment of immune defenses caused by immunosuppressive therapy is known to render patients prone to infection with viruses, some of which (herpes, Epstein–Barr and polyoma) are potentially oncogenic (Penn, 1979).

The neoplasms induced by certain carcinogens may be the result of the activation of a cellular oncogene. It has recently been recognized that some human oncogenes are related to the oncogenes of the retrovirus known as the Kirsten murine sarcoma virus. These human transforming genes have been detected in established tumor cell lines, and in unmanipulated human solid tumors such as colon, lung, pancreas, and embryonal rhabdomyosarcoma (Pulciani *et al.*, 1982). They are dominant transforming genes, and appear to be present in a variety of human tumors regardless of the clinical manifestations of the neoplasms.

CONCLUSION

In summary, chromosomal damage by radiation and/or antitumor agents is a risk factor for the development of neoplasia. The extent of chromosome damage and its repairability are probably controlled by genetic factors inherent in the individual at risk. Neoplasia is the end result of the multiple stages of initiation, promotion, and progression.

Effects on both T and B lymphocytes can alter immunological surveillance, possibly allowing the expression of cellular oncogenes or invasion by opportunistic viruses. The alteration, rearrangement or deletion of certain chromosomes after damage by irradiation or chemicals may allow for the expression of a cellular oncogene; during subsequent cell divisions an abnormal clone of cells could emerge with growth and selection advantage to produce leukemia or a solid tumor.

Acknowledgements

The authors are grateful to Mrs Bettie Sugar for her expert secretarial and editorial assistance and to Bryant E. Evans for his help in obtaining reference materials.

REFERENCES

Adams, F. H., Norman, A., Mello, R. S., and Bass, D. (1977). Effect of radiation and contrast media on chromosomes. Preliminary report. *Radiology,* **124,** 823.

Adler, K. R., Lempert, N., and Scharfman, W. B. (1978). Chronic granulocytic leukemia following successful renal transplantation. *Cancer,* **41,** 2206.

Alving, J., Jensen, M. K. and Meyer, H. (1977). Chromosome studies of bone marrow cells and peripheral blood lymphocytes from diphenylhydantoin-treated patients. *Mutation Research,* **48,** 361.

Antoine, J. L., Gerber, G. B., Leonard, A. *et al.* (1981). Correspondence. Chromosome aberrations induced in patients treated with telecobalt therapy for mammary carcinoma. *Radiation Research,* **86,** 171.

Arrighi, F. E. and Hsu, T. C. (1965). Experimental alteration of metaphase chromosome morphology. Effect of actinomycin D. *Experimental Cell Research,* **39,** 305.

Ashwood-Smith, M. J., and Grant, E. (1976). Chromosome damage produced by psoralan and ultraviolet light. *British Medical Journal,* **1,** 342.

Barańska, W. (1969). Chromosomal changes of *in vitro* cultured lymphocytes exposed to microwave irradiation. *Genetica Polonica,* **10,** 3.

Barański, S., Czerski, P., and Szmigielski, S. (1969). Microwave effects on mitosis, *in vivo* and *in vitro*. *Genetica Polonica,* **10,** 4.

Barlogie, B., Drewinko, B., Johnston, D. A., and Freireich, E. J. (1976). The effect of adriamycin on the cell cycle traverse of a human lymphoid cell line. *Cancer Research,* **36,** 1975.

Bastrup-Madsen, P., Nielsen, K., and Mose, C. B. (1971). Acute erythraemia (Diguglielmo's syndrome) after Thorotrast injection. *Acta Medica Scandinavica,* **189,** 349.

Bell, A. G. and Baker, D. G. (1965). X-irradiation-induced polyploidy in human leukocyte cultures. *Experimental Cell Research,* **38,** 144.

Bell, W. R., Whang, J. J., Carbone, P. P. *et al.* (1966). Cytogenetic and morphologic abnormalities in human bone marrow cells during cytosine arabinoside therapy. *Blood,* **27,** 771.

Bloom, A. D. and Tjio, J. H. (1964). *In vivo* effects of diagnostic X-irradiation on human chromosomes. *New England Journal of Medicine,* **270,** 1341.

Bloom, A. D., Neriishi, S., and Archer, P. G. (1968). Cytogenetics of the in-utero exposed of Hiroshima and Nagasaki. *Lancet,* **2,** 10.

Boice, J. D. Jr., Greene, M. H., Killen, J. Y. *et al.* (1983). Leukemia and preleukemia after adjuvant treatment of gastrointestinal cancer with methyl-CCNU. *New England Journal of Medicine,* **309,** 1076.

Booth, B. A., Moore, E. C., and Sartorelli, A. C. (1971). Metabolic effects of some tumor-inhibitory pyrimidine carboxyaldehyde thiosemicarbazones. *Cancer Research,* **31,** 228.

Boyd, J. T., Court Brown, W. M., Vennart, J., and Woodcock, G. E. (1966). Chromosome studies on women formerly employed as luminous-dial painters. *British Medical Journal,* **1,** 377.

Buckton, K. E., Jacobs, P. A., Court Brown, W. M., and Doll, R. (1962). A study of the chromosome damage persisting after X-ray therapy for ankylosing spondylitis. *Lancet,* **2,** 676.

Buckton, K. E., Langlands, A. O., and Woodcock, G. E. (1967). Cytogenetic change following Thorotrast administration. *International Journal of Radiation Biology,* **12,** 565.

Burch, P. R. J. (1964). Leukemogenesis in man. *Annals of the New York Academy of Sciences,* **114,** 213.

Cain, B. F. and Atwell, G. T. (1974). The experimental antitumor properties of three congeners of the acridylmethanesulphonanilide (AMSA) series. *European Journal of Cancer,* **10,** 539.

Canellos, G. P., DeVita, V. T., Arseneau, J. C. *et al.* (1975). Second malignancies complicating Hodgkin's disease in remission. *Lancet,* **1,** 947.

Cantolino, S. J., Schmickel, R. D., Ball, M., and Cisar, C. F. (1966). Persistent chromosomal aberrations following radioiodine therapy for thyrotoxicosis. *New England Journal of Medicine,* **275,** 739.

Caspersson, T., Zech, L., and Johansson, C. (1970). Differential binding of alkylating fluorochromes in human chromosomes. *Experimental Cell Research,* **60,** 315.

Chu, E. H. Y. (1965). Effects of ultraviolet radiation on mammalian cells II. Differential UV and X-ray sensitivity of chromosomes to breakage in 5-aminouracil synchronized cell populations. *Genetics,* **52,** 1279.

Cohen, M. M., Fruchtman, C. E., Simpson, S. J., and Martin, A. O. (1982). The cytogenetic response of Fanconi's anemia lymphoblastoid cell lines to various clastogens. *Cytogenetics and Cell Genetics,* **34,** 230.

Cohen, M. M., Gerbie, A. B., and Nadler, H. L. (1971). Chromosomal investigation in pregnancies following chemotherapy for choriocarcinoma. *Lancet,* **2,** 219.

Coleman, C. N., Williams, C. J., Flint, A. *et al.* (1977). Hematologic neoplasia in patients treated for Hodgkin's disease. *New England Journal of Medicine,* **297,** 1249.

Countryman, P. I. and Heddle, J. A. (1976). The production of micronuclei from chromosome aberrations in irradiated cultures of human lymphocytes. *Mutation Research,* **41,** 321.

Curtis, H. J. (1963). Biological mechanisms underlying the aging process. *Science,* **141,** 686.

da Silva Horta, J., Abbatt, J. D., da Motta, L. C., and Roriz, M. L. (1965). Malignancy and other late effects following administration of Thorotrast. *Lancet,* **2,** 201.

DiMarco, A., Arcamone, F., and Zunino, F. (1975). Daunomycin (Daunorubicin) and Adriamycin and structural analogues: Biological activity and mechanism of action. In *Antibiotics III. Mechanism of action of antimicrobial and anti-tumor agents* (eds J. W. Corcoran and F. E. Hahn). Berlin: Springer-Verlag, p. 101.

Drew, W. L., Mintz, L., Miner, R. C. *et al.* (1981). Prevalence of cytomegalovirus infection in homosexual men. *Journal of Infectious Diseases,* **143,** 188.

Evans, H. J. (1972). Actions of radiations on human chromosomes. *Physics in Medicine and Biology,* **17,** 1.

Faber, M. (1973). Follow-up of Danish Thorotrast cases. In *Proceedings of the Third International Meeting of the Toxicity of Thorotrast. Riso Report,* No. 294, 137.

Fischer, P., Pohl-Röling, J., and Pohl, E. (1971). Chromosome studies on persons exposed to increased levels of radon in the environment. Abstract No. 233, 4th International Congress of Human Genetics in Paris, France.

Fischer, P., Vetterlein, J., Pohl-Rüling, J., and Krepler, P. (1977). Cytogenetic effects of chemotherapy and cranial irradiation on the peripheral blood lymphocytes of children with malignant disease. *Oncology,* **34,** 224.

Fox, M. and Scott, D. (1980). The genetic toxicology of nitrogen and sulphur mustard. *Mutation Research,* **75,** 131.

Fraumeni, J. F. (1969). Constitutional disorders of man predisposing to leukemia and lymphoma. *National Cancer Institute Monograph,* **32,** 221.

Gange, R. W. and Jones, E. W. (1978). Kaposi's sarcoma and immunosuppressive therapy: an appraisal. *Clinical and Experimental Dermatology*, **3**, 135.

Gebhart, E. (1971). Experimentelle beiträge zum problem der lokalen achromasien (gaps). *Humangenetik*, **13**, 98.

Gebhart, E. (1974). Comparative studies on the distribution of aberrations on human chromosomes treated with busulphan *in vivo* and *in vitro*. *Humangenetik*, **21**, 263.

Goh, K. (1975). Total-body irradiation and human chromosomes. IV. Cytogenetic follow-up studies 8 and 10½ years after total-body irradiation. *Radiation Research*, **62**, 364.

Goh, K. (1981). Radioiodine treatment during prenancy: Chromosomal aberrations and cretinism associated maternal iodine-131 treatment. *Journal of the American Medical Women's Association*, **36**, 262.

Goh, K., Reddy, M. M., and Hempelmann, L. H. (1976). Chromosomal aberrations in lymphocytes of normal adults long after thymus irradiation. *Radiation Research*, **67**, 82.

Goldenberg, G. J., Vanstone, C. L., and Bihler, I. (1971). Transport of nitrogen mustard on the transport-carrier for choline in L5178Y lymphoblasts. *Science*, **172**, 1148.

Goodman, L. S., Wintrobe, M. M., Dameshek, W. *et al.* (1946). Nitrogen mustard therapy: Use of methyl-bis(beta-chloroethyl)amine hydrochloride and tris(beta-chloroethyl)amine hydrochloride for Hodgkin's disease, lymphosarcoma, leukemia and certain allied and miscellaneous disorders. *Journal of the American Medical Association*, **132**, 126.

Greenwood, B. M., Bradley-Moore, A. M., Palit, A., and Bryceson, A. D. M. (1972). Immunosuppression in children with malaria. *Lancet*, **1**, 169.

Hampel, K. E., Kober, B., Rösch, D. *et al.* (1966). The action of cytostatic agents on the chromosomes of human leukocytes *in vitro*. (Preliminary Communication.) *Blood*, **27**, 816.

Harder, H. C. and Rosenberg, B. (1970). Inhibitory effects of anti-tumor platinum compounds on DNA, RNA and protein synthesis in mammalian cells *in vitro*. *International Journal of Cancer*, **6**, 207.

Haverkos, H. W., and Curran, J. W. (1982). The current outbreak of Kaposi's sarcoma and opportunistic infections. *Ca-A Cancer Journal for Clinicians*, **32**, 330.

Hecht, F., and McCaw, B. K. (1977). Chromosome instability syndromes. In *Genetics of human cancer* (eds J. J. Mulvihill, R. W. Miller, and J. F. Fraumeni). New York: Raven Press, p. 105.

Hersh, E. M., Butler, W. T., Rossen, R. D. *et al.* (1970). *In vitro* studies of the human response to organ allografts. *Journal of Immunology*, **107**, 571.

Hilscher, W., and Reichelt, P. (1968)]. Untersuchungen an Samenpithel der Ratte nach Gabon von Endoxan und Natulan. *Beitraege zur Pathologischen Anatomie*, **137**, 452.

Hoover, R., and Fraumeni, J. F. (1973). Risk of cancer in renal transplant patients. *Lancet*, **2**, 55.

Ishihara, T., and Kumatori, T. (1966). Polyploid cells in human leukocytes following *in vivo* and *in vitro* irradiation. *Cytologia*, **31**, 59.

Jensen, M. K. (1967). Chromosome studies in patients treated with Azathioprine and Amethopterin. *Acta Medica Scandinavica*, **182**, 445.

Kamada, N., and Uchino, H. (1972). Preleukemic state in atomic bomb survivors, with special reference to retro- and prospective analysis. *Japanese Journal of Clinical Hematology*, **13**, 313.

Kamada, N., Kuramoto, A., Katsuki, T., and Hinuma, Y. (1979). Chromosome aberrations in B lymphocytes of atomic bomb survivors. *Blood,* **53,** 1140.

Kao-Shan, C. S., Micetich, K., Zwelling, L. A., and Whang-Peng, J. (1983). Cytogenetic effects of 4′([9-acridinyl]-amino)methanesulphon-*m*-anisidide(*m*-AMSA) on human lymphocytes *in vivo* and *in vitro.* In press.

Kapadia, S. B., Krause, J. R., Ellis, L. D., Pan, S. F., and Wald, N. (1980). Induced acute non-lymphocytic leukemia following long-term chemotherapy. A study of 20 cases. *Cancer,* **45,** 1315.

Karon, M., and Benedict, W. F. (1972). Chromatid breakage: Differential effect of inhibitors of DNA synthesis during G_2 phase. *Science,* **178,** 62.

Kaung, D. T., and Swartzendruber, A. A. (1969). Effect of chemotherapeutic agents on chromosomes of patients with lung cancer. *Disease of the Chest,* **55,** 98.

Kucerova, M. (1970). Chromosome aberrations after X-ray therapy. *Journal de Génétique Humaine,* **18,** 21.

Lambert, B., Ringborg, U., Harper, E., and Lindblad, A. (1978). Sister chromatid exchanges in lymphocyte cultures of patients receiving chemotherapy for malignant disorders. *Cancer Treatment Reports,* **62,** 1413.

Lawler, S. D., Millard, R. E., and Kay, H. E. M. (1970). Further cytogenetical investigations in polycythaemia vera. *European Journal of Cancer,* **6,** 223.

Lee, I. P., and Dixon, R. L. (1972). Effects of procarbazine on spermatogenesis determined by velocity sedimentation cell separation technique and serial mating. *Proceedings of the American Association for Cancer Research,* **13,** 63.

Léonard, A., and Deknudt, G. (1968). Chromosome rearrangements after low X-ray doses given to spermatogonia of mice. *Canadian Journal of Genetics and Cytology,* **10,** 119.

Li, F. P., Fine, W., Jaffe, N. *et al.* (1979). Offspring of patients treated for cancer in childhood. *Journal of the National Cancer Institute,* **62,** 1193.

Lisco, H., and Conard, R. A. (1967). Chromosome studies on Marshall Islanders exposed to fallout radiation. *Science,* **157,** 445.

Lloyd, D. C., Purrott, R. J., Dolphin, G. W. *et al.* (1976). A comparison of physical and cytogenetic estimates of radiation dose in patients treated with iodine-131 for thyroid carcinoma. *International Journal of Radiation Biology,* **30,** 473.

Malawista, S. E. (1971). Vinblastine: Colchicine-like effects on human blood leukocytes during phagocytosis. *Blood,* **37,** 519.

Manolov, G., Manolova, Y., Levan, A., and Klein, G. (1971). Experiments with fluorescent chromosome staining in Burkitt tumors. *Hereditas,* **68,** 235.

Marinello, M. J., Bloom, M. L., Doeblin, T. D., and Sandberg, A. A. (1980). Double minute chromosomes in human leukemia. *New England Journal of Medicine,* **303,** 704.

Matsuyama, S., Yen, F. S., Jarvik, L. F., and Fu, T. K. (1973). Marijuana and human chromosomes. *Genetics,* **74,** part 2, S175.

McMahon, B., and Levy, M. A. (1964). Prenatal origin of childhood leukemia; evidence from twins. *New England Journal of Medicine,* **270,** 1082.

Melnyk, J., Duffy, D. M., and Sparkes, R. S. (1971). Human mitotic and meiotic chromosome damage following *in vivo* exposure to methotrexate. *Clinical Genetics,* **2,** 28.

Meyne, J., and Lockhart, L. H. (1978). Cytogenetic effects of cis-platinum(II) diamminedichloride on human lymphocyte cultures. *Mutation Research,* **58,** 87.

Miller, O. J., Miller, D. A., and Warburton, D. (1973). Application of new staining techniques to the study of human chromosomes. *Progress in Medical Genetics,* **9,** 1.

Miller, R. C., Hill, R. B., Nichols, W. W., and Meadows, A. T. (1978). Acute and long-term cytogenetic effects of childhood cancer chemotherapy and radiotherapy. *Cancer Research,* **38,** 3241.

Mitelman, F., Nilsson, P. G., Brandt, L. *et al.* (1981). Chromosome pattern, occupation and clinical features in patients with acute nonlymphocytic leukemia. *Cancer Genetics and Cytogenetics,* **4,** 197.

Modan, B., and Lilienfeld, A. M. (1965). Polycythemia vera and leukemia – The role of radiation treatment. A study of 1222 patients. *Medicine,* **44,** 305.

Newman, A. J., and Gross, S. (1967). Turner's syndrome and congenital erythroid hyperplasia. *Lancet,* **1,** 449.

Nias, A. H. W., and Ockey, C. H. (1965). Change in chromosome number during continuous irradiation. *Nature,* **206,** 840.

Nofal, M. M., and Beierwaltes, W. H. (1964). Persistent chromosomal aberrations following radioiodine therapy. *Journal of Nuclear Medicine,* **5,** 840.

Norman, A., Adams, F. H., and Riley, R. F. (1978). Cytogenetic effects of contrast media and triiodobenzoic acid derivatives in human lymphocytes. *Radiology,* **129,** 199.

Nowell, P. C. and Hungerford, D. A. (1960). A minute chromosome in human chronic granulocytic leukemia. *Science,* **132,** 1497.

O'Donnell, J. F., Brereton, H. D., Greco, F. A. *et al.* (1979). Acute nonlymphocytic leukemia and acute myeloproliferative syndrome following radiation therapy for non-Hodgkin's lymphoma and chronic lymphocytic leukemia: Clinical studies. *Cancer,* **44,** 1930.

Ohama, K., and Kadotani, T. (1970). Cytologic effects of bleomycin on cultured human leukocytes. *Japanese Journal of Human Genetics,* **14,** 293.

Ohnuki, Y., Awa, A., and Pomerat, C. M. (1961). Chromosomal studies on irradiated leukocytes *in vitro. Annals of the New York Academy of Sciences.* **95,** 882.

Ohtsuru, M., Ishii, Y., Takai, S. *et al.* (1980). Sister chromatid exchanges in lymphocytes of cancer patients receiving mitomycin C treatment. *Cancer Research,* **40,** 477.

Patil, S. R., Corder, M. P., Jochimsen, P. R., and Dick, F. R. (1980). Bone marrow chromosome abnormalities in breast cancer patients following adjuvant chemotherapy. *Cancer Research,* **40,** 4076.

Pedersen-Bjergaard, J., Nissen, N. I., Sørensen, H. M. *et al.* (1980). Acute non-lymphocytic leukemia in patients with ovarian carcinoma following long-term treatment with treosulfan (dihydroxybusulfan). *Cancer,* **45,** 19.

Penn, I. (1979). Kaposi's sarcoma in organ transplant recipients: report of 20 cases. *Transplantation,* **27,** 8.

Pinedo, H. M., van Hemel, J. O., Vrede, M. A., and van der Sluys Veer, J. (1974). Acute myelofibrosis and chromosome damage after procarbazine treatment. *British Medical Journal,* **3,** 525.

Pochin, E. E. (1960). Leukemia following radioiodine treatment of thyrotoxicosis. *British Medical Journal,* **2,** 1545.

Portugal, M. A., Falkson, H. C., Stevens, K., and Falkson, G. (1979). Acute leukemia as a complication of long-term treatment of advanced breast cancer. *Cancer Treatment Reports,* **63,** 177.

Pulciani, S., Santos, E., Lauver, A. V. *et al.* (1982). Oncogenes in solid human tumors. *Nature,* **300,** 539.

Reddy, M. M., Goh, K. O., and Hempelmann, L .H. (1980). Induction of micronuclei in PHA-stimulated human lymphocyte cultures by therapeutic radiation. *Experientia,* **36,** 343.

Reddy, M. M., Goh, K. O., Logan, W. W., and Hempelmann, L. H. (1977). A study of T and B lymphocytes and chromosomes in breast irradiated mastitis patients. *Investigative Radiology,* **12,** 238.

Reeves, B. R., and Margoles, C. (1974). Preferential location of chlorambucil-induced breakage in the chromosomes of normal human lymphocytes. *Mutation Research*, **26**, 205.

Reeves, B. R., Pickup, V. L., Lawler, S. D. *et al.* (1975). A chromosome study of patients with uveitis treated with chlorambucil. *British Medical Journal*, **4**, 22.

Reich, E. (1964). Actinomycin: correlation of structure and function of its complexes with purines and DNA. *Science*, **143**, 684.

Riccardi, V. M., Sujansky, E., Smith, A. C., and Francke, U. (1978). Chromosomal imbalance in aniridia–Wilms' tumor association?: 11p interstitial deletion. *Pediatrics*, **61**, 604.

Richmond, J. Y., and Kaufman, B. N. (1969). Studies on busulfan (Myleran) treated leukocyte cultures. *Experimental Cell Research*, **54**, 377.

Rowley, J. D., Golomb, H. M., and Dougherty, C. (1977a). 15/17 translocation, a consistent chromosomal change in acute promyelocytic leukemia. *Lancet*, **1**, 549.

Rowley, J. D., Golomb, H.M., and Vardiman, J. (1977b). Nonrandom chromosomal abnormalities in acute nonlymphocytic leukemia in patients treated for Hodgkin disease and non-Hodgkin lymphomas. *Blood*, **50**, 759.

Sasaki, M. S., and Miyata, H. (1968). Biological dosimetry in atomic bomb survivors. *Nature*, **220**, 1189.

Schinzel, A., and Schmid, W. (1976). Lymphocyte chromosome studies in humans exposed to chemical mutagens: the validity of the method in 67 patients under cytostatic therapy. *Mutation Research*, **40**, 139.

Schmähl, D., Habs, M., Lorenz, M., and Wagner, T. (1982). Occurrence of second tumors in man after anticancer drug treatment. *Cancer Treatment Reviews*, **9**, 167.

Schmid, E., Dresp, J., Bauchinger, M. *et al.* (1980). Radiation-induced chromosome damage in patients after tumor therapy with 14 MeV, DT neutrons. *International Journal of Radiation Biology*, **38**, 691.

Schwartz, R. S. (1972). Immunoregulation, oncogenic viruses and malignant lymphomas. *Lancet*, **1**, 1266.

Schwartz, R. S. (1975). Another look at immunologic surveillance. *New England Journal of Medicine*, **293**, 181.

Setlow, R. B. (1978). Repair deficient human disorders and cancer. *Nature*, **271**, 713.

Sheibani, K., Bukowski, R. M., Tubbs, R. R. *et al.* (1980). Acute nonlymphocytic leukemia in patients receiving chemotherapy for nonmalignant diseases. *Human Pathology*, **11**, 175.

Sieber, S. M., and Adamson, R. H. (1975a). The clastogenic, mutagenic, teratogenic and carcinogenic effects of various antineoplastic agents. In *Pharmacological basis of cancer chemotherapy*. (Twenty-Seventh Annual Symposium on Fundamental Cancer Research, 1974), p. 401.

Sieber, S. M., and Adamson, R. H. (1975b). Toxicity of antineoplastic agents in man: chromosomal aberrations, antifertility effects, congenital malformation and carcinogenic potential. *Advances in Cancer Research*, **22**, 57.

Silverstein, M. N., Goldberg, J. D., and Balcerzak, S. P. (1979). The incidence of acute leukemia in a randomized clinical trial for polycythemia vera. *Blood*, **54**, (suppl.), 209a.

Skinner, M. D., and Schwartz, R. S. (1972). Immunosuppressive therapy. *New England Journal of Medicine*, **287**, 281.

Snaith, M. L., Holt, J. M., Oliver, D. O. *et al.* (1973). Treatment of patients with systemic lupus erythematosus including nephritis with chlorambucil. *British Medical Journal*, **2**, 197.

Soukup, S. W., Takacs, E., and Warkany, J. (1965). Chromosome changes in rat embryos following X-irradiation. *Cytogenetics*, **4**, 130.

Stenchever, M. A., Kunysz, T. J., and Allen, M. A. (1974). Chromosome breakage in users of marihuana. *American Journal of Obstetrics and Gynecology*, **118**, 106.
Stevenson, A. C., Bedford, J., Dolphin, G. W. *et al.* (1973). Cytogenetic and scanning study of patients receiving intra-articular injections of gold-198 and yttrium-90. *Annals of the Rheumatic Diseases*, **32**, 112.
Terasima, T., Yasukawa, M., and Umezawa, H. (1970). Breaks and rejoining of DNA in cultured mammalian cells treated with bleomycin. *Gann*, **61**, 513.
Theologides, A., Yarbro, J. W., and Kennedy, B. J. (1968). Daunomycin inhibition of DNA and RNA synthesis. *Cancer*, **21**, 16.
Thiery, J. P., Aurias, A., Dumont, J. *et al.* (1981). Acute nonlymphocytic leukemias following chemotherapy. Ultrastructural study of erythroblastic cell line and discussion of nuclear anomalies. *Blood Cells*, **7**, 341.
Tokunaga, M., Land, C. E., Yamamoto, T. *et al.* (1982). Brest cancer in Japanese A-bomb survivors. *Lancet*, **2**, 294.
Tolchin, S. F., Winkelstein, A., Rodnan, G. P. *et al.* (1974). Chromosome abnormalities from cyclophosphamide therapy in rheumatoid arthritis and progressive systemic sclerosis (scleroderma). *Arthritis and Rheumatism*, **17**, 375.
Tough, I. M., Buckton, K. E., Baikie, A. G., and Court Brown, W. M. (1960). X-ray induced chromosome damage in man. *Lancet*, **2**, 849.
Trübestein, G. K., and Citoler, P. (1973). Drei falle von Thorotrastspätschaden. *Medizinische Klinik*, **68**, 1442.
Umezawa, H. (1974). Chemistry and mechanism of action of bleomycin. *Federation Proceedings*, **33**, 2296.
Van Kaick, G., Lorenz, D., Muth, H., and Kaul, A. (1978). Malignancies in German Thorotrast patients and estimated tissue dose. *Health Physics*, **35**, 137.
Van Thiel, D. H., Sherins, R. J., Myers, G. H. Jr., and DeVita, V. T. Jr. (1972). Evidence for a specific seminiferous tubular factor affecting follicle stimulating hormone secretion in man. *Journal of Clinical Investigation*, **51**, 1009.
Vig, B. K. (1971). Chromosome aberrations induced in human leukocytes by the antileukemic antibiotic adriamycin. *Cancer Research*, **31**, 32.
Von Vormittag, W. (1974). Zytostatische immunodepressive therapie, chromosomale aberrationen und karzinogene wirkung. *Wiener Klinische Wochenschrift*, **86**, 69.
Voorhees, J. J., Janzen, M. K., Harrell, E. R., and Chakrabarti, S. G. (1969). Cytogenetic evaluation of methotrexate-treated psoriatic patients. *Archives of Dermatology*, **100**, 269.
Wald, N., Borges, W. H., Li, C. C. *et al.* (1961). Leukaemia associated with mongolism. *Lancet*, **1**, 1228.
Wanders, J., Wattendorff, A. R., Endtz, L. J. *et al.* (1981). Chronic myeloid leukemia in myasthenia gravis after long-term treatment with 6-mercaptopurine. *Acta Medica Scandinavia*, **210**, 235.
Warner, T. F. C. S., and O'Loughlin, S. (1975). Kaposi's sarcoma: a by-product of tumour rejection. *Lancet*, **2**, 687.
Weh, H. J., Zschaber, R., and Hossfeld, D. K. (1982). Double minute chromosomes: a frequent marker in leukemic patients with a previous history of malignant disease? *Cancer Genetics and Cytogenetics*, **5**, 279.
Whang-Peng, J., Leventhal, B. G., Adamson, J. W., and Perry, S. (1969). The effect of daunomycin on human cells *in vivo* and *in vitro*. *Cancer*, **23**, 113.
Whang-Peng, J., and Young, R. C. (1978). Cytogenetic studies in leukemia. In *The year in hematology, 1978* (eds R. Silber, J. LoBue, and A. S. Gordon). New York: Plenum Publishing Corporation, pp. 375–462.
Whang-Peng, J., Knutsen, T., O'Donnell, J. F., and Brereton, H. D. (1979). Acute

non-lymphocytic leukemia and acute myeloproliferative syndrome following radiation therapy for non-Hodgkin's lymphoma and chronic lymphocytic leukemia. *Cancer*, **44**, 1592.

Whang-Peng, J., Kao-Shan, C. S., Lee, E. C. *et al.* (1982). Specific chromosome defect associated with human small-cell lung cancer: Deletion 3p(14–23). *Science*, **215**, 181.

Yosida, T. H., and Hirumi, H. (1960). Cytological study on the effects of 8-azaguanine and related compounds on the Yoshida sarcoma cells. *Gann*, **51**, 345.

Yunis, J. J., and Ramsay, N. (1978). Retinoblastoma and subband deletion of chromosome 13. *American Journal of Diseases of Children*, **132**, 161.

Risk Factors and Multiple Cancer
Edited by B.A. Stoll
© 1984 John Wiley and Sons Ltd.

Chapter

5   B. HERITY

Role of Alcohol, Tobacco, and Socio-Economic Factors

Environmental factors are believed to influence the development of about 80% of common cancers (Higginson and Muir, 1977). Important environmental influences on cancer development include tobacco, alcohol, radiation, occupation, diet, sexual and reproductive factors, and infections. Socio-economic factors affect total lifestyle and, therefore, have an influence on exposure to risk factors and on potential for both primary and secondary prevention of cancer.

In this chapter, evidence for the effect of tobacco and alcohol both singly and in combination will be examined and the effect of socio-economic factors will be discussed. Intervention to reduce these risk factors will be explored.

TOBACCO

There is no dispute that the greatest single contribution to a reduction in mortality from cancer would be a decrease in tobacco consumption. The main effect would be on lung cancer but a decrease in incidence of mouth, pharynx, oesophagus, larynx, bladder, and to a lesser extent pancreas and kidney cancers would also follow. The evidence is derived from *in vitro* and *in vivo* laboratory studies and from epidemiological research (US Public Health Service, 1979, 1980, 1981).

Tobacco-related cancers result from the susceptibility of specific sites to tobacco smoke and tobacco juice constituents or their metabolites. In some sites there is direct contact with the carcinogens (e.g. mouth, pharynx, oesophagus, larynx, and lung) while in others (e.g. pancreas, bladder, and kidney) the organs are affected by tobacco compounds after they have been metabolized in the liver or target organs or both. The evidence suggests that direct contact has the greatest carcinogenic potential.

Certain facts have been established in relation to tobacco carcinogenesis. Cigarettes are the most harmful form of tobacco and the difference in risk between cigarettes and other forms of tobacco is most manifest in relation to lung, bladder, and pancreas cancers. Cigar and pipe smoking also increase the risk, especially for oral cancer, but the risk for lung cancer is considerably less than that from cigarettes. Chewing tobacco or other leaves such as betel which is common in South-East Asia is associated with high death rates from oral cancer (Mahboubi, 1977; Simarak *et al.*, 1977).

A marked dose–response relationship with tobacco consumption is well recognized. It is related to age at starting the habit, quantity consumed daily, depth of inhalation, and tar content of tobacco. The degree to which stopping smoking reduces risk is related to the 'dose' already received, but in general in one who has been smoking heavily for 20 years or longer, the risk following 10–15 years of abstinence from the habit, approaches that of a non-smoker.

ALCOHOL

It has been recognized for many years that heavy alcohol consumption is associated with cancers at certain sites, notably mouth, pharynx, oesophagus and larynx, and that primary liver cancer occurs more frequently in those with cirrhosis of the liver, whether of alcoholic or non-alcoholic aetiology. The evidence derives from studies of proportional mortality among alcoholics (Pell and d'Alonzo, 1973; Monson and Lyon, 1975; Hakulinen *et al.*, 1974; Nicholls *et al.*, 1974; Schmidt and de Lint, 1972); and from case-control studies of cancer (Wynder *et al.*, 1956, 1957a,b, 1976, 1977; Vincent and Marchetta 1963; Keller and Terris, 1965; Martinez, 1969; Wynder and Bross, 1961; Rothman and Keller, 1972; Wynder and Mabuchi, 1973; Schottenfeld *et al.*, 1974; Graham *et al.*, 1977; McMichael, 1978). An association of beer drinking with cancer of the large bowel has also been suggested (Sundby, 1967; Wynder and Shigematsu, 1967; Jensen, 1979; Dean *et al.*, 1979).

Ethanol in its pure form has not been shown to have carcinogenic effects in animals, although it may affect the genetic material in cultured cells (Harsanyi *et al.*, 1977; Obe and Ristow, 1979). Some alcoholic beverages have been shown to contain known carcinogens, e.g. nitrosamines (Bogovski *et al.*, 1974; Walker *et al.*, 1979) and perhaps other carcinogens not yet identified (Nagao *et al.*, 1981; Loquet *et al.*, 1981). Since the effect of alcohol in most studies has been shown to be related to total alcohol consumption and not to specific alcoholic drinks, either carcinogens must be present in all types of alcoholic beverages or else alcohol must act in a different manner to increase carcinogenesis.

Theories relating to the carcinogenic effect of alcohol are as follows:

1. It enhances the solubility of the carcinogen which passes with more facility through cellular membranes.
2. It alters liver metabolism by increasing production of carcinogens which are site specific, or decreasing ability to detoxify or inactivate carcinogens.
3. It alters the intracellular metabolism of epithelial cells at target sites.
4. It causes nutritional deficiencies which potentiate the effect of carcinogens.

Measurement of the effect of alcohol is confounded by tobacco consumption which is strongly correlated with alcohol use in most populations. Accurate assessment of the effect of alcohol is only possible when the effect of the generally high consumption of cigarettes by heavy alcohol users is controlled for. In studies where this has been done, excess head and neck cancer attributable to alcohol consumption has been demonstrated. However, most of these studies have not found a substantial group of heavy drinkers who do not smoke, so that very little evidence regarding the effect of heavy alcohol consumption in the absence of smoking is available.

It has been shown that light drinking has little or no effect in the absence of smoking but that heavy drinking allied to light smoking increases the risk for head and neck cancers (Wynder *et al.*, 1956; 1957a,b; 1977; Wynder and Bross, 1961; Vincent and Marchetta 1963; Keller and Terris, 1965; Feldman and Hazan, 1975; Herity *et al.*, 1981, 1982). The weight of the evidence to date points to a promoting effect of alcohol on tobacco carcinogenesis.

Excess mortality from lung cancer in heavy drinkers has been reported. However, a study which controlled for tobacco consumption showed that alcohol had little effect on lung cancer risk (Herity *et al.*, 1982). Table 1 shows the relative risks associated with drinking and smoking in a study of lung and larynx cancer patients in Ireland. In this study it was found that, whereas heavy alcohol consumption raised the risk of heavy smokers for larynx cancer, it had no such effect for lung cancer. The excess mortality from lung

Table 1 Relative risks and synergism for tobacco and alcohol consumption in cancers of the lung and larynx (From Herity *et al.*, 1982)

	Tobacco consumption	Alcohol consumption	
		Non-light	Heavy
Lung	*Non/light*	1	1.5
	Heavy	10.6	12.4
Larynx	*Non/light*	1.0	4.0
	Heavy	3.3	14.0

cancer among heavy drinkers was due to the association of heavy cigarette smoking with heavy alcohol consumption.

Some studies have shown a correlation between beer consumption and cancer of the large bowel. Three case-control studies distinguished between colon and rectal cancer; one from Japan (Wynder *et al.*, 1969) and one from the US (Graham *et al.*, 1978) found no relationship, and one (Wynder and Shigematsu, 1967) found excess risk for both sites related to beer consumption. Sundby (1967) found excess rectal cancer among beer drinkers in a follow-up study of approximately 1700 alcoholics in Norway. Studies of brewery workers in Copenhagen (Jensen, 1979) and Dublin (Dean *et al.*, 1979) found respectively no excess risk and a twofold excess of rectal cancer.

Potter *et al.* (1982) examined international correlations of beer consumption and age-standardized rectal cancer mortality for 29 countries and found a correlation coefficient of 0.77 in males and 0.75 in females. There was a weak negative correlation with wine drinking in both sexes and no correlation with total alcohol consumption. They also noted that the male : female ratio was about 1 : 1 in countries with low beer consumption and levelled off at around 1.9 : 1 for high consumption countries.

The evidence in relation to beer and large bowel cancer is no more than suggestive of an association, but the correlation coefficients of around 0.8 are similar to those derived for fat consumption and breast and bowel cancer; the association deserves further investigation both by epidemiological and laboratory studies.

Primary liver cancer is a rare disease in Western countries but is reported to occur in 10–30% of alcoholics who develop cirrhosis (Parker, 1957; Leevy *et al.*, 1964; Lee 1966). However, follow-up studies of mortality among alcoholics have not shown this excess risk (Monson and Lyon 1975; Schmidt and de Lint, 1972). The high incidence of hepatocellular carcinoma in Africa and South-East Asia, where chronic liver disease following hepatitis B infection is frequent, is supportive of the hypothesis that chronic liver disease of whatever aetiology predisposes to primary liver cancer but the mechanism of carcinogenesis is as yet obscure.

JOINT EFFECT OF TOBACCO AND ALCOHOL

The effect of any risk factor in disease may be expressed as the ratio of the risk in a group exposed to the risk factor to that in a non-exposed group. To study the joint effect of two risk factors (in this case of tobacco and alcohol), two concepts must be considered: (1) independent action of the risk factors; and (2) interaction between them which may be positive (i.e. synergistic), or negative (i.e. antagonistic). If the risk factors act independently the combined effect will be the sum of the individual effects; if there is synergism or antagonism the effect of both together will be respectively greater or less than the sum of the individual effects. Interaction between risk factors has been discussed in a number of recent papers (Rothman and Keller, 1972; Rothman, 1976; Hogan *et al.*, 1978; Saracci, 1980; Rothman *et al.*, 1980; Koopman, 1981; Flanders and Rothman, 1982).

Rothman and Keller (1972) examined the data of Keller and Terris (1965) and that of Wynder *et al.* (1957a) for evidence of interaction between the effects of alcohol and tobacco in cancer of the mouth. They concluded that the main effects were additive and independent, with a small synergistic effect. Herity *et al.* (1981) examined the interaction of smoking and drinking in 200 patients with head and neck cancer and 200 controls matched for age and sex, and found significant synergism for larynx cancer with a value of 2.5 (Table 1).

Flanders and Rothman (1982) studied the findings from the case-control studies of Wynder *et al.* (1976) and the Third National Cancer Survey (Williams and Horm, 1977) for evidence of interaction, and found 'moderate synergy of alcohol and tobacco' with a value of 1.5 for the data from the Third National Cancer Survey and 2.5 for that of Wynder and his colleagues. Feldman and Hazan (1975) found an index of interaction of 2.8 for tobacco and alcohol in head and neck cancer but it was not statistically significant.

From the evidence available at present, it appears that synergistic action between tobacco and alcohol has been convincingly demonstrated only for cancer of the larynx and is of the order of 1.5–2.5. This estimate would imply that the effect of tobacco and alcohol acting together is between 1½ and 2½ times greater than would be predicted if independent effects of the two risk factors were assumed.

SOCIO-ECONOMIC STATUS AND CANCER

Differences in cancer incidence and mortality by social class have been recognized for many years. Positive associations with breast and large bowel cancer and negative associations for lung, stomach, and cervix uteri cancers with high socio-economic status are well documented (Cutler and Young, 1975).

Social class is a widely used concept for ranking or stratifying a total population into subgroups which differ from each other in prestige, wealth, and power (Mausner and Bahn, 1974). Despite some discrepancies, it is a useful variable linking occupation, education, income, housing and behaviour albeit in a rather gross way, and is based on the assumption that the socio-cultural environment within which persons develop adaptive life patterns has a far-reaching influence on life experience.

The Registrar General's six social class categories based on occupation, are I. Professional; II. Intermediate; III. Non-manual and manual skilled; IV. Partly skilled; V. Unskilled; and VI. Other (students, armed forces, and

Table 2   Prevalence of cigarette smoking by sex and socio-economic group, 1972 and 1980, Great Britain (from Donaldson and Donaldson, 1983. Reproduced by permission of MTP.)

Socio-economic group	% Smoking cigarettes		% Change
	1972	1980	1972–80
Men			
1. Professional	33	21	−12
2. Employers and managers	44	35	− 9
3. Intermediate and junior non-manual	45	35	−10
4. Skilled manual and own account non-professional	57	48	− 9
5. Semi-skilled manual and personal service	57	49	− 8
6. Unskilled manual	64	57	− 7
All men:	52	42	−10

inadequately described occupations). An alternative method of classifying the population on the basis of occupation introduced in the UK in 1951 is to define 17 socio-economic groups (SEG) which are sometimes combined into six 'collapsed' categories (Table 2).

It is not surprising that lifestyle as measured by social class has an important influence on morbidity and mortality within a population. Way of life affects exposure to risk factors for disease, knowledge, attitudes, beliefs and values, and access to preventive medicine and medical care. In studying cancer risk, it is useful to analyse the effects of different lifestyle factors in order to try to identify the contribution of each one to total risk; in this way possibilities for prevention may be indicated. Occupation, income, area of residence and education are all indicators of social class and diet and behaviour are strongly influenced by socio-economic factors.

Occupation

For practical considerations, occupation is the most widely used measure of social class and since it is in general highly correlated with education, income and residence, it serves as a fairly reliable indicator of socio-economic status. Fox and Adelstein (1978), in an analysis of the 1970–72 occupational mortality statistics for England and Wales (Registrar General, 1978) discussed the difficulty in distinguishing between the influence of socio-economic group and occupation. A traditional method of separating the effect of occupation from that of 'lifestyle' has been to compare the mortality of men in certain occupations with that of their wives (Stevenson, 1923, 1928) but increasing numbers of women in employment, and the employment of women in the same or related occupations as their husbands (Fox and Adelstein 1978), has rendered this method less reliable than formerly. They suggest standardization for social class so that mortality rates in a specific occupational group are compared with those in the same socio-economic group (for example mortality among male medical doctors with that of all men in SEG 1). When this was done for mortality ratios for cancer in 25 occupational groups in England and Wales the results suggested that only 12% of the total variation was due to work environment and that 88% was due to social factors (Fox and Adelstein, 1978).

Estimates that less than 5% of cancer deaths in industrialized countries are due to occupation are generally accepted (Higginson and Muir, 1977, 1979; Wynder and Gori, 1977; Doll and Peto, 1981). Chapter 2 details recognized occupational cancers, but other cancers associated with work environment (although not usually termed occupational) are head and neck cancers associated with the sale and manufacture of alcohol, and skin cancer associated with exposure to sunlight in outdoor occupations.

It is noteworthy that many occupational cancers were recognized because they occurred at sites at which cancer is rare (e.g. liver, and nose and paranasal sinuses) and it is likely that some occupationally induced cancers at common sites have not yet been identified. There is still potential for recognition of such tumours by observant clinicians; clustering of cases within occupations and occurrence in a younger age group than in the general population are characteristics which may distinguish an occupational from a non-occupational aetiology in cancer.

Area of residence

Area of residence, another lifestyle factor influenced by social class, is regarded as a good indicator of economic resources. Although recognized as having an important effect on the incidence and outcome of communicable disease, it does not seem to have much effect on cancer incidence. Urban/rural differences have been described for lung cancer but, in general, cancer patterns within Europe do not show association with industrialization (Higginson and Muir, 1979).

There is no good evidence associating general air pollution with cancer although it may potentiate the effect of smoking (Haenzel *et al.*, 1962; Haenzel and Taueber, 1964; Buell and Dunn, 1967; Ford and Bialik, 1980). When population groups with a homogeneous lifestyle were studied, e.g. Mormons (Lyon *et al.*, 1976), urban/rural differences disappeared: it appears that area of residence must have minimal influence on the cancer risk of a population in comparison to other lifestyle factors with which it is associated.

Level of education and income

Educational measures of socio-economic status include number of years of full-time education, age at leaving school, type of educational establishment last attended full time, and qualifications gained. The main disadvantage of these measures up to the present has been that the majority of the population is concentrated in a single category but, with improved educational facilities they are likely to be more discriminating in future. Whereas area of residence or type of housing is regarded as an indicator of income, educational level is viewed as a sensitive indicator of attitudes and behaviour, particularly in relation to preventive medicine (Morgan, 1983).

Devesa and Diamond (1980) used data from the Third National Cancer Survey to study the association of breast and cervix cancer with income and education among white and black women in the US. Breast cancer showed a strong positive association with both variables in white women, but in black women with level of education only. This finding in black women may reflect an effect of postponement of first birth as education is pursued, whereas income is subject to modification at a later stage in life. Education had a stronger effect than income in reducing risk of breast cancer; the age-adjusted white : black relative risk (RR) of 1.20 was reduced to 1.16 with adjustment for income and to 1.09 with adjustment for education.

In cancer of the cervix, consistent negative associations were found with income and education, with relative risks greater than 4 between the highest and lowest categories; education had a particularly strong effect in women less than 44 years of age. Cancer of the cervix was significantly more common among blacks than whites but with adjustment for education, the age-adjusted racial RR of 1.82 was reduced to 1.53 and with adjustment for income to 1.27. It appears that in cancer of the cervix, income has a stronger effect than education.

Diet and nutrition

Diet may influence the incidence of cancer in many ways and, since it is affected by socio-economic considerations, it is not surprising that social class differences in diet-related cancers are apparent. In general, large bowel, breast, endometrium, ovary, and prostate cancers are associated with a high fat, high protein, low fibre dietary pattern, and are more common in the higher than lower socio-economic groups. Large bowel cancer is believed to be mediated through interaction between a high fat diet, the bile acids, and intestinal bacteria (Aries *et al.*, 1969; Hill *et al.*, 1971; Reddy and Wynder, 1973; Crowther *et al.*, 1976; MacDonald *et al.*, 1978) and Graham *et al.* (1978) found a protective effect from green and yellow vegetable consumption. The other so-called cancers of affluence are believed to be associated with an effect of a high fat diet on the production of hormones, and in the case of endometrial cancer with obesity (Benjamin and Romney, 1964).

On the other hand, stomach cancer is more common in the lower socio-economic groups, and in Western societies dietary deficiencies may be important. Association with diets low in fats, fresh fruit and vegetables and their related vitamins and minerals has been described (Graham *et al.*, 1972b; Hirayama, 1977; Wynder *et al.*, 1977). In Japan, milk and green and yellow vegetables have been associated with protection against stomach and lung cancer (Hirayama, 1977; MacLennan *et al.*, 1977) and Graham *et al.* (1981) found a protective effect for high vitamin A and C levels against cancer of the larynx. Peto *et al.* (1981) reviewed the evidence for a protective effect of vitamin A on cancer (see Chapter 12). It is also plausible that vitamin C is protective against the formation of carcinogens from ingested nitrates (Mirvish *et al.*, 1972; Weisburger 1977). Evidence then is accumulating for a protective effect of fresh fruit and vegetable consumption which is highly correlated with social class.

In the West, cancer of the oesophagus is strongly associated with tobacco and alcohol consumption, although in parts of Iran, the USSR, China and South Africa, local environmental factors may be important (Van Rensburg, 1981). However, dietary deficiencies have also been suspected in the aetiology of upper gastrointestinal tract cancer. Wynder *et al.* (1975b), in a study in Sweden, found an association between the Plummer–Vinson syndrome and cancer of the oesophagus, and with cancers of the mouth, pharynx, and oesophagus in a later study (Wynder *et al.*, 1977). They postulated that a factor common to the Plummer–Vinson syndrome and alcoholism, namely deficiency of iron and riboflavin, may predispose to the development of cancers of these sites. Laboratory studies lend some support to this thesis (Wynder and Klein, 1965).

There is then, during the last decade or so, an accumulation of evidence in relation to diet and cancer which is plausible in the light of the social class differences in common cancers which have been apparent for many years. It also fits in with epidemiological evidence of geographical differences in cancer rates, and with data from studies of migrant populations. In Western societies the cancer risk from over-nutrition is quantitatively of greater importance than that from deficiency states, and as an increasing proportion of Western populations reach satisfactory levels of subsistence the social class gradient in cancer rates decreases. This is already apparent in statistics relating to large bowel and breast cancer, and in falling rates of stomach cancer.

Other lifestyle factors

Other social class-related variables which have an important effect on cancer risk in women are age at first coitus, number of sexual partners, and age at first pregnancy. Carcinoma of the cervix uteri is commoner in SEG 5 than in the upper socio-economic groups, and is associated with early age at first sexual intercourse and multiple partners. Many factors are cited to explain the strong social class relationship of this cancer including unstable marriages, poor personal or sexual hygiene and poor medical care, and it is likely that all these factors play a part in the development of the disease.

Current suggestions of a viral or other infective aetiology would fit in with increased risk through poor hygiene and unstable sexual relationships, and delay in seeking screening or curative services will raise the incidence and mortality from invasive carcinoma of the cervix. Nutritional deficiencies such as low vitamin A levels may also predispose to the condition.

On the other hand delayed first pregnancy increases the risk for *breast* cancer (MacMahon *et al.*, 1970) and Christopherson (1964) noted that women in the lower socio-economic groups married on average two years later, and became pregnant four years later, than those in the upper SEGs. This factor has an effect in increasing breast cancer rates in the women in the upper socio-economic groups.

Uptake of preventive and curative medical services

Social class has a profound influence both on the perception of health problems and on action taken in relation to them. Goldthorpe *et al.* (1969) have described typical 'working-class' and 'middle-class' conceptions of life which are fundamental to the understanding of attitudes to all health problems including cancer. The main points made are that the 'middle-classes' see life in terms of opportunity open to individuals who have the responsibility and potential to make what they want of themselves; planning for the future is important, and present sacrifices are seen in the light of future gains. The 'working-class' conception of life is putting up with, and making the best of, what comes along and living in the present; in so far as action is seen to be effective, emphasis is placed on collective action, e.g. trade unionism, rather than on individual effort.

Rosenstock (1960) has discussed the determinants of health behaviour, and has analysed (Rosenstock, 1963) the conditions under which people take action leading to prevention of disease. In brief, action is related to the degree to which an individual believes he or she is susceptible to a given health problem, and the perceived seriousness of the condition should it occur. It is also affected by the perception of a particular course of action; if it is regarded as being painful, unpleasant or ineffective, it is unlikely to be undertaken. Furthermore, behaviour results from a conflict of competing motives, and in general, socio-economic motives take precedence over health ones, especially in the lower socio-economic groups. Behaviour can also result from pressure to conform to group norms (e.g. encouragement from friends, relatives or neighbours) rather than from concern about health.

These attitudes and beliefs have important implications in relation to primary and secondary prevention of cancer. Primary preventive strategies such as refraining from smoking, dietary modification and moderate alcohol consumption are all aimed at the avoidance of future ills rather than at any immediate advantage. Also the success of measures directed towards early diagnosis, such as breast examination, cervical smears, and tests for occult blood depends on their being seen as acceptable and effective actions against serious and relatively common conditions.

Kirscht *et al.* (1966) in a national study of health beliefs, found that cancer was perceived as serious and likely to occur; 31% of his sample placed cancer in the most serious category of worry. However, nearly 20% of his sample did not regard themselves as susceptible and almost 20% did not think that action in relation to cancer was effective. Belief in efficacy of cancer prevention and diagnosis was positively associated with education and income. Examples of social class effects on health behaviour are the marked decrease in cigarette smoking in men in the upper compared with the lower socio-economic groups, and the preferential uptake of cervical cytology by women in SEGs 1 and 2 (British Medical Journal, 1980).

Goldsen (1963) compared cancer patients with symptoms who delayed seeking diagnosis to those who presented early and found that the latter had higher occupational levels, higher income, and higher educational achievement. Linden (1969) and Berg *et al.* (1977) found a later stage at presentation for cancer patients in the lower compared to upper socio-economic groups. However, Berg *et al.* (1977) found that even when stage and treatment were controlled for, survival was worse for patients in the lower than in the higher social groups. The differences were minimal for early or late stage disease, but more treatment failures occurred in their 'indigent' group, for cancers of reasonable prognosis at all ages.

Berg and his colleagues speculate that perhaps immune deficits due to under-nutrition or in some cases excess consumption of alcohol may have been a factor in the poorer response to therapy of this group. Similar findings by Myers and Hankey (1982) of poorer survial among black than white cancer patients in the US were related to factors other than stage of disease. Evidence suggests that interaction between the many variables which contribute to socio-economic status must be important in determining cancer risk and survival.

PREVENTION

Tobacco and alcohol

The practical importance of examining the contribution of risk factors to the development of disease is to identify preventive measures for the community. Fairly reliable estimates of the cancer burden resulting from the use of tobacco and alcohol have been made. Doll and Peto (1981) estimated that 30% (range 25–40%) of cancer deaths in the US were due to cigarettes, and 3% (range 2–4%) due to alcohol. These figures were not mutually exclusive since most heavy drinkers smoked as well. Higginson and Muir (1979) estimated that 30% of male and 7% of female cancer deaths in the Birmingham region were due to tobacco and 5% of male and 3% of female cancer deaths were due to tobacco/alcohol; Wynder and Gori (1977) produced very similar figures for the US. These estimates are probably applicable to many industrialized societies.

It seems clear that reduction in tobacco consumption, in particular cigarette smoking, will result in a decrease in incidence and mortality from cancer in any community, with the major decrease being seen in lung cancer. In the case of head and neck cancer the interaction of tobacco and alcohol has important public health implications; if there is a strongly synergistic model removal of one exposure would eliminate or very greatly reduce the effect of the other. The evidence available to date is sparse, but it does appear that for oral cancer, tobacco and alcohol have largely independent effects with some synergism apparent. In cancer of the larynx, the synergistic effect is stronger, with alcohol and tobacco acting together producing 1½–2½ times the number of cases expected if independent effects were assumed. However, it seems that to prevent a large proportion of head and neck cancer in the community, removal of exposure to both risk factors would be necessary.

Action to control smoking has met with some success in countries where the habit has been widespread. It was estimated (WHO, 1979) that 35 million people in the US and 8 million in the UK had given up smoking. The decrease is particularly marked among men in SEGs 1 and 2 (Table 2). However, a very worrying feature is the growth of the smoking habit in developing countries due to the promotional efforts of the tobacco companies. The WHO report *Controlling the Smoking Epidemic* (1979) summarizes the current facts in relation to smoking, and makes recommendations for continued primary preventive action. Stratagems for control of smoking include public information and education programmes, legislation and restrictive measures, and smoking cessation programmes and action at both national and international level.

Since many persons continue to smoke in spite of the well recognized health hazard, research into less harmful smoking products is necessary. The development and acceptance of filter cigarettes since about 1960 and the production of lower tar cigarettes have resulted in lower death rates from lung cancer among younger men (Doll, 1974), and a decrease in the relative risk of lung and larynx cancer for long-term users of filter cigarettes (Wynder and Stellman, 1979; Wynder and Hoffman, 1979). Research into the components of tobacco and tobacco smoke has produced further information on the biological activity of these compounds, and changes in the production, cultivation, and curing of tobacco have altered the constitution of commercial cigarettes in the West (Wynder and Hoffman, 1982). Such developments have contributed to a reduction in risk of smoking-related cancers for those who continue to smoke and should be encouraged.

Public education about alcohol-related cancers has not been developed and could be included in smoking control programmes. The fact that alcohol can be safely used by most people, and that an appreciable cancer risk is only seen when consumption exceeds about 45 ml ethanol/day, may make the message more acceptable to the general public. However, it is well recognized that alcohol-related problems in any community are proportionate to *per capita* consumption and the marked increase in consumption of alcohol by young people is likely to lead to a concomitant rise in health problems in the future including an increase in alcohol-related cancers.

Socio-economic risk factors

Successful intervention to reduce cancer incidence and mortality due to socio-economic risk factors depends in the main on behaviour modification. The effect of area of residence or occupation is small compared with that of other lifestyle factors; even the best known of the occupationally induced cancers, namely lung cancer due to asbestos, is only slightly higher in non-smoking asbestos workers than in non-smokers in the general population (Selikoff *et al.*, 1968, 1980). Occupational cancers, however, are among those with the greatest potential for primary prevention and strict enforcement of statutory control of occupational carcinogens is essential.

The socio-economic variable which has the greatest effect on behaviour is educational level. Earlier statements (Royal College of Physicians, 1962) that medical doctors smoked less due to their special awareness of the health hazards of smoking were shown to be incorrect when later studies of university staff (Lynch, 1963; Herity *et al.*, 1976) and of students (Knopf and Wakefield, 1974) showed no differences in smoking habit between medical and non-medical personnel. Lynch's (1963) conclusion that fewer medical doctors smoke 'more because they are graduates than because they are medical' has been borne out by the fact that all men in SEGs 1 and 2 have reduced their smoking, not only medical doctors.

General improvements in educational opportunities in industrialized countries in recent years should produce populations who will be more receptive to information and education about health, and more motivated to undertake positive action in relation to it than previous generations. It could be argued that in terms of socio-economic risk factors, investment in general education has more to offer than investment in health services.

Nutritional deficiencies, particularly in heavy drinkers in whom alcohol may replace other food items, may interact with tobacco and alcohol.

Graham *et al.* (1981) found that men ingesting low amounts of vitamins A and C had approximately twice the risk of cancer of the larynx of those taking large amounts. Protective effects of vitamin A ingestion in other epithelial cancers have also been described (see above under diet). Dietary risk factors for cancer are not clearly identified; but risk is associated with patterns rather than with specific constituents of diet.

A diet which (a) provides energy requirements sufficient to maintain ideal body weight, (b) contains adequate protein and micronutrients, and (c) contains less total fat and meat and more fibre than generally consumed in Western industrialized societies, is likely to be consonant with minimum cancer incidence. It is clear that the scientific base for community intervention to reduce diet-related cancer is deficient, but general advice by clinicians to avoid obesity, to reduce fat consumption, and to consume fresh fruit and vegetables regularly (if followed by their patients) could result in a reduction in diet-related cancers in the community.

Risk factors associated with sexual and reproductive behaviour are not readily amenable to primary prevention strategies, and it is likely that at present the only justifiable preventive community intervention is population screening for cancer of the cervix. Provided that high risk women can be persuaded to attend screening clinics it is effective in reducing mortality from this disease. Screening for breast cancer is undergoing rigorous evaluation at present (de Waard *et al.*, 1978; Miller, 1980; Tabar and Gad, 1981; UK trial of early detection of breast cancer group, 1981).

CONCLUSION

The effect of tobacco, and to a lesser extent alcohol, on risk of cancer has been well documented; there is much less direct evidence of the influence of socio-economic factors and their complex interaction. Much interdisciplinary research remains to be done to establish where primary and secondary preventive strategies might be employed to reduce the impact of these factors on cancer incidence.

Statutory controls in relation to proven carcinogens such as tobacco or ocupational carcinogens must be enforced. In the case of tobacco, restriction of promotional advertising of products especially in the developing world is essential. Research into ways of changing behaviour to reduce exposure to lifestyle risk factors must also be pursued.

REFERENCES

Aries, V. C., Crowther, J. S., and Drasar, B. S. (1969). Bacteria and the etiology of cancer of the large bowel. *Gut,* **10,** 334.
Benjamin, F., and Romney, S. L. (1964). Disturbed carbohydrate metabolism in endometrial carcinoma. *Cancer,* **17,** 366.

Berg, J. W., Ross, R., and Latourette, H. B. (1977). Economic status and survival of cancer patients. *Cancer,* **39,** 467.

Bogovski, P., Walker, E. A., Castegnaro, M., and Pignatelli, B. (1974). Some evidence of the presence of traces of nitrosamines in cider distillates. In *N-nitroso compounds in the environment* (eds. P. Bogovski and E. A. Walker). Lyon: International Agency for Research on Cancer, p. 192.

Buell, P., and Dunn, J. E. (1967). Relative impact of smoking and air pollution on lung cancer. *Archives of Environmental Health,* **15,** 291.

Christopherson, W. M. (1964). The detection of asymptomatic cervical cancer. *Journal of the Irish Medical Association,* **55,** 160.

Cole, P., and Goldman, M. (1975). *Persons at high risk of cancer* (ed. J. Fraumeni), New York: Academic Press, p. 178.

Crowther, J. S., Drasar, B. S., MacLennan, R. *et al.* (1976). Faecal steroids and bacteria and large bowel cancer in Hong Kong by socioeconomic groups. *British Journal of Cancer,* **34,** 191.

Cutler, S. J., and Young, J. L. (1975). Third National Cancer Survey: Incidence data. *National Cancer Institute Monograph,* No. 41. Washington, DC: US Government Printing Office.

Dean, G., MacLennan, R., MacLoughlin, H., and Shelley, E. (1979). Causes of death of blue-collar workers at a Dublin brewery, 1954–73. *British Journal of Cancer,* **40,** 581.

Devesa, S., and Diamond, E. (1980). Association of breast cancer and cervical cancer incidences with income and education among whites and blacks. *Journal of the National Cancer Institute,* **65,** 515.

de Waard, F., Rombach, J. J., and Colette, H. J. A. (1978). The DOM project for breast cancer screening in the city of Utrecht. In *Screening in cancer* (ed. A. B. Miller). Geneva: UICC Technical Report, No. 40, p. 183.

Doll, R. (1974). Surveillance and monitoring. *International Journal of Epidemiology,* **3,** 305.

Doll, R., and Peto, R. (1981). Avoidable risks of cancer in the US. *Journal of the National Cancer Institute,* **66,** 1193.

Donaldson, R. J., and Donaldson, L. J. (1983). *Essential community medicine.* Lancaster: MTP Press, p. 85.

Editorial (1980). High risk groups and cervical cancer. *British Medical Journal,* **281,** 629.

Feldman, J. G., and Hazan, M. (1975). A case-control investigation of alcohol, tobacco and diet in head and neck cancer. *Preventive Medicine,* **4,** 444.

Flanders, W. D., and Rothman, K. J. (1982). Interaction of alcohol and tobacco in laryngeal cancer. *American Journal of Epidemiology,* **115,** 371.

Ford, A., and Bialik, O. (1980). Air pollution and urban factors in relation to cancer mortality. *Archives of Environmental Health,* **35,** 350.

Fox, A. J., and Adelstein, A. M. (1978). Occupational mortality: work or way of life? *Journal of Epidemiology and Community Health,* **32,** 73.

Goldsen, R. K. (1963). Patient delay in seeking cancer diagnosis: behavioural aspects. *Journal of Chronic Diseases,* **16,** 427.

Goldthorpe, J., Lockwood, D., Bechoffer, F., and Plath, J. (1969). *The affluent worker in the class structure,* Cambridge: Cambridge University Press, p. 118.

Graham, S., Dayal, H., Rohrer, T. *et al.* (1977). Dentition, diet, tobacco and alcohol in the epidemiology of oral cancer. *Journal of the National Cancer Institute,* **59,** 1611.

Graham, S., Dayal, H., Swanson, M. *et al.* (1978). Diet in the epidemiology of cancer of the colon and rectum. *Journal of the National Cancer Institute,* **61,** 709.

Graham, S., Mettlin, C., Marshall, J. *et al.* (1981). Dietary factors in the epidemiology of cancer of the larynx. *American Journal of Epidemiology*, **113**, 675.

Graham, S., Schotz, W., and Martino, P. (1972a). Alimentary factors in the epidemiology of gastric cancer. *Cancer*, **4**, 927.

Graham, S., Schotz, W., and Martino, P. (1972b). Alimentary factors in the epidemiology of cancer of the colon and rectum. *Journal of the National Cancer Institute*, **61**, 709.

Haenzel, W., and Taueber, K. E. (1964). Lung cancer mortality as related to residence and smoking histories. II. White females. *Journal of the National Cancer Institute*, **32**, 803.

Haenzel, W., Loveland, D. B, and Sirken, M. G. (1962). Lung cancer mortality as related to residence and smoking histories. I. White males. *Journal of the National Cancer Institute*, **28**, 947.

Hakulinen, T., Lehtimaki, L., Lehtonen, M., and Teppo, L. (1974). Cancer morbidity among two male cohorts with increased alcohol consumption in Finland. *Journal of the National Cancer Institute*, **52**, 1711.

Harsanyi, Z., Granek, I. A., and MacKenzie, D. W. (1977). Genetic damage induced by ethyl alcohol in aspergillus nidulans. *Mutation Research*, **48**, 51.

Herity, B. A., Bourke, G. J., and Wilson-Davis, K. (1976). A study of the smoking habits of medical and non-medical university staff. *Journal of the Irish Medical Association*, **69**, 163.

Herity, B., Moriarty, M., Bourke, G. J., and Daly, L. (1981). A case-control study of head and neck cancer in the Republic of Ireland. *British Journal of Cancer*, **43**, 177.

Herity, B., Moriarty, M., Daly, L. *et al.* (1982). The role of tobacco and alcohol in lung and larynx cancer. *British Journal of Cancer*, **46**, 961.

Higginson, J., and Muir, C. S. (1977). Determination de l'importance des facteurs environnementaux dans le cancer humain: Role de l'epidemiologie. *Bulletin du Cancer* (Paris), **64**, 365.

Higginson, J., and Muir, C. S. (1979). Environmental carcinogenesis: Misconceptions and limitations to cancer control. *Journal of the National Cancer Institute*, **63**, 1291.

Hill, M. J., Drasar, B. S., Aries, V., and Hawksworth, G. (1971). Bacteria and aetiology of cancer of large bowel. *Lancet*, **1**, 95.

Hirayama, T. (1977). Changing patterns of cancer in Japan with special reference to the decrease in stomach cancer mortality. In *Origins of human cancer* (eds H. H. Hiatt, J. D. Watson, and J. A. Winston). New York: Cold Spring Harbor Laboratory, p. 55.

Hogan, M. D., Kupper, L. L., Most, B. M., and Haseman, J. K. (1978). Alternatives to Rothman's approach for assessing synergism (or antagonism) in cohort studies). *American Journal of Epidemiology*, **108**, 60.

Jensen, O. M. (1979). Cancer morbidity and causes of death among Danish brewery workers. *International Journal of Cancer*, **23**, 454.

Keller, A. Z., and Terris, M. (1965). The association of alcohol and tobacco with cancer of the mouth and pharynx. *American Journal of Public Health*, **55**, 1578.

Kirscht, J. P., Haefner D. P., and Kegeles, S. S. (1966). A national study of health beliefs. *Journal of Health and Human Behaviour*, **7**, 248.

Knopf, A., and Wakefield, J. (1974). Effect of medical education on smoking behaviour. *British Journal of Preventive and Social Medicine*, **28**, 246.

Koopman, J. S. (1981). Interaction between discrete causes. *American Journal of Epidemiology*, **113**, 716.

Lee, F. I. (1966). Cirrhosis and hepatoma in alcoholics. *Gut*, **7**, 77.

Leevy, C. M., Gellene, R., and Ning, M. (1964). Primary liver cancer in cirrhosis of the alcoholic. *Annals of the New York Academy of Science*, **114**, 1026.

Linden, G. (1969). The influence of social class in the survival of cancer patients. *American Journal of Public Health*, **59**, 267.

Loquet, C., Toussaint, G., and Le Talaer, J. Y. (1981). Studies on mutagenic constituents of apple brandy and various alcoholic beverages collected in Western France, a high incidence area for oesphageal cancer. *Mutation Research*, **88**, 155.

Lynch, G. W. (1963). Smoking habits of medical and non-medical university staff. Changes since R.C.P. report. *British Medical Journal*, **1**, 852.

Lyon, J. L., Klauber, M. R., Gardner, J. W., and Smart, C. R. (1976). Cancer incidence in Mormons and non-Mormons in Utah. 1966–70. *New England Journal of Medicine*, **294**, 129.

MacDonald, I. A., Webb, G. R., and Mahony, D. E. (1978). Fecal, hydroxy-steroid dehydrogenase activities in vegetarian Seventh-day Adventists, control subjects and bowel cancer patients. *American Journal of Clinical Nutrition*, **31**, 5233.

MacLennan, R., Da Costa, J., Day, N. E. *et al.* (1977). Risk factors for lung cancer in Singapore Chinese, a population with high female incidence rates. *International Journal of Cancer*, **20**, 854.

MacMahon, B., Cole, P., Lin, T. M. *et al.* (1970). Age at first birth and breast cancer risk. A summary of an international study. *Bulletin of the World Health Organization*, **43**, 209.

Mahboubi, E. (1977). The epidemiology of oral cavity, pharyngeal and oesophageal cancer outside of North America and Western Europe. *Cancer*, **40**, 1879.

Martinez, I. (1969). Factors associated with the cancer of the oesphagus, mouth and pharynx in Puerto Rico. *Journal of the National Cancer Institute*, **42**, 1069.

Mausner, J. S., and Bahn, A. K. (1974). Epidemiology: An introductory text. Philadelphia: W. B. Saunders, p. 51.

McMichael, A. J. (1978). Increases in laryngeal cancer in Britain and Australia, in relation to tobacco and alcohol consumption trends. *Lancet*, **1**, 1244.

Miller, A. B. (1980). National breast cancer screening gets underway. *Canadian Medical Association Journal*, **122**, 243.

Mirvish, S. S., Wallcave, L., Eagen, M. (1972). Ascorbate–nitrate reaction. Possible means of blocking the promotion of carcinogenic *N*-nitroso compounds. *Science*, **177**, 65.

Monson, D. R., and Lyon, J. L. (1975). Proportional mortality among alcoholics, *Cancer*, **36**, 1077.

Morgan, M. (1983). Measuring social inequality: Occupational classifications and their alternatives. *Community Medicine*, **5**, 125.

Myers, M., and Hankey, B. (1982). Cancer patient survival in the United States. In *Cancer epidemiology and prevention* (eds. D. Schottenfeld and J. F. Fraumeni). Philadelphia: W. B. Saunders, p. 173.

Nagao, T., Takahaski, V., Wakabayaski, K., and Sugimura, T. (1981). Mutagenicity of alcoholic beverages, *Mutation Research*, **88**, 147.

Nicholls, P., Edwards, O., and Kyle, E. (1974). Alcoholics admitted to four hospitals in England. II General and cause-specific mortality. *Quarterly Journal of Studies in Alcohol*, **35**, 841.

Obe, G., and Ristow, H. (1979). Mutagenic, cancerogenic and teratogenic effects of alcohol. *Mutation Research*, **65**, 229.

Parker, R. G. F. (1957). The incidence of primary hepatic carcinoma in cirrhosis. *Proceedings of the Royal Society of Medicine*, **50**, 145.

Pell, S., and d'Alonzo, C. A. (1973). A five-year mortality study of alcoholics. *Journal of Occupational Medicine*, **15**, 120.

Peto, R., Doll, R., Buckley, J. D., and Sporr, M. B. (1981). Can dietary beta-carotene materially reduce human cancer rates? *Nature*, **290**, 201.

Potter, J. D., McMichael, A. J., and Hartshorne, J. M. (1982). Alcohol and beer consumption in relation to cancers of bowel and lung: an extended correlation analysis. *Journal of Chronic Diseases*, **35**, 833.

Reddy, B. S., and Wynder, E. L. (1973). Large bowel carcinogenesis: Fecal constituents of populations with diverse incidence rates of colon cancer. *Journal of the National Cancer Institute*, **50**, 1437.

Registrar General (1978). *Occupational Mortality 1970–72*. Decennial Supplement. London: HMSO.

Rosenstock, I. M. (1960). What research in motivation suggests for public health. *American Journal of Public Health*, **50**, 295.

Rosenstock, I. M. (1963). Public response to cancer screening and detection programmes. Determinants of health behaviour. *Journal of Chronic Diseases*, **16**, 407.

Rothman, K. J. (1976). The estimation of synergy or antagonism. *American Journal of Epidemiology*, **103**, 506.

Rothman, K., and Keller, A. (1972). The affect of joint exposure to alcohol and tobacco on risk of cancer of the mouth and pharynx. *Journal of Chronic Disease*, **25**, 711.

Rothman, K. J., Greenland, S., and Walker, A. M. (1980). Concepts of interaction. *American Journal of Epidemiology*, **112**, 467.

Royal College of Physicians (1962). *Smoking and health*. London: Pitman, p. 41.

Saracci, R. (1980). Interaction and synergism. *American Journal of Epidemiology*, **112**, 465.

Schmidt, W., and de Lint, J. (1972). Causes of death of alcoholics. *Quarterly Journal of Studies in Alcohol*, **33**, 171.

Schottenfeld, D., Gantt, R. C., and Wynder, E. (1974). The role of alcohol and tobacco in multiple primary cancers of the upper digestive systems, larynx and lung. A progressive study. *Preventive Medicine*, **3**, 277.

Selikoff, I. J., Hammond, E. C., and Churg, J. (1968). Asbestos exposure, smoking and neoplasia. *Journal of the American Medical Association*, **204**, 106.

Selikoff, I. J., Seidman, H., and Hammond, E. C. (1980). Mortality effects of cigarette smoking among amosite asbestos factory workers. *Journal of the National Cancer Institute*, **65**, 507.

Simarak, S., de Jong, V. W., Breslow, N. *et al.* (1977). Cancer of the oral cavity, pharynx, larynx and lung in North Thailand: case-control study and analysis of cigar smoke. *British Journal of Cancer*, **36**, 130.

Stevenson, T. H. C. (1923). The social distribution of mortality from different causes in England and Wales 1910–12. *Biometrika*, **XV**, 382.

Stevenson, T. H. C. (1928). The vital statistics of wealth and poverty. *Journal of the Royal Statistical Society*, **XCI**, 207.

Sundby, P. (1967). *Alcoholism and mortality*. Publication No. 6. Oslo: National Institute for Alcohol research, p. 82.

Tabar, L., and Gad, A. (1981). Screening for breast cancer – the Swedish Trial. *Radiology*, **138**, 219.

UK Trial of Early Detection of Breast Cancer Group (1981). Trial of early detection of breast cancer: description of method. *British Journal of Cancer*, **44**, 618.

US Public Health Service (1979). *Smoking and Health. A report of the Surgeon General of the Public Health Service*. Washington, DC: US Department of Health and Human Services, Office on Smoking and Health.

US Public Health Service (1980). *Smoking and Health. The health consequences of smoking for women*. Washington, DC: US Department of Health and Human Services, Office on Smoking and Health.

US Public Health Service (1981). *The health consequences of smoking – the changing cigarette.* Washington, DC: US Department of Health and Human Services, Office on Smoking and Health.

Van Rensburg, S. J. (1981). Epidemiologic and dietary evidence for a specific nutritional predisposition of esophageal cancer. *Journal of the National Cancer Institute,* **67,** 243.

Vincent, R. G., and Marchetta, F. (1963). The relationship of the use of tobacco and alcohol to cancer of the oral cavity, pharynx or larynx. *American Journal of Surgery,* **106,** 501.

Walker, E. A., Castegnard, M., Garren, L. *et al.* (1979). Intake of volatile nitrosamines from consumption of alcohols. *Journal of the National Cancer Institute,* **63,** 947.

Weisburger, J. H. (1977). Vitamin C and prevention of nitrosamine formation, *Lancet,* **2,** 607.

Williams, R. R., and Horm, J. W. (1977). Association of cancer sites with tobacco and alcohol consumption and socioeconomic status of patients; interview study from the Third National Cancer Survey. *Journal of the National Cancer Institute,* **58,** 525.

World Health Organization (1979). *Controlling the smoking epidemic.* Report of the WHO Expert Committee on Smoking Control. Geneva: WHO, pp. 39–40, 53–66.

Wynder, E., and Bross, I. J. (1961). A study of aetiological factors in cancer of the oesophagus, *Cancer,* **14,** 389.

Wynder, E. L., and Gori, G. B. (1977). Contribution of the environment to cancer incidence: an epidemiologic exercise. *Journal of the National Cancer Institute,* **58,** 825.

Wynder, E. L., and Hoffman, O. (1979). Tobacco and health. A societal challenge. *New England Journal of Medicine,* **300,** 894.

Wynder, E. L., and Hoffman, D. (1982). Tobacco. In *Cancer epidemiology and prevention* (eds D. Schottenfeld and J. Fraumeni). Philadelphia: W. B. Saunders, pp. 287–288.

Wynder, E. L., and Klein, V. E. (1965). Possible role of riboflavin deficiency in epithelial neoplasm. I. Epithelial changes of mice in simple deficiency. *Cancer,* **18,** 167.

Wynder, E. L., and Mabuchi, K. (1973). Etiological and environmental factors in esophageal cancer. *Journal of the American Medical Association.* **226,** 1546.

Wynder, E. L., and Shigematsu, T. (1967). Environmental factors of cancer of the colon and rectum. *Cancer,* **20,** 1520.

Wynder, E. L., and Stellman, S. D. (1979). Impact of long-term filter cigarette usage on lung and larynx cancer risk: a case-control study. *Journal of the National Cancer Institute,* **62,** 471.

Wynder, E. L., Bross, I. J., and Day, E. (1956). A study of environmental factors in cancer of the larynx. *Cancer,* **9,** 86.

Wynder, E. L., Bross, I., and Feldman, R. M. (1957a). A study of etiological factors in cancer of the mouth. *Cancer,* **10,** 1300.

Wynder, E. L., Cooey, L. S., Mabuchi, K., and Mushinski, M. (1976). Environmental factors in cancer of the larynx, a second look. *Cancer,* **38,** 1591.

Wynder, E., Dodo, H., Bloch, D. *et al.* (1969). Epidemiologic investigation of multiple primary cancer of the upper alimentary and respiratory tracts. 1. A retrospective study. *Cancer,* **24,** 730.

Wynder, E. L., Hultberg, J., Jacobson, F., and Bross, I. D. J. (1957b). Environmental factors in cancer of the upper alimentary tract – a Swedish study with special reference to Plummer–Vinson (Patterson–Kelly) syndrome. *Cancer,* **19,** 470.

Wynder, E. L., Mushinski, M. I., and Spivak, J. C. (1977). Tobacco and alcohol consumption in relation to the development of multiple primary cancers. *Cancer*, 1872.

Risk Factors and Multiple Cancer
Edited by B.A. Stoll
© 1984 John Wiley and Sons Ltd.

Chapter

6 M. J. HILL and M. H. THOMPSON

Role of Endogenous Carcinogens

The literature on chemical carcinogenesis is mainly devoted to the study of chemicals present in the environment or produced during industrial processes, but it is possible that endogenous carcinogens may be equally important. These carcinogens may be divided into two main classes; (a) those which are synthesized by the body and are essential to the normal function of the human organism; (b) those which are formed coincidentally and are, therefore, not essential to the human host.

In the first group, the most prominent agents are the steroid hormones, cholesterol and bile acids. These are all essential to the host, but become important in carcinogenesis when the host is eating a diet which is 'abnormal' by historical criteria and in comparison with that eaten by the vast majority of the world population. The second group includes *N*-nitroso compounds, certain amino acid metabolites, faecal mutagens and retoxified hepatic conjugates; these are not essential to the host but may be produced in harmful amounts under certain exceptional conditions. This chapter will review the various classes of endogenous carcinogens and their possible role in human cancer.

ENDOGENOUS CARCINOGENS

Several classes of compounds produced in the human body have been shown to be tumour promoters or initiators in animals, or to be mutagenic in *in vitro* studies. Many of these are truly endogenous, but others are produced by the metabolic action of bacteria inhabiting the digestive or urogenital tract, and so might strictly be considered as exogenous. For the purposes of this review these bacterial metabolites will be treated as endogenous since they are formed as a result of the synergistic relationship between the host and his bacterial flora.

The endogenous carcinogens include steroids, nitrogen compounds, biliary conjugates, and unidentified mutagenic products of bacterial metabolism. In the group of steroid compounds, the three major classes of endogenous products thought to be implicated in carcinogenesis are the steroid hormones, bile acid metabolites and cholesterol. The first two classes are thought to be tumour promoters but cholesterol is considered by some to be carcinogenic (Hieger, 1958) or premutagenic (Kelsey and Pienta, 1979). In the group of nitrogen compounds the *N*-nitroso derivatives and ethionine are tumour initiators; tryptophan metabolites may also be tumour initiators, but tyrosine metabolites are tumour promoters.

The group of biliary conjugates includes glucuronide and glutathione conjugates of polycyclic aromatic hydrocarbon (PAH) metabolites derived from tobacco tar and air pollutants; the aglycones released are potential mutagens and likely to be tumour initiators. The unidentified mutagens found in faeces may be bacterial metabolites of unknown precursors and are direct-acting mutagens. Although much less work has been done on metabolites with antitumour activity, this is a field of growing interest. The various groups of endogenous carcinogens will be discussed in turn, followed by the antitumour agents.

Steroid hormones

Interest in the possible role of steroid hormones in human carcinogenesis was aroused by the success of endocrine therapy in the treatment of cancers of the breast, prostate, and endometrium. Endocrine ablation has also been shown to cause regression of tumours of the breast or other sites in animals and has been reviewed by Huggins (1967).

Lacassagne (1932) was the first to demonstrate the carcinogenicity of oestradiol in male mice given subcutaneous implants and subsequent reports have been reviewed by Furth (1975). The various animal models used to demonstrate the carcinogenicity of steroid oestrogens include subcutaneous implant of oestradiol in male rats to induce breast cancer (Lacassagne, 1932); subcutaneous implant of oestradiol in castrated female mice to induce endometrial cancer (Noble *et al.*, 1967); female rats treated with polycyclic aromatic hydrocarbons followed by removal of the pituitaries to demonstrate oestrogen-dependence of mammary tumours (Huggins, 1967); subcutaneous implants of oestrogens in male or gonadectomized female Syrian hamsters to induce renal tumours (Kirkman, 1957); subcutaneous injection of oestradiol in an oily vehicle in mice to induce local sarcomas (Olivi *et al.*, 1965).

Only a proportion of human breast cancers are oestrogen-dependent (see Chapter 10) but most oestrogen-dependent tumours contain oestrogen receptors (McGuire *et al.*, 1975) both in female and in male breast cancer (Everson *et al.*, 1980). Remission of human oestrogen-dependent tumours can be achieved not only by ablation therapy (adrenalectomy, hypophysectomy or oophorectomy) but also by the administration of anti-oestrogens. Steroid hormones may also be implicated in tumorigenesis at other sites. Hormonal control of prostatic cancer is indicated by tumour regression following orchiectomy or the administration of pharmacological doses of oestrogen.

Cholesterol

The apparent carcinogenicity of cholesterol was first demonstrated by Hieger (1949). In a series of experiments, cholesterol was shown to be weakly carcinogenic by the production of tumours at the site of injection of the compound suspended in an oily vehicle. This observation proved difficult to repeat, and Bischoff and Bryson carried out a series of studies (Bischoff, 1969) which suggested that the tumours were due to solid state carcinogenesis associated with the deposition at the injection site of cholesterol crystals from the supersaturated solutions employed.

Not all authorities accept this view, and Fieser (1954) for example, thought that it was inconceivable that a compound so widely distributed in the body could be carcinogenic, and postulated that a contaminant was responsible for this activity. Of the possible oxidation products, he selected 5-cholesten-3-one as the most likely candidate, since it should be highly reactive at the C-4 position. However, this compound was later shown not to be carcinogenic in rats and marsh mice.

An alternative oxidation product is cholesterol-α-epoxide which together with its hydration product cholestriol and the parent cholesterol, were tested for carcinogenicity and cocarcinogenicity in the rat colon by Reddy and his colleagues (Reddy and Watanabe, 1979) but found to be inactive. They were also shown to be inactive in the *Salmonella* mutagenesis assay, but in an alternative *in vitro* test, cholesterol-α-epoxide was shown to be able to transform hamster embryo cells (Kelsey and Pienta, 1979). Thus the question of cholesterol carcinogenicity remains unresolved.

Cruse *et al.* (1978) reported that large bowel cancer could be induced experimentally in rats by dietary supplements of cholesterol, and large bowel cancer mortality in humans has been reported to be associated with high cholesterol intake by Cruse *et al.* (1979) and by Liu *et al.* (1979), although the association reported by Drasar and Irving (1973) was only weak compared with that with other dietary components. Reddy and Watanabe (1979) could detect no carcinogenicity or tumour-promoting activity in cholesterol in their experimental model of colon cancer.

Bile acids

Interest in the bile acids as possible carcinogens was first aroused by the independent reports by Cook and Haslewood (1933) and by Wieland and

Dane (1933) that deoxycholic acid could be pyrolysed to the potent carcinogen 20-methylcholanthrene via a dehydronorcholene intermediate. Later it was shown that deoxycholic acid, when suspended in an oily vehicle and painted on the skin of mice, was carcinogenic (Cook *et al.*, 1940; Salaman and Roe. 1956). It is now known that the oily vehicle contained a carcinogen and that the deoxycholic acid was acting as a tumour promoter.

Subsequent studies have shown that deoxycholic acid is mutagenic in bacteria (Jensen *et al.*, 1951), comutagenic in the *Salmonella* mutagenesis assay (Silverman and Andrews, 1977; Wilpart *et al.*, 1983), and mutagenic in *Drosophila* (Demerec, 1948). More recently, deoxycholic acid has been shown to possess tumour-promoting activity in the *N*-methyl-*N*-nitroso-*N*-nitro-guanidine (MNNG) model of colon cancer (Narisawa *et al.*, 1974). In this model, rats are treated with intrarectal injections of MNNG (a potent locally) acting carcinogen) and then compounds to be tested for tumour-promoting activity are instilled into the rectum; at the end of the experiment the number of colon tumours is determined as a measure of the promoting effect of the test compound.

The primary bile acids, cholic acid and chenodeoxycholic acid, have no promoting activity in germ-free animals but have weak activity in conventional animals. The secondary bile acids, deoxycholic acid and lithocholic acid, are active either in germ-free or conventional animals; the activity of the primary bile acids in conventional animals is probably due to their metabolism to the secondary bile acids by the gut bacteria.

Lithocholic acid has also been shown to be cocarcinogenic in the MNNG model (Narisawa *et al.*, 1974), comutagenic in the *Salmonella* mutagenesis assay (Silverman and Andrews, 1977; Wilpart *et al.*, 1983), and mutagenic in the hamster embryo cell transformation test (Kelsey and Pienta, 1979). A number of other bile acids, including apocholic acid and bisnor-5-cholenic acid have been shown to be carcinogenic on the mouse skin (Lacassagne *et al.*, 1961, 1966).

N-nitroso compounds

The *N*-nitroso compounds are a potent group of carcinogens which have proved to be active in *all* animal species in which they have been tested. While there is no clear proof that they are active in humans, there is no good reason for suspecting that humans are uniquely resistant to their carcinogenic effects (Magee and Barnes, 1967; Olajos, 1978). They are formed by the action of nitrite on a suitable nitrogen compound; secondary amines give *N*-nitrosamines, alkylureas give *N*-nitroso ureas, and amides give *N*-nitrosamides. The reaction is acid catalysed with a pH optimum of 2 for *N*-nitrosamine formation (Mirvish, 1975), 3 to 3.5 for *N*-nitrosamides, and more acid pH values for alkyl ureas. Their formation has been demonstrated

Table 1 Formation of *N*-nitroso compounds by bacterial action

Reference	Observation
Sander (1968)	*N*-nitrosation at neutral pH values in the presence of bacteria but not in their absence
Hawksworth and Hill (1971)	Confirmed Sander (1968). Further extended the range of bacteria tested. Needed growing cultures, but reaction may be non-enzymic. Only a proportion of *E. coli* able to carry out the reaction
Collins-Thompson *et al.* (1972)	Repeated much of above. Reaction did not need growing cultures and was not destroyed by autoclaving so non-enzymic
Klubes *et al.* (1972)	Repeated much of the first two references above. Concluded that there was more than one mechanism; partly enzymic and partly non-enzymic
Brooks *et al.* (1972)	*N*-nitrosation *in vivo* by *Proteus* spp. in urine
Ishiwata *et al.* (1975)	*N*-nitrosation by bacteria in saliva
Coloe and Heywood (1976)	Wide variation in ability of *E. coli* to catalyse *N*-nitrosation in urine *in vitro*. Studied kinetics of the reaction
Kunisaki *et al.* (1976)	Studied *N*-nitrosation by *E. coli* and concluded that it was enzymic
Yang *et al.* (1977)	Studied *N*-nitrosation by bacteria and concluded that it was non-enzymic
Tannenbaum *et al.* (1978)	Demonstrated *N*-nitrosation by bacteria in saliva and that live organisms were necessary
Ruddell *et al.* (1978)	Demonstrated *N*-nitrosation by bacteria in gastric juice
Kunisaki and Hayashi (1979)	Studied *N*-nitrosation by resting cells of *E. coli* B and concluded that it was enzymic

by an acid catalysed reaction in the normal acid stomach (Fine *et al.*, 1977).

Sander (1968) showed that the *N*-nitrosation reaction could be catalysed by bacteria at neutral pH values, and so *N*-nitroso compounds could potentially be formed wherever bacteria, nitrite and a suitable nitrosatable amino compound were present together in the body; this observation has been confirmed since by many groups (Table 1). Studies of the pharmacology of nitrate (Hill, 1979; Bartholomew *et al.*, 1979), showed that dietary nitrate is excreted mainly in the urine, but is also secreted in saliva, sweat, tears, gastric

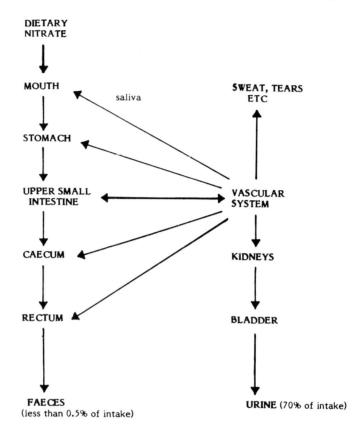

Figure 1   The metabolism and route of excretion of dietary nitrate.

juice and probably also in colonic and vaginal secretions (Figure 1). The formation of *N*-nitroso compounds has been demonstrated or claimed in saliva, normal gastric juice, the achlorhydric stomach, the infected urinary bladder, the colon, and the infected vagina (Table 2).

Although *N*-nitroso ureas and *N*-nitrosamides are proximate carcinogens and act at the site to which they are exposed, the *N*-nitrosamines require activation and so tend to act at distant sites. These depend on the nature of the parent secondary amines and on the animal species used, but not in general on the route of administration (Table 3). Thus, it is impossible to deduce the likely site of action of an *N*-nitrosamine in humans from its site of action in rodents; it is equally impossible to rule out any site as a possible target on the basis of the animal data. Although a great deal of information is available on the carcinogenicity of volatile *N*-nitrosamines, there have been

Table 2 Sites of the body where the *in vivo* formation of *N*-nitroso compounds has been demonstrated

Site	Special conditions	Reference
Saliva	*In vitro*	Tannenbaum *et al.* (1978) Ishiwata *et al.* (1975)
Stomach	Normal Achlorhydric	Fine *et al.* (1977) Ruddell *et al.* (1978)
Urinary bladder	Bacterially infected In association with bilharzia	Brooks *et al.* (1972) Hicks *et al.* (1977) Radomski *et al.* (1978) Hicks *et al.* (1977)
Colon	Normal In ureterosigmoidostomy	Wang *et al.* (1978)
Cervix	Women with *Trichomonas vaginalis* infection	Allsobrook *et al.* (1975)

Table 3 The target of various *N*-nitrosamines in different animal species (Magee and Barnes, 1967)

N-nitrosamine	Animal species	Target organ
Dimethylnitrosamine	Rat Hamster	Kidney Liver
Diethylnitrosamine	Mouse Rat	Liver Liver
Dibutylnitrosamine	Mouse Rat	Urinary bladder Urinary bladder
n-Butylethylnitrosamine	Mouse Rat	Forestomach Oesophagus
N-Nitrosopiperidine	Rat Hamster	Oesophagus Lung
N-Nitrosomopholine	Rat Hamster	Liver Lung
N-Nitrosopiperazine	Mouse Rat	Lung Oesophagus
N-Nitrososarcosine ethylester	Rat	Forestomach

few studies of the non-volatile analogues (e.g. *N*-nitroso peptides) as they are much more difficult to assay.

Metabolites of tryptophan

Dunning *et al.* (1950) showed that while rats fed 2-acetylaminofluorene (AAF) do not develop bladder tumours, a high incidence of such tumours was induced in rats fed AAF together with tryptophan or indole. This was confirmed and extended by Boyland *et al.* (1954) who showed that tryptophan could be replaced by indole or by indole acetic acid but that the AAF could not be replaced by compounds known to be carcinogenic in the human bladder such as benzidine or 2-naphthylamine.

On the basis of the initial studies it was concluded that tryptophan and its metabolites were acting as tumour promoters since AAF is a known carcinogen. However, Dyer and Morris (1961) showed that AAF was causing a disturbance of tryptophan metabolism; from this, and since AAF does not

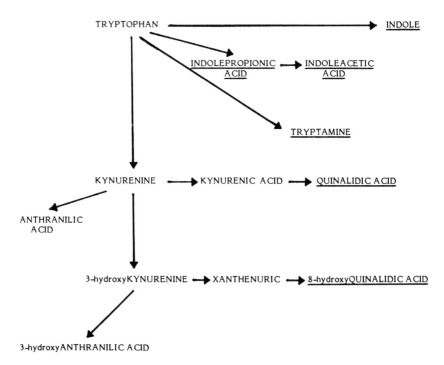

Figure 2   The pathways of tryptophan metabolism. Metabolites underlined are only produced by bacterial action.

cause bladder tumours, it was concluded that the tryptophan metabolites were acting as carcinogens and that AAF was merely causing a favourable disturbance of tryptophan metabolism.

This led to other tests of carcinogenicity being applied to tryptophan metabolites. Figure 2 illustrates the pathways of tryptophan metabolism and Table 4 summarizes the positive results of carcinogenicity tests on tryptophan metabolites. The subject has been extensively reviewed by Bryan (1971). The metabolite pathways illustrated in Figure 2 are carried out in the liver and the intermediates are excreted in urine. The same pathways have been illustrated in bacteria and so it is possible that the same metabolites may be produced by the bacteria in the gut and excreted in the urine. The tryptophan metabolites are not mutagenic in the *Salmonella* mutagenesis assay (Bowden *et al.*, 1976).

Another group of tryptophan metabolites which may be of interest is the skatole group. They are produced in large amounts in the colon, and methods for their analysis have been reported. However, their mutagenicity and possible role as carcinogens has not yet been assessed.

Tyrosine metabolites

Tyrosine is metabolized in the body to a range of phenolic acids and finally to the volatile phenolic compounds phenol, *p*-cresol, and 4-ethylphenol. These are absorbed from the colon, conjugated as glucuronides or sulphates, and excreted in the urine. In normal healthy persons 50–100 mg of volatile phenols are excreted in urine per day, more than 80% of which is *p*-cresol and most of the remainder is phenol (Table 5). Only small amounts of 4-ethyl phenol are normally present in urine.

The amount of urinary volatile phenol (UVP) depends on the amount of dietary protein and on the intestinal transit time (Cummings *et al.*, 1979), but

Table 4   Evidence that metabolites of tryptophan are carcinogenic, mutagenic or cocarcinogenic

Test system	Metabolites which gave positive reactions
2-Acetylaminofluorene-treated rats	Tryptophan, indole, indoleacetic acid
Bladder implantation test (Allen *et al.*, 1957)	3-Hydroxykynurenine, 3-hydroxyanthranilic acid, 8-hydroxyquinaldic acid, xanthenuric acid, kynurenine, quinaldic acid
Cultured mammalian cell mutagenesis (Kuznezova, 1969)	3-Hydroxykynurenine, 3-hydroxyanthranilic acid

can be reduced to very low amounts by any procedure which decreases the opportunity for bacterial metabolism, or which decreases the number of bacteria (such as antibiotics, colonic wash-out, an elemental diet or total colectomy). Apparently the production of UVP takes place in the right colon, since resection of the bowel to remove a tumour of the sigmoid colon or rectum does not have a profound effect on the amount of UVP excretion.

Boutwell and Bosch (1959) showed that both phenol and *p*-cresol acted as tumour promoters when applied to the skin of mice treated with 7,12-dimethylbenzanthracene as tumour initiator. The tumour-promoting activity of phenols was later confirmed by Wynder and Hoffmann (1968) and by Boutwell (1967).

Ethionine

Ethionine, the *S*-ethyl analogue of methionine, is produced by a range of bacterial species (including *Escherichia coli*) when grown in a mineral salts medium supplemented with glucose, methionine, and sulphate. The ethionine was not incorporated into bacterial protein but was formed as the free amino acid in the culture supernate (Fisher and Mallette, 1961).

Table 5   The daily excretion of urinary volatile phenols in normal healthy humans and in persons undergoing various surgical or medical treatments

Subject group	Urinary volatile phenols (mg/day)			
	Phenol	*p*-Cresol	Total	C/P*
Normal healthy Britons living in London	11.3	56.8	68.1	5.0
Danes living in Copenhagen	11.9	82.0	93.9	6.9
Danes living in Them	17.1	46.3	63.4	2.7
Finns living in Helsinki	17.3	53.6	70.9	3.1
Finns living in Perrikala	10.5	57.9	68.4	5.5
Patients with small bowel colonization	46.5	93.7	140.2	2.0
Patients with total colectomy	5.0	1.2	6.2	0.2
Patients with left hemi-colectomy	4.8	56.7	61.5	12.0
Patients given pre-operative bowel preparation	2.4	19.2	21.6	8.0
Normal healthy Britons consuming 140 g protein/day			108.1	
60 g protein/day			74.1	

*C/P = ratio of *p*-cresol to phenol.

The carcinogenicity of ethionine was reviewed by Farber (1963) and its mode of action has been the subject of much research. Ethionine competes with methionine in the production of S-adenosyl analogues; S-adenosyl-ethionine accumulates while the important general methylating agent S-adenosyl methionine is depleted. There are also effects on RNA synthesis; the activity of RNA polymerase is decreased and the level of ATP is severely depleted in the presence of ethionine, both of these effects being reversed by treatment with exogenous adenine. Ethionine interferes with the maturation of r-RNA by inhibiting its methylation and also induces changes in the level of methylation of t-RNA and of DNA. These are all undoubtedly important in the toxicity of ethionine but its mechanism of carcinogenicity is still unclear.

Hydrolysis of conjugated carcinogens

Polycyclic aromatic hydrocarbons (PAHs) present in the environment and ingested or inhaled are detoxified in the liver, usually via hydroxylation followed by conjugation as the sulphate, glucuronide or glutathione derivative. They are subsequently secreted in the bile.

A wide range of bacterial species produces β-glucuronidase and this is important in the enterohepatic circulation of PAHs (Smith, 1966). The hydroxylated PAHs released are not carcinogenic or mutagenic, but may be further activated to direct acting carcinogens or mutagens by the cellular enzymes of the colonic mucosa. Furthermore, under certain conditions an active intermediate is formed during the hydrolysis which is able to bind to DNA (Kinoshita and Gelboin, 1978) and so may be important in carcinogenesis. Renwick and Drasar (1976) demonstrated that while a high proportion of gut bacterial strains could hydrolyse glucuronide conjugates of PAHs, certain strains of human faecal organisms (principally *Clostridia*) could dehydroxylate the hydroxylated PAHs and so regenerate the parent carcinogen.

Faecal mutagens

Bruce and his colleagues first reported the presence of a mutagen in ether extracts of faeces from male volunteers eating a Western diet (Bruce *et al.*, 1977). The mutagen was detected using the *Salmonella* mutagenesis assay. Its activity was high when the subject ate a diet rich in beef and was low when a high fibre diet was eaten. Initial studies indicated that it was an N-nitroso compound (Bruce *et al.*, 1979), and a number of volatile N-nitroso compounds were detected in faeces (Wang *et al.*, 1978). Later, this postulate was withdrawn and the mutagen has now been identified as the glycerol ether of dodeca-(1,3,5,7,9)-pentenyl-l-ol (Hirai *et al.*, 1983).

The observation of the faecal mutagen has been confirmed by many groups (reviewed by Venitt, 1982) but the relevance of the observation to human carcinogenesis has still to be assessed. Most of the studies have involved single assays on single stool samples; it is essential to carry out dose–response assays in order to confirm the presence of mutagen.

Endogenously formed tumour inhibitors

A great deal of attention has been devoted to the identification of exogenous inhibitors of carcinogenesis (such as vitamins A, C, and E and the polyphenolic compounds from cruciferous vegetables) but little attention has been given to the production of such compounds endogenously. However, a number of studies on lignans have shown anti-cancer properties.

Lignans are normally present in higher plants, in man, and in several animals. The principal lignans found in humans, enterolactone and enterodiol, are formed from dietary precursors by the bacterial flora of the intestinal tract (Adlercreutz *et al.*, 1981). The amounts are correlated with the amount of dietary fibre (Adlercreutz *et al.*, 1982) particularly that from grain, nuts, and legumes. The biological function of lignans is unknown but they have been shown to have anti-cancer properties (McDaniel and Cole, 1972; Hartwell, 1976; Barclay and Perdue, 1976).

ENDOGENOUS CARCINOGENS IN HUMAN CANCER

Endogenous carcinogens have been implicated in the causation of cancers at a wide range of sites, principally the digestive tract, urogenital tract, and the breast. The quality of the evidence varies considerably between sites. In many cases the sites are those which may be especially affected by a Western lifestyle.

Colorectal cancer

Colorectal cancer is one of the diseases of Western civilization, being common in North America, north-west Europe, and Australasia and relatively rare in rural populations in Africa, Asia, and the Andean countries of South and Central America. Within Europe it is more common in the north and west than in the south and east, and the same is true of the British Isles. It is more common in urban than in rural areas, and in many countries its incidence is correlated with socio-economic class. The epidemiology of colorectal cancer has been reviewed recently by Correa (1978) and by Jensen (1980).

Studies of migrants between and within countries, and of religious groups within countries indicate that the incidence of colorectal cancer in a population is determined by environmental rather than by genetic factors (see Chapter 8). Also, the cultural or 'personal' environment (e.g.diet, smoking

Table 6   Dietary factors associated with large bowel cancer

Dietary item	Association	Type of study	Reference
Meat	Causal	Populations	Armstrong and Doll, 1975
		Case-control	Haenszel *et al.*, 1973
Animal protein	Causal	Populations	Armstrong and Doll, 1975
		Populations	Gregor *et al.*, 1969
		Populations	Drasar and Irving, 1973
Fat	Causal	Populations	Gregor *et al.*, 1969
		Populations	Drasar and Irving, 1973
		Populations	Armstrong and Doll, 1975
		Case-control	Wynder and Shigematsu, 1967
		Case-control	Pernu, 1960
		Case-control	Dales *et al.*, 1978
		Case-control	Phillips, 1975
Fibre	Protective	Case-control	Modan *et al.*, 1975
		Case-control	Dales *et al.*, 1978
		Populations	IARC Working Party, 1977
	Causal	Case-control	Haenszel *et al.*, 1973
		Populations	Hill *et al.*, 1979
Beer	Causal	Populations	Enstrom, 1977
		Populations	IARC Working Party, 1977
Milk	Protective	Populations	IARC Working Party, 1977
Vitamins A and C	Protective	Case-control	Bjelke, 1974
Ammonia	Causal		

or the use of other drugs, personal hygiene habits) may be much more important than the physical or 'shared' environment (e.g. climate, geographical location, air pollution). It is generally agreed that diet is an important aetiological agent but there is disagreement regarding the particular type of diet most strongly associated with the disease (Table 6). Since searches for dietary or other exogenous carcinogens correlated with the risk of developing colorectal cancer have not been notably successful, Aries *et al.* (1969) have postulated that the carcinogens or tumour promoters responsible for the high incidence of the disease were produced *in situ* in the colon from benign substrates, the concentrations of which were determined by the diet.

A wide range of possible substrates has been examined (Table 7) based on the assumption that the substrates were provided by dietary meat. Other postulated dietary factors might moderate the rate of production (e.g. dietary fibre) or the rate of action (e.g. vitamin C) of the carcinogens, rather than

Table 7   Range of possible substrates for bacterial production of carcinogens in the human colon

Dietary component	Item	Product
Protein	Methionine	Ethionine
	Basic amino acids (lysine, arginine, ornithine)	Cyclic secondary amines giving N-nitrosamines
	Phenolic amino acids (tyrosine, phenylalanine)	Volatile phenols (p-cresol, phenol)
	Tryptophan	Range of metabolites with tumour-promoting properties
	All amino acids	Ammonia
Fat	Lecithin	Dimethylamine, giving dimethylnitrosamine
	Bile acids	Tumour-promoting metabolites
	Cholesterol	Metabolized to tumour initiator

provide substrates for their production. The evidence for the relative importance of the various substrates has been reviewed elsewhere (Hill, 1977, 1981) and strongly supports a role for bile acids (Hill, 1980). This evidence (Table 8) comes from studies of populations, case-control studies, studies of patient groups at high risk of developing large bowel cancer and from studies of animal models.

Large bowel carcinogenesis is a multistage process and a hypothesis of the mechanism of carcinogenesis based on the histopathological adenoma–carcinoma sequence suggested by Morson (1974), has been proposed (Hill *et al.*, 1978). On this hypothesis, adenomas are caused by environmental factors E1 (Figure 3) acting on previously normal mucosal tissue. These adenomas remain small unless exposed to further environmental factors (E2) which cause adenomas to grow. Further factors (C) cause increasingly severe epithelial dysplasia and ultimately neoplasia, in adenomatous tissue.

The rate of increase in severity of dysplasia appears to depend on the amount of adenomatous tissue, a high proportion of large adenomas having foci of malignancy compared with only a small proportion of small adenomas. Recent attempts to define the role of bile acid metabolites in colorectal carcinogenesis indicate that they probably have no role in the initial formation of adenomas but may be important in determining the rate of adenoma

Table 8   The evidence that bile acids are important in colorectal carcinogenesis

Type of study	Conclusion
Metabolic ward studies	FBA concentration is related to the amount of dietary fat
Carcinogenesis studies	Bile acids are tumour promoters in the rat colon and are comutagenic in microbial mutagenesis assays
Animal models of human colorectal cancer	Dietary manipulations which alter the FBA concentration have a parallel effect on the number of colorectal tumours
Comparison of populations in various parts of the world	The mean FBA concentration in a population is correlated with the incidence of colorectal cancer
Comparison of populations within a country	The mean FBA concentration in a population is correlated with the incidence of colorectal cancer
Case-comparison studies	The FBA concentration in patients with colorectal cancer (especially early cancer and in the left colon) is higher than in patients with non-malignant bowel disease
Studies of patients at high risk	The FBA concentration is correlated with adenoma size (which is correlated with risk of malignancy) and with the severity of epithelial dysplasia in chronic ulcerative colitis (which is related to the risk of malignancy)

growth and perhaps also in the development of increasing epithelial dysplasia (Hill, 1981; 1982).

Faecal mutagens have also been implicated in the causation of colorectal cancer, but the evidence is difficult to assess. The temporal variation in mutagen activity in faeces from a person is much greater than the variation in activity between persons. Consequently, studies of populations which show a correlation between faecal mutagen activity and colorectal cancer incidence (Ehrich *et al.*, 1979; Reddy *et al.*, 1980) are inconclusive, as also are studies which show no correlation (Correa *et al.*, 1981).

Metabolites produced by the hydrolysis of conjugates of polycyclic aromatic hydrocarbons have been implicated by Renwick and Drasar (1976). These metabolites are likely to be released in the caecum and so might be the cause of cancer of the right colon, but it is difficult to rationalize their involvement in cancer of the sigmoid colon or rectum. *N*-nitroso compounds have been implicated by others, but attempts by experienced workers to detect volatile *N*-nitrosamines in faeces have failed (Archer *et al.*, 1981).

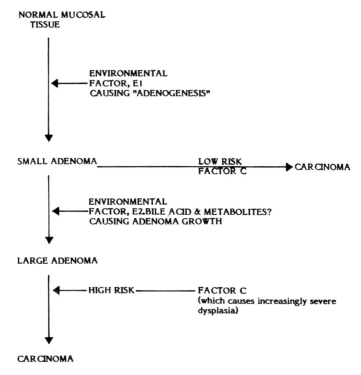

Figure 3   The postulated mechanism of the adenoma–carcinoma sequence in colorectal carcinogenesis. (Based on Hill *et al.*, 1978.)

Breast cancer

The incidence of cancer of the breast in a population is highly correlated with
the incidence of colorectal cancer (Drasar and Irving, 1973; Hill, 1975) and
like colorectal cancer, the disease incidence is correlated with the intake of
dietary fat (Drasar and Irving, 1973; Armstrong and Doll, 1975; DeWaard,
1975; Carroll, 1981). The epidemiology of the disease has been reviewed by
McMahon *et al.* (1973), DeWaard (1979), Carroll (1981) and DeWaard *et al.*
(1981); their observations are summarized in Table 9.

   The aetiology of breast cancer in premenopausal women differs from that
in postmenopausal women in that the latter appears to be more strongly
related to diet. There is no evidence that the link between postmenopausal
breast cancer and diet is due to ingested carcinogens, and a currently popular
hypothesis is that postmenopausal oestrogen-dependent cancers are stimulated by the effect of diet on the endogenous production of carcinogens
together with an effect on tissue susceptibility to carcinogens (Figure 4).

Table 9   The epidemiology of cancer of the breast

Geographic distribution	Common in N. America, Europe, and Australasia Rare in Africa, Asia, and South America
Migrant studies	Children of migrants have an incidence similar to that of their new homeland
Variation of incidence with age	Possibly two types; postmenopausal is related to diet, premenopausal is not
Relation to diet	Correlated with dietary fat
Relation to hormone status	Correlated with early menarche and late menopause Inversely related to age at first pregnancy and to parity
Relation to other cancer sites	Geographically correlated with cancers of the colon, endometrium, and ovary Related in multiple primaries to cancers of the colon and endometrium

Oestrogen production is known to be related to obesity and to total body fat (Lipsett, 1975); both of these are correlated with breast carcinogenesis and both are correlated with dietary fat and total energy intake.

All breast cancers are believed to contain oestrogen receptors but the density of receptors is much higher in oestrogen-dependent tumours (Jensen,

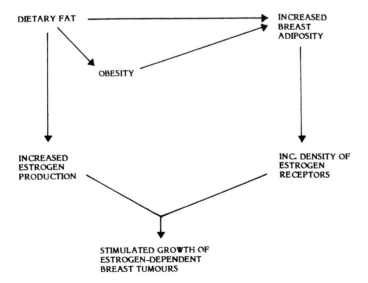

Figure 4   A postulated mechanism for the relation between diet and cancer of the breast.

1975); the density of oestrogen receptors is related to breast adiposity, which is itself related to diet. Thus, diet is related to oestrogen-receptor density; it is also related to circulating oestrogen levels and rates of oestrogen synthesis and thereby is related to the rate of growth of oestrogen-dependent breast tumours.

Goldgraber *et al.* (1958) noted that women who had had a colectomy for ulcerative colitis were at decreased risk of breast cancer. The close epidemiological correlation between breast and colorectal cancer (Carroll, 1981), and the observation that gut bacteria were capable of producing oestrogen analogues from faecal steroids both *in vitro* and *in vivo* in the rat and guinea pig (Goddard and Hill, 1972, 1974), led to the suggestion that the gut bacteria might be involved in breast carcinogenesis as an alternative source of oestrogen analogues (Hill *et al.*, 1971). In support of this hypothesis, Murray *et al.* (1980) showed that the organisms potentially capable of producing these metabolites were carried by a higher proportion of breast cancer cases compared with controls. Papatestas *et al.* (1982) showed that the faecal concentration of bile acids and neutral steroids (cholesterol, coprostanol and coprostanone) was much higher in breast cancer cases than in controls.

Endometrial cancer

Cancer of the endometrium shows a strong geographical association with cancer of the large bowel and cancer of the breast. In addition, patients who have had an endometrial carcinoma resected are at above average risk of developing breast or colorectal cancer. The epidemiology of endometrial cancer has been reviewed by McMahon (1974), Wynder *et al.* (1966) and by Elwood *et al.* (1977) who showed its relation to obesity, dietary fat, early menarche, late menopause, hypertension, and previous cancer of the breast or ovary.

This evidence indicates a possible causative role for oestrogens in endometrial cancer and this is supported by the observation that oestrogen replacement therapy is associated with an increased risk of endometrial cancer (Mack *et al.*, 1976; Antunes *et al.*, 1979). The endometrium contains oestrogen and progesterone receptor sites (Siiteri *et al.*, 1974) and the use of oral contraceptive agents is associated with an increased risk of endometrial cancer in some studies (Silverberg and Makowski, 1975).

Armstrong (1977) has produced a unified hypothesis, based on the thesis that endometrial cancer is caused by exposure to excessive oestrogen levels, especially of oestrone. He suggested that excess dietary fat causes excess oestrogen production, and also caused obesity, early menarche, late menopause, and hypertension; the correlation of these latter factors with endometrial carcinogenesis would then be secondary to the association with dietary fat.

Ovarian cancer

The aetiology of cancer of the ovary has been reviewed by Lingeman (1974) and various risk factors discussed by Berg and Lamp (1981). The mean age at diagnosis is close to that at menopause; ovarian cancer is not associated with obesity, early menarche or late menopause but is associated with low parity. Although there are many histological types of ovarian cancer, epithelial carcinomas account for more than 90% of the cases in white Americans (Berg and Lamp, 1981). Ovarian cancer is associated with breast cancer both geographically and in studies of second primaries; ovarian cancer is followed by breast cancer 4.4 times as often as expected, and breast cancer follows ovarian cancer twice as often as expected (Schottenfeld and Berg, 1971).

In another study of second primary neoplasms following ovarian cancer (Reimer *et al.*, 1978), there was an increased risk of cancer of the endometrium, breast, and colon. This indicates a possible role for steroid hormones, and this conclusion is supported by the observation that women treated with oestrogens as hormone replacement therapy are at increased risk of ovarian cancer (Hoover *et al.*, 1977). However, a role for steroid hormones in the causation of ovarian cancer has not been clearly established.

Prostatic cancer

The epidemiology of cancer of the prostate was reviewed by Wynder *et al.* (1971) and by Franks (1973). The disease is highly correlated with dietary fat (Armstrong and Doll, 1975), and with the incidence of cancer of the colon (Hill, 1975). Prostatic cancer may respond to orchiectomy and to pharmacological doses of oestrogen and suggests a possible role for steroid hormones as tumour promoters in prostatic carcinogenesis.

It has been hypothesized that a sexually transmitted agent might also be implicated in the causation of this cancer; the oncogenic virus theory is based on the observed relationship between the risk of prostatic cancer and sexual activity, and on the observed association between prostatic cancer and cervical cancer in marriage partners. A study of Catholic priests in which the incidence of prostatic cancer was higher than expected from the general male population does not support this hypothesis (Ross *et al.*, 1981).

Gastric cancer

Gastric cancer is very common in East Asia, the Andean countries of South America, Eastern Europe, Finland and Iceland and is much less common in Western Europe, Australasia, and North America. Throughout the world the incidence is falling; in England gastric cancer was the commonest cancer in 1930–40 but is now only the fourth commonest. Within the British Isles the disease is most common in Scotland and Ireland and is least common in south-east and eastern England.

The histopathological classification of gastric cancer described by Lauren (1965) may be useful in studying the aetiology of the disease. Lauren classified gastric cancers as intestinal, diffuse or mixed and later studies (Correa *et al.*, 1970; Munoz and Asvall, 1971) indicated that while the incidence of the diffuse type was similar in all countries, the differences in incidence of the disease between countries or between regions were due to differences in the incidence of the intestinal type of disease. The intestinal type could then be thought of as the 'epidemic type' while the diffuse type was more associated with familial or genetic factors. This has been discussed in reviews (Correa, 1982; Day, 1981).

The intestinal type of the disease is associated with a number of precursor lesions and Correa *et al.* (1975) postulated a histopathological sequence in which the first step was gastric atrophy, followed by atrophic gastritis, then intestinal metaplasia with increasing degrees of dysplasia and finally neoplasia (Figure 5). Gastric atrophy is accompanied by decreased acid secretion and eventually achlorhydria, and this has two results. The absence of gastric acid

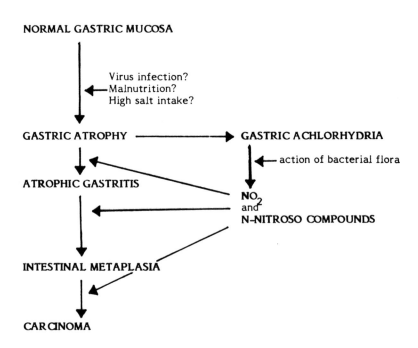

Figure 5   A postulated mechanism of gastric carcinogenesis. (Based on Correa *et al.*, 1975.)

permits the establishment of a resident bacterial flora (Drasar *et al.*, 1969) and under these conditions nitrate is reduced to nitrite and *N*-nitroso compounds are formed (Ruddell *et al.*, 1976). In addition gastric achlorhydria is accompanied by bile reflux (DuPlessis, 1965; Capper *et al.*, 1966; Rhodes *et al.*, 1969).

Both pernicious anaemia and Polya partial gastrectomy are accompanied by gastric achlorhydria and carry an increased risk of gastric cancer. It has been hypothesized that *N*-nitroso compounds formed endogenously in the achlorhydric stomach are responsible for the high incidence of gastric cancer in pernicious anaemia (Ruddell *et al.*, 1978) or after Polya partial gastrectomy (Schlag *et al.*, 1980).

A role for refluxed bile acids has also been suggested (Lowenfels, 1978). The bile salts present in bile are conjugated and relatively non-toxic, but the bacterial flora of the achlorhydric stomach is capable of releasing free bile acids from their conjugates (Domello *et al.*, 1980); the free bile acids, and particularly deoxycholic acid can cause mucosal damage (Shiner, 1970). Lowenfels (1978) has suggested that the released free bile acids might cause gastritis in the atrophic mucosa (one of the early steps in gastric carcinogenesis) and may also act as tumour promoters in the final stages of the disease.

Biliary tract and gallbladder cancer

The epidemiology of cancer of the gallbladder and biliary tract has been reviewed by Fraumeni (1975). The major risk factor is gallstones (which are present in the gallbladder of 80–90% of females and 60% of males with gallbladder cancer) and consequent bacterial infection of the bile. Approximately 70% of all patients with gallstones have bacterial infections of the bile and anaerobic bacteria (usually *Clostridium perfringens* or *Bacteroides fragilis*) can be isolated from a high proportion of these (England and Rosenblatt, 1977; Shimada *et al.*, 1977).

Since the organisms most commonly isolated (*E. coli*, enterococci, *Klebsiella* spp., and the anaerobes already cited) are rich in β-glucuronidase, it is possible that they are able to hydrolyse the conjugates of polycyclic aromatic hydrocarbons (PAH) secreted in the bile; the anaerobes are also able to deconjugate and further degrade bile acids. Lowenfels (1978) has suggested that bile acid metabolites are important in the causation of cancer of the gallbladder and biliary tree, but it is not known whether the gallstones and biliary infections are secondary to the carcinoma or vice versa.

Welton *et al.* (1979) have carried out a prospective study of patients known to be typhoid carriers (and who would, therefore, have *Salmonella typhi* colonization of the biliary tract) and the long-term typhoid carriers were found to have a greatly increased risk of cancer of the biliary tract. *Salmonella typhi* does not metabolize bile salts but produces β-glucuronidase; if the relationship between biliary infection and biliary tract cancer is causal, it is more likely to be due to hydrolysis of PAH conjugates than to bile salt metabolism.

Cancer of the urinary bladder

Many chemicals encountered in the dye industry have been associated with bladder cancer but it is likely that the vast majority of bladder cancers are not caused by industrial exposures. Many lines of evidence had linked the causation of these non-industrial bladder cancers to tryptophan metabolites. The experiments of Dunning *et al.* (1950) on the effect of dietary tryptophan on bladder carcinogenesis in AAF-treated rats have been described earlier in the chapter. Several groups of workers (Boyland and Williams, 1956; Benassi *et al.*, 1963) have demonstrated elevated amounts of tryptophan metabolites in the urine of bladder cancer patients compared with controls. In addition, patients with non-industrial bladder cancer, to whom loading doses of tryptophan were given, showed abnormal metabolism of tryptophan.

The hypothesis has been reviewed by Bryan (1971), but recently doubt has been cast on the causality of the relationship. Teulings *et al.* (1978) noted that high levels of tryptophan metabolites were present in the urine of 36% of bladder cancer patients but also in 67% of renal cancer patients. In bladder cancer the elevated concentrations of tryptophan metabolites were associated with tumours which obstructed the outflow of urine from the kidneys. Patients with untreated bladder cancers and elevated levels of tryptophan metabolites had lower levels after treatment of the tumour. They concluded that the high levels of tryptophan metabolites were the result of the presence of the tumour rather than the cause of it.

The urine is the major route of excretion of nitrate and also of nitrosatable amino compounds, and in urinary tract infection there is, therefore, the possibility of N-nitroso compound formation; this has been demonstrated by Radomski *et al.* (1978), Hicks *et al.* (1977), and Brooks *et al.* (1972) in humans and by Hawksworth and Hill (1974) in animals. It has been suggested that N-nitroso compounds formed by bacteria might be responsible for the high incidence of bladder cancer associated with bilharzial infection; infection of the bladder with mixed populations of bacteria are common secondary to bilharzial infection and these have been shown to produce N-nitroso compounds in large quantities (Hicks *et al.*, 1977).

CONCLUSION

It is possible to construct hypotheses implicating endogenously produced carcinogens in the causation of cancer at a number of sites in the body. The strongest evidence implicates bile acids as aetological agents in colorectal cancer and steroid hormones in the causation of cancers of the breast and endometrium. There is also evidence that steroid hormones may be associated with cancers of prostate, ovary and colon. (In addition, cancers of the breast and prostate have a therapeutic association with steroid hormones.)

N-nitroso compounds have been implicated in gastric carcinogenesis and also in the bladder cancer associated with bilharzia. If these associations can be confirmed, the risk of these cancers may be reduced by prophylactic treatment of patients at risk with effective scavengers of nitrite (ascorbic acid is the most widely cited agent on the basis of its *in vitro* activity). Similarly, confirmation of the association between biliary tract infection and gallbladder cancer would suggest that chronic typhoid carriers be treated more energetically.

While there are many ways in which cancers due to endogenously produced carcinogens might be involved in human carcinogenesis, so far it has not been clearly demonstrated that any of the mechanisms are of substantial importance.

REFERENCES

Adlercreutz, H., Fotsis, T., and Heikkinen, R. *et al.* (1981). Diet and urinary excretion of lignans in female subjects. *Medical Biology,* **59,** 259–261.

Adlercreutz, H., Heikkinen, R., Woods, M. *et al.* (1982). Excretion of the lignans enterolactone and enterodiol and of equol in omnivorous and vegetarian post menopausal women and in women with breast cancer. *Lancet,* **2,** 1295–1298.

Allen, M. J., Boyland, E., Dukes, C. E. *et al.* (1957). Cancer of the urinary bladder induced in mice with metabolites of aromatic amines and tryptophan. *British Journal of Cancer,* **2,** 212.

Allsobrook, A. J. R., Du Plessis, L S., Harington, J. S. *et al.* (1975). In *N-nitroso compounds in the environment* (eds P. Bogovski and E. A. Walker). Lyon: IARC, pp. 197–199.

Antunes, C. M. F., Strolley, P. D., Rosenstein, N. D. *et al.* (1979). Endometrial cancer and estrogen use. Report of a large case-control study. *New England Journal of Medicine,* **300,** 9–13.

Archer, M. C., Saul, R. L., Lee, L. J., and Bruce, W. R. (1981). Analyses of nitrate, nitrite and nitrosamines in human feces. In *Gastrointestinal cancer: endogenous factors* (eds W. R. Bruce *et al.*). New York: Cold Spring Harbor Press, pp. 321–330.

Aries, V. C., Crowther, J. S., Drasar, B. S. *et al.* (1969). Bacteria and the etiology of cancer of the large bowel. *Gut,* **10,** 334–335.

Armstrong, B. (1977). The role of diet in human carcinogenesis with special reference to endometrial cancer. In *Origins of human cancer* (eds H. Hiatt, J. Watson, and J. Winsten). New York: Cold Spring Harbor Lab. pp. 557–566.

Armstrong, B. and Doll, R. (1975). Environmental factors and the incidence and mortality from cancer in different countries with special reference to dietary practice. *International Journal of Cancer,* **15,** 617–631.

Barclay, A. S., and Perdue, R. E. (1976). Distribution of anti cancer activity in higher plants. *Cancer Treatment Reports,* **60,** 1081–1113.

Bartholomew, B., Butt, A., Caygill, C. *et al.* (1979). The origin of urinary nitrates. *Proceedings of the Nutrition Society,* **38,** 124.

Benassi, C. A., Perissonotto, B., and Allegri, G. (1963). The metabolism of tryptophan in patients with bladder cancer and other urological disorders. *Clinical Chimica Acta*, **8**, 822–831.

Berg, J. W., and Lamp, J. G. (1981). High risk factors in gynaecological cancer. *Cancer*, **48**, 429–441.

Bischoff, F. (1969). Carcinogenic effects of steroids. *Advances in Steroid Research*, **7**, 165–244.

Bjelke, E. (1974). Epidemiological studies of cancer of the stomach, colon and rectum. *Scandinavian Journal of Gastrology*, **9** (Suppl. 31), 1.

Boutwell, R. K. (1967). In *Phenolic compounds and metabolic regulation* (ed J. B. Finkle and V. C. Runeckles). New York: Appleton-Century-Crofts.

Boutwell, R. K., and Bosch, D. K. (1959). The tumour-promoting action of phenol and related compounds on the mouse skin. *Cancer Research*, **19**, 413–427.

Bowden, J. P., Chung, K. T., and Andrews, A. W. (1976). Mutagenic activity of tryptophan metabolites produced by rat intestinal microflora. *Journal of the National Cancer Institute*, **57**, 921–924.

Boyland, E., Harris, J., and Horning, E. S. (1954). Induction of carcinoma of the bladder in rats with acetamidofluorene. *British Journal of Cancer*, **8**, 647.

Boyland, E., and Williams, D. C. (1956). The metabolism of tryptophan in patients suffering from cancer of the bladder. *Biochemical Journal*, **64**, 578–582.

Brooks, J. B., Cherry, W. B., Thacker, L., and Alley, C. C. (1972). Analysis by gas chromatography of amines and nitrosamines produced *in vivo* and *in vitro* by *Proteus mirabilis*. *Journal of Infectious Diseases*, **126**, 143–153.

Bruce, W. R., Varghese, A. J., Furrer, R., and Land, P. C. (1977). In *Origins of human cancer* (eds H. Haiatt, J. Watson, and J. Winsten). New York: Cold Spring Harbor Lab., pp. 1641–1646.

Bruce, W. R., Varghese, A. J., Wang, S., and Dion, P. (1979). The endogenous production of nitroso compounds in the colon and cancer at that site. In *Naturally occurring carcinogens/mutagens and modulators of carcinogenesis* (eds E. C. Miller *et al.*). Tokyo: Japan Scientific Societies Press, pp. 221–228.

Bryan, G. T. (1971). The role of urinary tryptophan metabolites in the etiology of bladder cancer. *American Journal of Clinical Nutrition*, **24**, 841–847.

Capper, W. M., Airth, G. R., and Kirby, T. O. (1966). A test of pyloric regurgitation. *Lancet*, **2**, 621–623.

Carroll, K. K. (1981). Influence of diet on mammary cancer. *Nutrition and Cancer*, **2**, 232–236.

Collins-Thompson, D. L., Senn, P., Aris, B., and Schwinghamer, L. (1972). Non-enzymic *in vitro* formation of nitrosamines by bacteria isolated from meat products. *Canadian Journal of Microbiology*, **18**, 1968–1971.

Coloe, P. J., and Heywood, N. J. (1976). The importance of prolonged incubation for the synthesis of dimethyl nitrosamine by enterobacteria. *Journal of Medical Microbiology*, **9**, 211–224.

Cook, J. W., and Haslewood, G. A. D. (1933). Conversion of a bile acid into a hydrocarbon derived from 1,2 benzanthracene. *Chemistry and Industry*, **ii**, 758–759.

Cook, J. W., Kennaway, E. L., and Kennaway, N. B. (1940). Production of tumours in mice by deoxycholic acid. *Nature*, **145**, 627.

Correa, P. (1978). Epidemiology of polyps and cancer. In *The pathogenesis of colorectal cancer*. (ed B. C. Morson) London: Saunders. pp. 126–152.

Correa, P. (1982). Epidemiology of gastric cancer and its precursor lesions. In *Gastrointestinal cancer* (eds J. De Coss and P. Sherlock). Amsterdam: Martinus Nijhoff, pp. 119–130.

Correa, P., Cuello, C., and Duque, E. (1970). Carcinoma and intestinal metaplasia of the stomach in Colombian migrants. *Journal of the National Cancer Institute*, **44**, 297–306.

Correa, P., Haenszel, W., Cuello, C. *et al.* (1975). A model for gastric cancer epidemiology. *Lancet*, **2**, 58–60.

Correa, P., Paschal, J., Pizzolato, P. *et al.* (1981). In *Gastrointestinal cancer: endogenous factors* (eds W. R. Bruce, P. Correa, M. Lipkin, S. Tannenbaum, and T. Wilkins). New York: Cold Spring Harbor Lab. Press, pp. 119–128.

Cruse, P., Lewin, M. and Clark, C. G. (1979). Dietary cholesterol is cocarcinogenic for human colon cancer. *Lancet*, **1**, 752–755.

Cruse, P., Lewin, M., Ferulano, G., and Clark, C. G. (1978). Cocarcinogenic effects of dietary cholesterol in experimental colon cancer. *Nature*, **276**, 822–824.

Cummings, J. H., Hill, M. J., Bone, E. S. *et al.* (1979). The effect of meat protein with and without dietary fibre on colonic function and metabolism II. Bacterial metabolites in faeces and urine. *American Journal of Clinical Nutrition*, **32**, 2094–2101.

Dales, L. G., Friedman, G. D., Ury, H. K. *et al.* (1978). A case-control study of relationships of diet and other traits to colorectal cancer in American blacks. *American Journal of Epidemiology*, **109**, 132–144.

Day, D. (1981). Histopathology of gastric cancer. In *Gastric cancer* (eds J. Fielding, C. Newman, C. Ford, and B. Jones). Oxford: Pergamon Press, pp. 95–110.

Demerec, M. (1948). Mutations induced by carcinogens. *British Journal of Cancer*, **2**, 114–117.

DeWaard (1975). Breast cancer incidence and nutritional status with particular reference to body weight and height. *Cancer Research*, **35**, 3351–3356.

DeWaard, F. (1979). Premenopausal and postmenopausal breast cancer: one disease or two? *Journal of the National Cancer Institute*, **63**, 549–552.

DeWaard, F., Poortman, J., and Collette, B. (1981). Relationship of weight to the promotion of breast cancer after menopause. *Nutrition and Cancer*, **2**, 237–240.

Doll, R. (1969). The geographical distribution of cancer. *British Journal of Cancer*, **23**, 1–8.

Domello, F. L., Reddy, B. S., and Weisburger, J. H. (1980). Microflora and deconjugation of bile acids in alkaline reflux after partial gastrectomy. *American Journal of Surgery*, **140**, 291–295.

Drasar, B. S., and Irving, D. (1973). Environmental factors and cancer of the colon and breast. *British Journal of Cancer*, **27**, 167–172.

Drasar, B. S., Shiner, M., and McLeod, G. M. (1969). The bacterial flora of the gastrointestinal tract in healthy and achlorhydric persons. *Gastroenterology*, **56**, 71–77.

Dunning, W. F., Curtis, M. R., and Maun, M. E. (1950). The effect of added dietary tryptophan on the occurrence of 2-acetylaminofluorene-induced liver and bladder cancer in rats. *Cancer Research*, **10**, 454.

DuPlessis, D. J. (1965). Pathogenesis of gastric ulceration. *Lancet*, **1**, 974–978.

Dyer, N. H., and Morris, H. P. (1961). An effect of N-2-fluorenylacetamide on the metabolism of tryptophan in rats. *Journal of the National Cancer Institute*, **26**, 315.

Ehrich, M., Aswell, J. E., Van Tassell, R. L. *et al.* (1979). Mutagens in the faeces of 3 South African populations at different levels of risk for colon cancer. *Mutation Research*, **64**, 231–240.

Elwood, J. M., Cole, P., Rothman, K. J., and Kaplan, S. D. (1977). The epidemiology of endometrial cancer. *Journal of the National Cancer Institute*, **59**, 1055–1060.

England, D. M., and Rosenblatt, J. E. (1977). Anaerobes in human biliary tracts. *Journal of Clinical Microbiology*, **6**, 494–570.

Enstrom, J. E. (1977). Colorectal cancer and beer drinking. *British Journal of Cancer*, **35**, 674–683.

Everson, R. B., Lippman, M. E., Thompson, E. B. *et al.* (1980). Clinical correlations of steroid receptors and male breast cancer. *Cancer Research*, **40**, 991–997.

Farber, E. (1963). Ethionine carcinogenesis. *Advances in Cancer Research*, **7**, 383.

Farber, E., McConomy, J., Franzen, B. *et al.* (1967). Interaction between ethionine and rat liver RNA and protein *in vivo*. *Cancer Research*, **27**, 1761–1772.

Fieser, L. F. (1954). Some aspects of the chemistry and biochemistry of cholesterol. *Science*, **119**, 710–716.

Fine, D. H., Ross, R., Rounbehler, D. P. *et al.* (1977). Formation *in vivo* of volatile *N*-nitrosamines in man after ingestion of cooked bacon and spinach. *Nature*, **265**, 753–755.

Fisher, J. F., and Mallette, M. F. (1961). The natural occurrence of ethionine in bacteria. *Journal of General Physiology*, **45**, 1–13.

Franks, L. M. (1973). Etiology, epidemiology and pathology of prostatic cancer. *Cancer*, **32**, 1092–1095.

Fraumeni, J. F. (1975). Cancers of the pancreas and biliary tract; epidemiological considereations. *Cancer Research*, **35**, 3437–3446.

Furth, J. (1975). Hormones as etiological agents in neoplasia. In *Cancer. A comprehensive treatise*. Volume I (ed F. Becker). New York: Plenum Press, pp. 75–120.

Goddard, P., and Hill, M. J. (1972). Degradation of steroids by intestinal bacteria. IV. the aromatisation of ring A. *Biochimica Biophysica Acta*, **280**, 336–342.

Goddard, P., and Hill, M. J. (1974). The *in vivo* metabolism of cholesterol by gut bacteria in the rat and guinea pig. *Journal of Steroid Biochemistry*, **5**, 569–572.

Goldgraber, M. B., Humphreys, E. M., Kirsner, J. B., and Palmer, W. L. (1958). Carcinoma and ulcerative colitis, a clinical-pathologic study. II Statistical analysis. *Gastroenterology* **34**, 840–846.

Gregor, O., Toman, R., and Pruscova, F. (1969). Gastrointestinal cancer and nutrition. *Gut*, **10**, 1031–1034.

Haenszel, W., Berg, J. W., Segi, M. *et al.* (1973). Large bowel cancer in Hawaiian Japanese. *Journal of the National Cancer Institute*, **51**, 1765–1779.

Hartwell, J. L. (1976). Types of anticancer agents isolated from plants. *Cancer Treatment Reports*, **60**, 1031–1067.

Hawksworth, G. M., and Hill, M. J. (1971). Bacteria and N-nitrosation of secondary amines. *British Journal of Cancer*, **25**, 520–526.

Hawksworth, G. M., and Hill, M. J. (1974). The *in vivo* formation of N-nitrosamines in the rat bladder and their subsequent absorption. *British Journal of Cancer*, **29**, 353–358.

Hicks, R. M., Walters, C. L., Elsebai, I. *et al.* (1977). Demonstration of nitrosamines in human urine: Preliminary observations on a possible etiology for bladder cancer in association with chronic urinary tract infections. *Proceedings of the Royal Society of Medicine*, **70**, 413–416.

Hieger, I. (1949). Carcinogenic activity of lipoid substances. *British Journal of Cancer*, **3**, 123.

Hieger, I. (1958). Cholesterol carcinogenesis. *British Medical Bulletin*, **14**, 159–160.

Hill, M. J. (1975). The etiology of colon cancer. *Critical Reviews in Toxicology*, **4**, 31–82.

Hill, M. J. (1977). Bacterial factors. *Topics in Gastroenterology*, **5**, 45–64.

Hill, M. J. (1979). *In vivo* bacterial N-nitrosation and its possible role in human cancer. In *Naturally occurring carcinogens-mutagens and modulators of carcinogenesis* (eds E. C. Miller, I. Hirono, T. Sugimura, and S. Takayama). Tokyo: Japan Scientific Societies Press, pp. 229–240.

Hill, M. J. (1980). The aetiology of colorectal cancer. In *Recent advances in gastrointestinal pathology* (ed. R. Wright). London: Saunders, pp. 297–310.

Hill, M. J. (1981). Metabolic epidemiology of large bowel cancer. In *Gastrointestinal cancer* (eds J. DeCosse and P. Sherlock). The Hague: Martinus Nijhoff, pp. 187–226.

Hill, M. J. (1982). Genetic and environmental factors in human colorectal cancer. In *Colon carcinogenesis* (eds R. Malt and R. Williamson). Lancaster: MTP, pp. 73–81.

Hill, M. J., Goddard, P., and Williams, R. E. O. (1971). Gut bacteria and etiology of cancer of the breast. *Lancet*, **2**, 472–473.

Hill, M. J., Maclennan, R., and Newcombe, J. (1979). Diet and large bowel cancer in three socioeconomic groups in Hong Kong. *Lancet*, **1**, 436.

Hill, M. J., Morson, B. C., and Bussey, H. J. R. (1978). Etiology of adenoma–carcinoma sequence in large bowel. *Lancet*, **1**, 245–247.

Hirai, N., Kingston, D. G., Van Tassell, R. L., and Wilkins, T. D. (1983). Structure elucidation of a potent mutagen from human feces. *Journal of the American Chemical Society*, **104**, 6149–6150.

Hoover, R., Gray, L. A., and Fraumeni, J. F. (1977). Stilbestrol (diethylstilbestrol) and the risk of ovarian cancer. *Lancet*, **2**, 533–534.

Huggins, C. (1967). Endocrine-induced regression of cancers. *Science*, **156**, 1050–1054.

IARC Working Party (1977). Dietary fibre, transit time, faecal bacteria, steroids and colon cancer in two Scandinavian populations. *Lancet*, **2**, 207–211.

Ishiwata, H., Boriboon, P., Nakamura, Y. *et al.* (1975). Studies on *in vivo* formation of nitroso compounds. *Journal of the Food and Hygiene Society (Japan)*, **16**, 234–239.

Jensen, E. V. (1975). Estrogen-receptors in hormone-dependent breast cancer. *Cancer Research*, **35**, 3362–3364.

Jensen, K. A., Kirk, I., Kilmarg, G., and Westergaard, M. (1951). Chemically induced mutations in neurospora. Cold Spring Harbor Symposium on Quantitative Biology, **16**, 245–261.

Jensen, O. M. (1980). Epidemiology of colorectal cancer. In *Colorectal cancer* (ed. K. Welvaart, L. Blumgart, and J. Kreuning). The Hague: Leiden University Press, pp. 3–14.

Kelsey, M. I., and Pienta, R. J. (1979). Transformation of hamster embryo cells by cholesterol-α-epoxide and lithocholic acid. *Cancer Letters*, **6**, 143–149.

Kinoshita, N., and Gelboin, H. (1978). β-glucuronidase catalysed hydrolysis of benzo-[a]-pyrene-3-glucuronide and binding to DNA. *Science*, **199**, 307–309.

Kirkman, H. (1957). Steroid tumorigenesis. *Cancer*, **10**, 757–764.

Klubes, P., Cerna, I., Rabinowitz, A. E. *et al.* (1972). Factors affecting the dimethylnitrosamine formation from simple precursors by rat intestinal bacteria. *Food and Cosmetic Toxicology*, **10**, 757–767.

Kunisaki, N., and Hayashi, M. (1979). Formation of *N*-nitrosamines from secondary amines and nitrite by resting cells of *Eschericia coli* B. *Applied Environmental Microbiology*, **37**, 279–282.

Kunisaki, N., Matsuura, H., and Hayashi, M. (1976). Formation of *N*-nitrosodimethylamine by *Eschericia coli*. *Journal of the Food and Hygiene Society (Japan)*, **17**, 314–319.

Kuznezova, L. E. (1969). Mutagenic effect of 3 hydroxykynurenine and 3 hydroxyanthranilic acid. *Nature (London)*, **222**, 454–485.

Lacassagne, A. (1932). Apparition de cancers de la mamelle chez la souris male, soumise a des injections de folliculine. Induced mammary cancers in male mice using purified estrogens. *Comptes Rendues,* **195,** 630.

Lacassagne, A., Buu-Hoi, N. P., and Zajdela, F. (1961). Carcinogenic activity of apocholic acid. *Nature,* **190,** 1007–1008.

Lacassagne, A., Buu-Hoi, N. P., and Zajdela, F. (1966). Carcinogenic activity *in situ* of further steroid compounds. *Nature,* **209,** 1026–1027.

Lauren, P. (1965). The two histological main types of gastric carcinoma: diffuse and so-called intestinal type. *Acta Pathologica et Microbiologica Scandinavica,* **64,** 31–49.

Lingeman, C. H. (1974). Etiology of cancer of the human ovary: A review. *Journal of the National Cancer Institute,* **53,** 1603–1618.

Lipsett, M. B. (1975). Hormones, nutrition and cancer. *Cancer Research,* **35,** 3559–3361.

Liu, K., Moss, M., Persky, V. *et al.* (1979). Dietary cholesterol, fat and fibre and colon-cancer mortality. *Lancet,* **2,** 782–785.

Lowenfels, A. (1978). Does bile promote extra-colonic cancer? *Lancet,* **2,** 239–241.

McDaniel, P. B., and Cole, J. R. (1972). Antitumour activity of *Bursera schlectendalii:* isolation and structure determination of two new lignans. *Journal of Pharmaceutical Science,* **61,** 1992–1994.

McGuire, W. L., Carbone, P. P., and Vollmer, E. P. (eds) (1975). *Estrogen receptors in human breast cancer.* New York: Raven Press.

Mack, T. M., Pike, M. C., Henderson, B. E. *et al.* (1976). Estrogens and endometrial cancer in a retirement community. *New England Journal of Medicine,* **293,** 1262–1267.

McMahon, B. (1974). Risk factors for endometrial cancer. *Gynecologic Oncology,* **2,** 122–129.

McMahon, B., Cole, P., and Brown, J. (1973). Etiology of human breast cancer: a review. *Journal of the National Cancer Institute,* **50,** 21–42.

Magee, P. N., and Barnes, J. M. (1967). Carcinogenic N-nitroso compounds. *Advances in Cancer Research,* **10,** 163–246.

Mirvish, S. S. (1975). Formation of *N*-nitroso compounds: chemistry, kinetics and *in vivo* occurrence. *Toxicology and Applied Pharmacology,* **31,** 325–351.

Modan, B., Barell, V., Lubin, F. *et al.* (1975). Low-fiber intake as an etiologic factor in cancer of the colon. *Journal of the National Cancer Institute,* **55,** 15–18.

Morson, B. C. (1974). The polyp-cancer sequence in the large bowel. *Proceedings of the Royal Society of Medicine,* **67,** 451–457.

Munoz, N., and Asvall, J. (1971). Time trends of intestinal and diffuse types of gastric cancer in Norway. *International Journal of Cancer,* **8,** 144–157.

Murray, W. R., Blackwood, A., Calman, K. C., and Mackay, C. (1980). Fecal bile acids and clostridia in patients with breast cancer. *British Journal of Cancer,* **42,** 856–860.

Narisawa, T., Magadia, N., Weisburger, J., and Wynder, E. L. (1974). Promoting effect of bile acids on colon carcinogenesis after intrarectal instillation of *N*-methyl-*N*-nitro-*N*-nitroso-guanidine in rats. *Journal of the National Cancer Institute,* **53,** 1093–1097.

Noble, R. L., Beer, C. T., and McIntyre, R. W. (1967). Biological effects of dihydrovinblastine. *Cancer,* **20,** 885.

Olajos, E. J. (1978). Comparative toxicology of N-nitroso compounds and their carcinogenic potential to man. *Exotoxicology and Environmental Safety,* **2,** 317–367.

Olivi, M., Barbieri, G., and Paoletti, I. (1965). Ripetibilita di un esperimento: ala incidenza di sarcomi sottocutanei nei topi del C57BL-Cb/Se substrain sottoposti a iniezioni oleose di benzoato de estradiolo. *Lavon 1st Anal. Univ. Perugia,* **25,** 97.

Papatestas, A. E., Panvelliwalla, D., Tarttar, P. I. *et al.* (1982). Fecal steroid metabolites and breast cancer risk. *Cancer,* **49,** 1201–1205.

Pernu, J. (1960). An epidemiological study on cancer of the digestive organs and respiratory system. *Annales Medicinae Internae Fenniae,* **49,** 1–117.

Phillips, R. L. (1975). Role of life style and dietary habits in risk of cancer among 7th Day Adventists. *Cancer Research,* **35,** 3513–3522.

Radomski, J. L., Greenwald, D., Hearn, W. L. *et al.* (1978). Nitrosamine formation in bladder infections and its role in the etiology of bladder cancer. *Journal of Urology,* **120,** 48–50.

Reddy, B. S., Sharma, C., Darby L. *et al.* (1980). Metabolic epidemiology of large bowel cancer. Fecal mutagens in high and low risk populations for colon cancer. *Mutation Research,* **72,** 511–522.

Reddy, B. S., and Watanabe, K. (1979). Effect of cholesterol metabolites and promoting effect of lithocholic acid in germ free and conventional F344 rats. *Cancer Research,* **39,** 1521–1524.

Reimer, R. R., Hoover, R., Fraumeni, J. F., and Young, R. C. (1978). Second primary neoplasm following ovarian cancer. *Journal of the National Cancer Institute,* **61,** 1195–1197.

Renwick, A. G., and Drasar, B. S. (1976). Environmental carcinogens and large bowel cancer. *Nature,* **263,** 234–235.

Rhodes, J., Baruardo, D., Phillips, S. *et al.* (1969). Increased reflux of bile into the stomach in patients with gastric ulcer. *Gastroenterology,* **57,** 241–252.

Ross, R. K., Deapen, D. M., Casagrande, J. T. *et al.* (1981). A cohort study of mortality from cancer of the prostate in Catholic Priests. *British Journal of Cancer,* **43,** 233–235.

Ruddell, W. S., Blendis, L. M., and Walters, C. L. (1976). Nitrite and thiocyanate in gastric juice. *Gut,* **17,** 401.

Ruddell, W. S. J., Bone, E. S., Hill, M. J., and Walters, C. L. (1978). Pathogenesis of gastric cancer in pernicious anemia. *Lancet,* **1,** 521–523.

Salaman, M. H., and Roe, F. J. C. (1956). Further tests for tumour-initiating activity: *N,N*-di-(2-chloroethyl)-*p*-aminophenylbutyric acid (CB 1348) as initiator of skin tumour formation in the mouse. *British Journal of Cancer,* **10,** 363–379.

Sander, J. (1968). Nitrosaminsynthese durch Bakterien. *Hoppe Seyler's Zeitschrift für Physiologische Chemie,* **349,** 429–432.

Schlag, P., Bockler, R., Ulrich, H. *et al.* (1980). Are nitrite and *N*-nitroso compounds in the gastric juice risk factors for carcinoma of the operated stomach? *Lancet,* **1,** 727–729.

Schottenfeld, D., and Berg, J. (1971). Incidence of multiple primary cancers IV. Cancers of the female breast and genital organs. *Journal of the National Cancer Institute,* **46,** 161–170.

Shimada, K., Inamatsu, T., and Uamashiro, M. (1977). Anaerobic bacteria in biliary disease in elderly persons. *Journal of Infectious Diseases,* **135,** 850–854.

Shiner, M. (1970). In *Bile salt metabolism* (eds L. Schiff, J. B. Carey, and J. M. Dietschy). Thomas, Springfield, p. 41.

Silverberg, S. G., and Makowski, E. L. (1975). Endometrial carcinoma in young women taking oral contraceptive agents. *Obstetrics and Gynecology,* **46,** 503–506.

Silverman, S. J., and Andrews, A. W. (1977). Bile acids: Co-mutagenic activity in the Salmonella-mammalian-microsome mutagenicity test. *Journal of the National Cancer Institute,* **59,** 1557–1559.

Siiteri, P. K., Schwarz, B. E., and MacDonald, P. G. (1974). Estrogen receptors and estrone hypothesis in relation to endometrial and breast cancer. *Gynecologic Oncology,* **2,** 228–238.

Smith, R. L. (1966). The biliary secretion and enterohepatic circulation of drugs and other organic compounds. *Progress in Drug Research*, **9**, 300–360.

Tannenbaum, S. R., Archer, M. C., Wisbok, J. S., and Bisop, W. W. (1978). Nitrosamine formation in human saliva. *Journal of the National Cancer Institute*, **60**, 251–253.

Teulings, F., Peters, H., Hop, W. *et al.* (1978). A new aspect of the urinary excretion of tryptophan metabolites in patients with cancer of the bladder. *International Journal of Cancer*, **21**, 140–146.

Venitt, S. (1982). Faecal mutagens in the aetiology of colonic cancer. In *Colonic carcinogenesis* (eds R. Malt and R. Williamson). Lancaster: MTP Press, pp. 59–72.

Wang, T., Kakizoe, T., Dion, P. *et al.* (1978). Volatile nitrosamines in normal human faeces. *Nature*, **276**, 280–282.

Welton, J. C., Marr, J. S., and Fiedman, S. M. (1979). An association between hepatobiliary cancer and the typhoid carrier state. *Lancet*, **1**, 791–794.

Wieland, H., and Dane, E. (1933). The constitution of bile acids III the place of attachment of the side chain. *Hoppe Seyler's Zeitschrift für Physiologische Chemie*, **219**, 240–244.

Wilpart, M., Mainguet, P., Maskens, A., and Roberfroid, M. (1983). Mutagenicity of 1,2-dimethylhydrazine towards *Salmonella typhimurium*, co-mutagenic effect of secondary bile acids. *Carcinogenesis*, **4**, 45–48.

Wynder, E. L., and Hoffmann, D. (1968). Experimental tobacco carcinogenesis. *Science*, **162**, 862–871.

Wynder, E. L., and Shigematsu, T. (1967). Environmental factors of cancer of the colon and rectum. *Cancer*, **20**, 1520–1561.

Wynder, E. L., Mabuchi, K., and Whitmore, W. F. (1971). Epidemiology of cancer of the prostate. *Cancer*, **28**, 344–360.

Wynder, E. L., Scher, G. C., and Mantel, N. (1966). An epidemiological investigation of cancer of the endometrium. *Cancer*, **19**, 489–520.

Yang, H. S., Okun, J. D., and Archer, M. C. (1977). Non-enzymatic microbial acceleration of nitrosamine formation. *Journal of Agriculture and Food Chemistry*, **25**, 1181–1183.

Part 2

Markers of cancer risk

Risk Factors and Multiple Cancer
Edited by B.A. Stoll
© 1984 John Wiley and Sons Ltd.

Chapter

7   W. H. BUTLER and H. ELIZABETH DRIVER

Clinical Significance of Preneoplasia

INTRODUCTION

Preneoplasia, the changes which occur before the emergence of overt neoplasia, includes prebenign as well as premalignant conditions. Consideration of preneoplastic conditions (either clinical or experimental) is made difficult by the lack of a precise definition of the term, and in this chapter we consider clinical preneoplasia to encompass two distinct, yet overlapping conditions – predisposing diseases and premalignant lesions.

Predisposing diseases are considered here to be those in which there is an increased risk of the patient developing a malignant neoplasm, although the underlying defect, if identified, may not bear any obvious relation to the site of the eventual neoplasm. There may be no morphologically recognizable preneoplastic lesion, or the malignant neoplasm may arise at a site remote from any other specific lesion. In contrast, in the diseases classed here as premalignant, there is a morphologically recognizable lesion present at the site of later development of a malignant neoplasm.

The premalignant lesion is not necessarily an obligate antecedent for malignant neoplasia. Its significance lies in the fact that it indicates an increased risk of developing malignant neoplasia, which is much more likely to supervene at that site than in adjacent morphologically normal tissue. It is, however, likely that malignant neoplasms at many sites arise *de novo* in morphologically normal tissue without any premalignant phase having been recognized.

The importance of recognizing potentially predisposing or premalignant conditions is obvious in the early detection and treatment of cancer, and the use of such terms is justifiable for pragmatic reasons in clinical practice. However, when one considers experimental models of carcinogenesis, designation of a lesion as preneoplastic is useful only if a mechanistic significance can be accorded to the lesion in the stages of development of neoplasia.

PREDISPOSING CONDITIONS

Predisposing diseases encompass a diverse group of conditions in which there is an increased chance of the patient developing a malignant neoplasm, although the neoplasm does not always arise in a morphologically identifiable premalignant lesion. Probably the best examples of predisposing diseases are the chromosome 'instability' syndromes such as xeroderma pigmentosum, ataxia telangiectasia, Fanconi's anaemia, and Bloom's syndrome. These are discussed also in Chapter 9.

In most cases of xeroderma pigmentosum the cells are unable to carry out excision repair of ultraviolet-damaged DNA, so that light-induced skin cancer develops by the age of 20 years. The defect may, however, not be complete, and ranges from 50% in some individuals to 90% in others (Cleaver and Bootsma, 1975). A small number of cases are defective in post-replication DNA repair, so it could be argued that although there is no morphologically recognizable lesion in xeroderma pigmentosum, there are various genetic defects which could be regarded as premalignant (Gianelli and Pawsey, 1976).

Ataxia telangiectasia (AT) is another autosomal recessive condition and is characterized by progressive cerebellar ataxia, dilated blood vessels in the eye, and immune deficiencies. Patients with AT are excessively sensitive to X-rays and their levels of radiation-induced and spontaneously occurring chromosomal aberrations are abnormally high. Repair defects after chemical damage are also a feature of AT, so patients would be expected to have an increased sensitivity to environmental carcinogens.

In Fanconi's anaemia there are various skeletal and connective tissue disorders as well as haematological abnormalities which eventually lead to the patient's death. As in ataxia telangiectasia, cells from affected individuals show more spontaneous chromosome aberrations than do normal ones, and it appears that there is a defect in the repair of cross-links. Patients with Fanconi's anaemia commonly develop myelomonocytic leukaemias (Bloom *et al.*, 1966) and also squamous cell carcinomas (Kennedy and Hart, 1982), particularly of the anogenital and oral mucosae but also of the vulva, cervix, skin, and oesophagus. There is also a relatively high incidence of hepatocellular neoplasms among patients with Fanconi's anaemia. Of a series of 300 cases, 9 developed hepatocellular neoplasms, 7 acute leukaemia and 5 some other neoplasm (Obeid *et al.*, 1980).

Peutz–Jegher's syndrome is associated with an increased risk of malignant neoplasms other than those arising in colonic polyps. An increased incidence of tumours of the skin, ovary, uterus, and breast has been found, and sometimes multiple tumours may occur, in particular, bilateral breast carcinoma (Trau *et al.*, 1982). It is likely that an underlying disorder comparable to the chromosome instability syndromes predisposes to the development of malignant neoplasia at sites other than the colon. Peutz–Jegher's syndrome can, therefore, be regarded as a predisposing disease and also as a premalignant one with respect to the colon.

Down's syndrome is also associated with an increase in the incidence of various leukaemias and myeloproliferative disorders. These are not preceded by a morphologically recognizable premalignant lesion, although there is of course an underlying genetic defect. How the increase in neoplastic change is mediated is not known.

In diabetes, there is a biochemically recognizable lesion. Diabetic females (though not males) carry a twofold risk of developing carcinoma of the pancreas (MacMahon, 1982), so it could be argued that diabetes is a predisposing disease in females, but not in males.

Tuberous sclerosis (epiloia) is a familial condition inherited as an autosomal dominant in which hamartomatous connective tissue malformations occur in the dermis, kidneys, lungs, and heart. A relatively high proportion of cases develop renal sarcoma, particularly liposarcoma, but papillary adenomas are also seen (Inglis, 1954). In addition, tumours of the retinal glial cells (phakomas) may be seen.

A similar autosomal dominant condition, which is perhaps more properly regarded as a premalignant disease, is Von Recklinghausen's neurofibromatosis. The neurofibromata in the peripheral nerves, particularly in the limbs, may occasionally undergo sarcomatous change, but the most commonly occurring neoplasms are of the central nervous system (Kramer, 1971). In a review of 48 cases of Von Recklinghausen's disease who also had acoustic neurinomas and multiple meningiomas, 45% had associated gliomas, mostly in the cerebrum (Rodriguez and Berthrong, 1966). Ependymomas are frequently seen in the spinal cord (see Chapter 16).

It appears that diseases which can predispose to the development of neoplasia may range from a minor genetic defect to a complex syndrome of morphologically recognizable lesions.

PREMALIGNANT CONDITIONS

If one defines premalignant conditions as those in which a discrete lesion is recognizable prior to the development of a malignant neoplasm at that site, then a range of morphologically diverse pathological conditions is encompassed. Hyperplasia, metaplasia, dysplasia, and benign neoplasia are the generally accepted precursors of malignancy, but atrophy, inflammation, and sometimes the processes of repair and regeneration also, may be premalignant.

It should be stressed that it is not merely the presence of the morphological lesion itself which predisposes to the development of malignancy, but the site at which it occurs and the existence of other predisposing factors. For example, hyperplasia of the mucous glands of the bronchi is diagnostic of chronic bronchitis but is almost never premalignant. On the other hand, hyperplasia in the ducts of the breast (epitheliosis) may be regarded as the first event in the sequence of changes leading to breast carcinoma (Wellings *et al.*, 1975) and is considered by some authors to represent the most common premalignant condition in the human breast (Jensen *et al.*, 1976). It seems probable that in order to undergo malignant transformation, a dysplastic change must have occurred, rather than a purely hyperplastic one, although epitheliosis is certainly the antecedent lesion. In mice, hyperplastic alveolar nodules appear to precede the development of mammary tumours (DeOme *et al.*, 1959).

Oesophageal carcinoma

Carcinoma of the oesophagus can be preceded by three quite distinct morphological and aetiological premalignant states. First is the Plummer–Vinson syndrome, in which there is an iron-deficiency anaemia associated with atrophy of the oesophageal mucosa and, in such cases, carcinoma of the upper part of the oesophagus may develop. Second is Barrett's oesophagus (ulceration of the oesophageal mucosa, usually associated with stricture or hiatus hernia) and this is associated with adenocarcinoma of the lower part of the oesophagus.

The third premalignant condition is the chronic inflammation of the oesophagus found very commonly in populations in which the incidence of carcinoma of the oesophagus is high, such as in the Transkei, Japan, China, and Iran. In these populations the oesophagitis is generally found in the middle and lower oesophagus, but it is rarely seen in the precardial mucosa (Rasmussen, 1976). On the other hand, in patients with gastric reflux, a condition common throughout the world, the resultant oesophagitis is usually confined to the precardial region and these people do not have an increased risk of developing oesophageal squamous carcinoma, although they may rarely develop adenocarcinoma. Therefore, one cannot describe oesophagitis as a premalignant disease without any further qualification: the site of the lesion, the population referred to, and the existence of other social and dietary factors must also be defined.

Oesophageal carcinoma has been extensively studied in north-western China (Yang, 1980), where it is known to have been endemic for at least 2000 years and where a temple has been built to the 'Throat-God'. An epidemiological survey in north-west China begun in 1959 encompassed 181 counties with a total population of approximately 50 million centred around Linxian. Deaths due to carcinoma of the oesophagus totalled around 20% of the total deaths in this province. A study of 858 resected carcinomas showed 58.3% to be located in the middle third of the oesophagus, 38.9% in the lower third, and only 2.8% in the upper third. Of the total number 90.6% were squamous cell carcinomas.

Mass cytological surveys of different geographical areas disclosed a close correlation between the incidence of oesophageal dysplasia and that of oesophageal carcinoma, the average age of patients with severe dysplasia being seven to eight years younger than that of cancer patients. A series of 105 patients with mild dysplasia were followed up over eight years: 15.2% progressed to severe dysplasia, 40% remained unchanged, and 44.8% returned to normal. Of 79 patients with severe dysplasia, 26.6% progressed to carcinoma.

Despite considerable research on oesophageal carcinoma and its precursor lesions, the aetiology of the disease is still uncertain, as are the factors which influence progression of the premalignant lesions to carcinoma. The primary causative agents may be nitrosamines, either derived directly from food or synthesized in the gastrointestinal tract by the action of micro-organisms on secondary amines and nitrites. However, the only evidence for this is experimental, in that certain nitrosamines are known oesophageal carcinogens. Nutritional deficiencies, particularly of vitamins A and C may contribute, but there is no increased risk of oesophageal carcinoma in other poorly nourished countries such as India.

Other likely causative factors in China and other high-risk areas of the world are the mycotoxins, some of which have been demonstrated to be carcinogens in experimental systems. Mouldy corn meal and pickles fed to rats (Yang, 1980) induced epithelial hyperplasia and dysplasia of the oesophagus, as well as tumours of the stomach and other organs. However, the experiments in China did not demonstrate an increase in carcinoma of the oesophagus, probably as a result of the experimental design. A synergistic effect between the moulds found in corn meal and pickles, and nitrosamines present in these and other foods, is suggested by the Chinese feeding experiments.

A dramatic increase in the number of deaths from oesophageal cancer has recently been reported in black males in Washington DC (Pattern *et al.*, 1981). The major aetiological factor in this population appears to be alcohol, which was estimated to be causally associated with around 80% of the cases. Cigarette smoking also appears to increase the risk of developing carcinoma of the oesophagus.

It is clear that oesophagitis is an important premalignant lesion preceding squamous carcinoma of the oesophagus, but it seems to apply only in some populations and the factors influencing the progression of the premalignant lesion to cancer seem to vary from one high risk region to another. Additional experimental evidence implying that oesophagitis is a premalignant condition is that primates dosed with methyl nitrosourea (MNU) at subcarcinogenic doses over relatively short periods have developed oesophagitis. However, the production of an inflammatory lesion by MNU may be quite separate from its carcinogenic action (Correa, 1982).

Gastric carcinoma

Atrophy is another pathological change where the site of the lesion is important in determining predisposition to malignancy. Many organs undergo atrophy as a normal effect of ageing, as seen in the genitalia of the postmenopausal woman. Atrophy of the testis occurs in a variety of conditions, including avitaminosis, senility, hypothyroidism and disorders of the pituitary and hypothalamus. Muscle undergoes atrophy if it is not used for a long period or if the motor nerve supply is interrupted. However, these changes do not themselves increase the incidence of malignant neoplasia, and atrophy cannot be generally regarded as a premalignant change.

In contrast, atrophy of the gastric mucosa (chronic atrophic gastritis) is a well-recognized precursor of gastric carcinoma. There are several types of chronic gastritis but not all of them are preneoplastic. Autoimmune chronic gastritis, which occurs in patients with pernicious anaemia, causes damage to the parietal cells and, therefore, results in a diffuse distribution of the lesion in the corpus and fundus, leaving the antrum intact. This type of gastritis is frequently accompanied by atrophy and intestinal metaplasia and carries a relatively high risk of gastric carcinoma. On the other hand, the hypersecretory chronic gastritis seen in patients with duodenal or peptic ulceration is not accompanied by atrophy or by intestinal metaplasia and the risk of carcinoma is not increased.

The third type of chronic gastritis is that seen in those parts of the world where the risk of gastric carcinoma is high. This lesion is multifocal, involving the antrum and corpus, and undergoes a progression of changes to carcinoma. Haenszel *et al.* (1976) studied the incidence of chronic atrophic gastritis in three areas of Colombia with high, intermediate, and low incidence of gastric cancer and found that in the high risk area, 75% of the population developed gastritis by 45 years, whereas in the other two areas, the incidence of gastritis was considerably lower. The area of the stomach affected was found to be significant: the people with a high risk of gastric cancer in the Colombian survey all had multifocal atrophic gastritis involving both the antrum and the corpus. Purely antral gastritis, generally associated with gastric ulcer but not with carcinoma, was not seen in this population, nor was the autoimmune type seen in pernicious anaemia.

As early as 1883, Kupffer described islets of intestinal glands in the gastric mucosa of patients with gastric carcinoma. Intestinal metaplasia is now established as a premalignant lesion preceding the development of intestinal-type gastric carcinoma. Imai *et al.* (1971) compared the incidence of carcinoma of the stomach and intestinal metaplasia in Japanese and US populations, and demonstrated a positive correlation. In resected specimens, intestinal-type carcinomas are frequently seen to be arising in areas of intestinal metaplasia. A continuum of change from normal gastric mucosa, through atrophic gastritis and intestinal metaplasia to dysplasia and on to gastric carcinoma has been demonstrated (Haenszel *et al.*, 1976), the complete sequence of events taking many years.

In the Colombian study, Correa *et al.* (1976) calculated the probability of each of the precursor lesions undergoing progression to a more advanced lesion in this sequence. The percentage probability of each transition occurring varied greatly from area to area. In the high risk area of Narino, 74% of the population underwent transition from normal gastric mucosa to a superficial gastritis; of these 67% then progressed to atrophic gastritis and 38% of these progressed to intestinal metaplasia. An estimated 19% would undergo the entire sequence of changes from normal gastric mucosa to intestinal metaplasia. However, in the low risk areas, while 70% of the population underwent the initial transition from normal gastric mucosa to superficial gastritis, only 8% reached the stage of intestinal metaplasia. (Correspondingly fewer people progressed to atrophic gastritis.) The factors influencing each transition are not clear although the nitrate content of well-water in the area appeared to be a factor in the Colombian study.

In recent years the overall incidence of gastric carcinoma has been falling in most countries, particularly among the white population of the USA. This fall is due to reduction in the number of intestinal-type carcinomas, the incidence of diffuse or infiltrative-type carcinomas remaining static. So far no precursor lesions have been identified for this latter type of carcinoma. It is interesting to note that while a relatively high proportion of patients exhibiting intestinal metaplasia go on to develop gastric carcinoma, the small intestine itself relatively rarely develops malignant neoplasia.

Carcinoma of the colon

Polyps in the colon are widely regarded as potentially premalignant. However, only a small proportion of so-called polyps actually represent a premalignant lesion while 90% merely represent hyperplasia and cannot be regarded as preneoplastic. However, a minority of polyps are benign i.e. colonic adenomas and represent the precursor tissue from which colorectal carcinomas develop (Fenoglio and Pascal 1982).

Development of malignant change within adenomas has been demonstrated. Initially, the malignant change may be confined to the mucosa (carcinoma *in situ*) but later it may reach the submucosa and become truly invasive. The likelihood of malignant change occurring in an adenoma is largely dependent on size and, in general, carcinoma is more likely to develop in the larger, sessile lesions with papillary features.

Patients with familial polyposis have a large number of adenomatous polyps and it appears that in these people, all the carcinomas arise in pre-existing lesions. Carcinoma has also been shown to arise occasionally in Peutz–Jegher's polyps and in juvenile polyps (Fenoglio and Pascal, 1982). It seems that invasive carcinoma is less likely to supervene in polyps in which there is a prominent lympho-plasmacytic infiltrate with well-formed germinal centres surrounding the malignant focus, suggesting that host reaction plays an important role in modifying invasion.

Deschner and her colleagues (Deschner, 1981; Deschner and Lipkin, 1975; Deschner and Maskens, 1981) have described three stages in the alteration of mucosal crypts towards neoplasia. Normally the proliferative activity is confined to the lower two-thirds of the crypt, with the predominant zone of DNA synthesis in the basal third. In stage I abnormality, the proliferative zone expands towards the luminal surface but the major zone of DNA synthesis remains in the lower third. This alteration has been found in normal-appearing mucosa of patients with familial polyposis, in their relatives and in patients with colonic adenomas and carcinomas.

In stage II abnormality, the major zone of DNA synthesis has shifted up to the middle and upper thirds of the crypts. Patients with this defect represent a high risk group. There is a further abnormality (stage III) which occurs in patients with a history of colonic adenoma or carcinoma; this is the presence of isolated crypts with abnormally high levels of DNA synthesis. These hyperactive crypts are thought to have a selective advantage over normal glands, allowing earlier expression of neoplastic transformation.

Mice treated with 1,2-dimethylhydrazine (DMH) show all three stages of abnormal proliferation and DNA synthesis prior to the development of adenomas (Deschner, 1978). In contrast, in DMH-treated BD IX rats there is a *downward* shift of the dominant zone of DNA synthesis and a resultant endophytic tumour growth with potential for microinvasion. It seems that the direction of the proliferative shift determines the type of tumour to be formed. Thus, for carcinoma of the colon, both a premalignant lesion (the adenomatous polyp) and a predisposing lesion (the shift in proliferation and DNA synthesis in the crypts) have been identified.

Patients with long-standing ulcerative colitis also have an increased risk of developing carcinoma of the colon but it seems that the premalignant lesion in these cases is an area of dysplasia in flat, non-hyperplastic epithelium, rather than in a polyp.

Cervical carcinoma

Carcinoma of the cervix similarly shows a premalignant lesion with a continuum of change from mild to severe dysplasia, to carcinoma *in situ* and finally (in a proportion of cases) to invasive carcinoma (Christopherson, 1977). This series of changes is undisputed, although the factors which cause dysplasia and control progression from one stage to the next are not clear.

The role of the potentially oncogenic venereal infections such as herpes simplex 2 (HSV$_2$), cytomegalovirus (CMV), and human papilloma virus (HPV) has been extensively investigated (see Chapter 3). As infections caused by these viruses and cervical neoplasia are all covariables of promiscuity, statistical associations inevitably exist between them and determining a causative role is difficult, particularly as infection is frequently subclinical.

Recent work (Reid *et al.*, 1982) suggests that infection by the human papillomavirus may precede the development of cervical neoplasia, and the oncogenicity of the papillomavirus *in vivo* and *in vitro* makes such suggestions plausible. Bovine (Jarrett, 1978), rabbit (Syverton, 1952), and mastomys (Muller and Grissmann, 1978) papillomaviruses induce cancer in the appropriate species.

Hepatocarcinoma

Another contentious infectious disease in the aetiology of carcinoma is hepatitis B virus (HBV). Blumberg and London (1982) stress the role of HBV in the aetiology of hepatocarcinoma and consider that almost all such carcinomas are associated with HBV infection. Case-control studies have shown that 90% of patients with hepatocarcinoma who live in areas where HBV is endemic have high antibody titres against components of the virus. Controls living in these areas have a lower incidence of high antibody titre.

Direct evidence for the involvement of HBV in liver cancer comes from Summers's work (Summers *et al.*, 1978) in which he extracted HBV–DNA base sequences from 9 of 11 liver carcinomas collected from patients with positive antibody titres to HBV. However, HBV infection may be a predisposing factor in the aetiology of hepatocarcinoma rather than the sole causative agent.

The role of cirrhosis in the development of hepatocarcinoma has long been disputed. In countries with a low incidence of hepatocarcinoma, the carcinoma is usually associated with cirrhosis, but in areas of high incidence, carcinoma occurs in the absence of cirrhosis (Anthony, 1979). There is now increasing evidence that the association between HBV infection and hepatocellular carcinoma is independent of the presence of cirrhosis (Ohaki *et al.*, 1983), although the situation is inevitably confused by the fact that infection with HBV frequently does result in post-hepatitic macronodular cirrhosis. In non-tropical areas, micronodular (alcoholic, nutritional) cirrhosis is far more common than the macronodular pattern and appears to have no association with carcinoma except that in long-standing alcoholic cirrhosis, the pattern may change to macronodular and then carries a higher risk of malignancy (Lee, 1966).

In animal experiments, many agents are capable of producing both a cirrhotic lesion and carcinoma, but these two effects may be quite unrelated. It seems probable that cirrhosis, with the associated repeated cell loss and regeneration, acts as a non-specific enhancer of carcinogenesis.

The carcinogen aflatoxin may be important in the development of liver cancer. It is a well-documented carcinogen for most of the species in which it has been tested, and man is known to be susceptible to the acute toxic action of this compound. Extensive epidemiological studies in many areas of the world have demonstrated a good correlation between daily aflatoxin intake through food and the incidence of hepatocarcinoma (Gibson and Chan, 1972; Van Rensburg *et al.*, 1974; Peers and Linsell, 1973). The dose–response characteristics indicate a male–female difference with a no-effect level in the order of 5 µg/day intake. It is possible that HBV infection, resulting in liver injury and a reparative response, as well as cirrhosis, represent predisposing conditions resulting in increased susceptibility of the liver to direct causative agents such as the aflatoxins.

Other cancers

In contrast to the colon, carcinomas of the urinary bladder do not always arise in benign papillary neoplasms. They may arise in non-papillary areas of the urothelium, although carcinomas do occur more commonly in bladders which are also affected by papillary neoplasms (Brawn, 1982). The more common precursors of invasive bladder carcinoma seem to be areas of atypical hyperplasia and a non-papillary carcinoma *in situ*.

A recent study of 500 cases of breast cancer (Simpson *et al.*, 1982) has shown a bimodal age–frequency distribution of epitheliosis, with the first, large peak in the premenopausal group, a trough in the 56–60 year rank and a second, much lower peak in the elderly. Compared with those of a normal population, the cancerous breasts of the premenopausal group contained an excessive amount of epitheliosis, whereas in the postmenopausal patients, incidence of epitheliosis was only slightly above normal. It seems likely that carcinoma arises in foci of epitheliosis, but at the menopause any non-cancerous areas of epitheliosis regress. These authors consider that the epitheliosis present in the breasts of elderly breast cancer patients in fact represents indolent autonomous neoplasm.

Metaplasia may occur without being premalignant. Smoking induces metaplasia in both the larynx and the bronchus, to a much greater extent in the larynx, yet it is in the bronchus that most tumours occur. The incidence for carcinoma of the bronchus has increased with the number of people smoking yet no change has been detected in the incidence of carcinoma of the larynx.

EXPERIMENTAL ASPECTS

To understand the early stages of neoplastic development, we will examine experimental models for the events preceding overt malignancy. Most of the systems studied in experimental carcinogenesis have relied upon chemically induced neoplasia. As chemical carcinogens are toxic to the target cells where neoplasia is induced, problems arise in distinguishing toxic and reactive processes from those specifically related to the neoplasia.

Many systems have been used to study the development of neoplasms in organs such as liver, kidney, bladder, colon, skin, and mammary gland. Much of the work describes associations of lesions with eventual carcinoma but little is devoted to their biological properties related to autonomy and growth. This section will discuss some of the experimental data.

Chapter 1 describes the concept of two-stage carcinogenesis which arose from work in the skin of mice (Rous and Kidd, 1941; Berenblum and Shubik, 1947). This work showed clearly that a non-carcinogenic dose of a carcinogen 'initiated' the skin to which it was applied and a non-carcinogenic 'promoter' caused tumours to develop at the site of application. These concepts have been adapted to other systems, primarily the liver (Peraino *et al.*, 1971; Solt *et al.*, 1977), but it is debatable whether the multiple and variable insults to a liver which undoubtedly modify the incidence of frank neoplasia, are truly comparable to the original experiments in mouse or rabbit skin.

This chapter will describe some model systems which have been studied to elucidate the early changes during carcinogenesis. They each demonstrate the difficulty of interpreting findings within tissues which are able to undergo compensatory reparative processes.

A system which employs a single insult and the subsequent development of 100% incidence of malignant neoplasm is the rat kidney exposed to dimethyl-nitrosamine. Magee and Barnes (1962) showed that long term survivors of an LD_{50} of dimethylnitrosamine (DMN) resulted in renal neoplasm in the rat. Dietary modification allowed the animals to survive a much higher dose of DMN (the LD_{50} can be increased from 30–60 mg/kg) and 100% of the survivors of this higher dose developed renal tumours. These tumours were shown to be mesenchymal and predominantly vascular (Hard and Butler, 1970a). The development of the tumours was studied in detail and it was shown that at 24 hours a lesion was present in the interstitium of the renal cortex. Hypercellular foci developed in the cortex composed of atypical cells as well as an inflammatory reaction. The subsequent development of the hypercellular foci was described up to the recognition of the overt malignant neoplasm (Hard and Butler, 1970b). Therefore after a single dose of DMN an irreversible change had been induced which resulted in a morphological lesion in the renal cortex as early as 24 hours and in the inevitable sequel of malignant neoplasm of the renal cortex.

While there is a continuity of effect in that the early toxic damage and proliferative response occur in the same population, there is uncertainty about the biological characteristics of the abnormal cells. Should the early lesions be considered to be already a neoplasm or merely preneoplastic? In order for the population of abnormal cortical fibrocytes to be considered as neoplastic it is necessary to demonstrate autonomy.

This problem has been investigated by Hard and his colleagues who have shown that it is possible to isolate from the rat kidney, as early as 24 hours, cells which will have some of the properties of transformed cells (Hard, 1982). The clear demonstration of transformation *in vitro* may require up to five subcultures. Such results may be interpreted either as showing that the cells isolated from the kidney require further changes to become transformed, or that they require five subcultures to be recognized by the techniques currently available.

A further question is whether the abnormal cells observed in the kidney correspond with the transformed cells grown in culture. At present there is no unequivocal marker for the cells *in vivo* that can also be demonstrated *in vitro*. However, cytological studies suggest that such a correspondence is present (Hard *et al.*, 1971). These studies indicate that a very early irreversible change has occurred and that the designation 'premalignant' in mechanistic terms is inappropriate.

The experimental induction of transitional cell carcinoma of the urinary bladder has demonstrated many of the problems of interpretation of early lesions. Hicks and Wakefield (1972) have suggested that atypical hyperplasia observed in the bladder epithelium in such experiments should be considered preneoplastic, as the regime results in 100% incidence of carcinoma. This is, however, an operational diagnosis similar to that used in diagnostic pathology and is not based on an understanding of mechanism. Similar atypical hyperplasia may be induced by the cytotoxic agent cyclophosphamide (Koss, 1967), but these lesions rapidly resolve (D. M. Creasy, personal communication) and should be considered to be reactive hyperplasia.

Reactive hyperplasia of bladder epithelium may result from causes such as infection, calculi or chemical injury, which alone will not necessarily lead to carcinoma. Although bladder calculi are associated with a low incidence of papilloma in the rat, the early hyperplasia is probably reactive to injury and infection. However, if the epithelium is further exposed to a carcinogen a carcinoma is more likely to result. The hyperplasia may be fertile ground for induction of carcinoma, as in the case of liver described below, but is premalignant.

Markers of irreversible change have been sought in the bladder but without success. Such markers include the absence of alkaline phosphatase (Kunze *et al.*, 1975) and the ingrowth of capillaries into the epithelium (Hicks and Choisaniec, 1978). Another observed change is the induction of pleomorphic villi but these are found also following treatment with cyclophosphamide (Fukushima *et al.*, 1981), which is non-carcinogenic for the bladder in the experimental system used. It is of interest in this connection that patients with pleomorphic microvilli appear to be at greater risk of developing a recurrence of bladder papillomas and carcinoma (Herd and Williams, 1983). Thus, there is some evidence that the experimental studies of bladder neoplasia in rodents are correlated with prospective studies in humans.

A similar correlation has been attempted in colonic neoplasia. It is widely accepted that in man adenocarcinoma arises in an adenomatous polyp and Madara *et al.* (1983) have described a similar sequence in rats treated with dimethylhydrazine. However, if the adenomatous polyps are indeed benign neoplasia. As discussed above, Deschner and Maskens (1981) have described fails to answer the question as to whether a transitional stage precedes neoplasia. As described above, Deschner and Maskens (1981) have described three stages of alteration of the proliferative activity of the colonic crypts which may be mechanistically related to the subsequent neoplasm, but a morphological lesion prior to the development of the polyp is not described.

Many studies have investigated the sequence of events leading to the development of hepatocarcinoma in rats and have attempted, without success, to characterize populations of preneoplastic cells. The earlier studies in this field used toxic carcinogens such as 4-dimethylaminoazo benzene and 2-acetylaminofluorine (2-AAF). These compounds induce marked oval cell and biliary proliferation, and parenchymal cell nodular hyperplasia. In an analogy with the cirrhotic human liver, nodular hyperplasia was considered to be a premalignant lesion (Farber, 1973).

It is now recognized that such lesions are not in themselves preneoplastic as, even when induced by the carcinogen 2-AAF, most nodules of hyperplasia would resolve unless the carcinogen regime were continued (Teebor and Becker, 1971). It has been shown that a choline-deficient diet will also produce focal nodular hyperplasia in the rat but not hepatocarcinoma unless a carcinogen is also given to the animal (Newberne *et al.*, 1966). Under these circumstances the liver is more susceptible to the carcinogen but the nodular hyperplasia is a reactive response to hepatocyte damage.

Other studies have utilized the less toxic but more active carcinogens nitrosomorpholine (Bannasch, 1968) and aflatoxin (Butler *et al.*, 1981). With both of these compounds relatively short-term treatment, between 6 and 10 weeks, is sufficient to induce 100% incidence of carcinoma. At the time of irreversible change (that is at the end of exposure to the carcinogen) a spectrum of lesions is present in the liver. These range from basophilic foci, clear cell areas of glycogen storage, and small proliferative foci of hepatic parenchymal cells. Many of the foci have starvation-resistant glycogen, reduced glucose-6-phosphatase, and increased glucose-6-phosphate dehydrogenase.

Bannasch (1968) considered these foci to be the putative preneoplastic lesions and Emmelot and Scherer (1980) have studied the kinetics and time/dose characteristics of their appearance. It is of interest that many of the lesions studied by the latter are produced in systems that do not result in carcinoma and hence may represent only a response to the acute toxicity of the carcinogen.

Currently, the most commonly used marker for the identification of putative preneoplastic lesions in the rat liver is γ-glutamyl transpeptidase (γ-GT). This enzyme has been reported as occurring within focal areas of hepatocytes corresponding to those with glycogen retention and reduction of glucose-6-phosphatase (Butler *et al.*, 1981). However, the studies of Neal (personal communication) have shown that while many basophilic foci are positive for γ-GT, others are not, and in the normal lobular liver many areas are positive for γ-GT. Neal *et al.* (1981) have suggested that the increased levels of γ-GT represent a protective mechanism by which populations of parenchymal cells are able to survive and proliferate in the presence of a toxic agent.

The presence of foci with altered enzymatic patterns has been studied mainly in the rat. Our studies have shown that many of the features appear also in the mouse, except for the presence of γ-GT-positive cells which have been reported only from long-term feeding of safrole (Lipsky *et al.*, 1980). Hepatocarcinoma may be readily induced in the mouse by a single neonatal dose of diethylnitrosamine and during the development of the carcinoma a wide range of lesions is present, none of which is positive for γ-GT. This suggests that the continued presence of a toxic agent is required for the induction of γ-GT, lending support to the views of Neal *et al.* (1981).

While these studies have been attempting to find markers for preneoplastic cells, little information has been forthcoming about the biological properties of the different cell populations related to growth. Attempts have been made to isolate cell populations from livers after treatment with carcinogens. Judah *et al.* (1977) have reported that following six week's feeding of aflatoxin, which induces an irreversible change, populations of γ-GT-positive cells may be cultured which are resistant to the toxic action of aflatoxin. Also Hanigan and Pitot (1982) have isolated γ-GT-positive cells from livers of animals fed 2-AAF. The problem remains, however, as to the origin of the γ-GT-positive cells within the liver and their relationship to the developing neoplasm.

So far, the attempts at prolonged tissue culture with the demonstration of transformed epithelium, similar to the kidney system described above, have been unsuccessful. Therefore, at the time of irreversible change, we do not know whether the lesion is a carcinoma *in situ* or whether the cell population represents incomplete neoplasia requiring progression through multiple stages to complete neoplasm, i.e. carcinoma.

Until such basic information is available, it will be difficult to interpret the detailed studies of hepatocarcinogenesis in which the stages of 'initiation' and 'promotion' are described (Peraino *et al.*, 1971; Solt *et al.*, 1977). In studies on the skin, the carcinogen was applied directly to the site of initiation and followed by application of the promoter to the same site. The mechanism by which chemicals produce these two apparent effects is still not understood. There are considerable problems in a mechanistic interpretation of a multiple stage model following systemic administration of either two carcinogens and/or hepatectomy. It is difficult to distinguish between the direct effects of chemicals on a cell population from an indirect action mediated through an effect by host homoeostasis on the growth and survival of malignant transformed cells.

From this discussion of the investigations of the early stages of carcinogenesis the question may be asked 'What is premalignant neoplasia?' Without an understanding of the mechanisms of carcinogenesis, such a term encompasses a wide range of phenomena of a disparate nature. Preneoplasia, if it has a mechanistic meaning, should describe a lesion consisting of a population of cells which are partially transformed. This lesion in itself may be irreversible but requires the acquisition of a further change before the lesion becomes complete neoplasia. Such a lesion must be distinguished from physiological reactive responses such as compensatory focal hyperplasia of the liver which is reversible but in which the cells are more susceptible to the action of a carcinogen.

A consideration of preneoplasia in these terms relates to the process of 'initiation'. However, until it is possible to identify the growth characteristics of 'initiated' cells and the mechanism of 'promotion' it is unwise to describe the wide range of phenotypically altered cells in response to carcinogen treatment as 'preneoplastic'. In mechanistic terms, as opposed to clinical operational usage, the designation of 'premalignant neoplasia' is, therefore, not justified.

CONCLUSION

A wide range of morphologically recognizable premalignant lesions exists, but the factors which control their progression to malignant neoplasia are poorly understood. Benign neoplasms rarely undergo malignant change (e.g. uterine leiomyomata very rarely become sarcomatous). Premalignant lesions are much more commonly dysplastic or atrophic in nature.

Carcinoma *in situ* can be regarded as the first step in the presentation of an invasive malignant tumour. This stage probably exists for all malignant neoplasms, but is not often detected sufficiently early before some local invasion has occurred. It is relatively commonly seen in the skin, in the cervix, in colonic adenomatous polyps and in the breast and stomach, but is almost certainly a universal precursor of invasive neoplasia, even though it may often go undetected.

REFERENCES

Anthony, P. P. (1979). Hepatic Neoplasms. In *Pathology of the liver* (eds R. N. M. MacSween, P. P. Antony, and P. J. Scheuer). London: Churchill Livingstone.

Bannasch, P. (1968). The cytoplasm of hepatocytes during carcinogenesis; electron and light microscopical investigations of the nitrosomorpholine – intoxicated rat liver. In *Recent results in cancer research*, Vol. 19. Berlin: Springer-Verlag.

Berenblum, I., and Shubik, P. (1947). The role of croton oil applications, associated with a single painting of a carcinogen in tumour induction of mouse's skin. *British Journal of Cancer*, **1**, 379.

Bloom, G. E., Warner, S., Gerald, P. S., and Diamond, L. K. (1966). Chromosomal abnormalities in constitutional aplastic anaemia. *New England Journal of Medicine*, **274**, 8.

Blumberg, B. S., and London, W. T. (1982). Hepatitis B virus: Pathogenesis and prevention of primary cancer of the liver. *Cancer*, **50**, 1657.

Brawn P. N. (1982). The origin of invasive carcinoma of the bladder. *Cancer*, **50**, 515.

Butler, W. H., Hempsall, V., and Stewart (1981). Histochemical studies on the early proliferative lesion induced in the rat liver by aflatoxin. *Journal of Pathology*, **133**, 325.

Christopherson, W. M. (1977). Dysplasia, carcinoma *in situ* and microinvasive carcinoma of the uterine cervix. *Human Pathology*, **8**, 489.

Cleaver, J. E., and Bootsma, D. (1975). Xeroderma pigmentosum: biochemical and genetic characteristics. *Annual Review of Genetics*, **9**, 19.

Correa, P. (1982). Precursors of gastric and oesophageal cancer. *Cancer*, **50** (suppl.), 2554.

Correa, P., Cuello, C., Duque, E. *et al.* (1976). Gastric cancer in Colombia III: natural history of precursor lesions. *Journal of the National Cancer Institute*, **57**, 1027.

DeOme, K. B., Faulkin, L. J., Bern, H. A., and Blair, P. B. (1959). Development of mammary tumours from hyperplastic alveolar nodules transplanted into gland-free mammary fat pads of female C3H mice. *Cancer Research*, **19**, 515.

Deschner, E. E. (1978). Early proliferative defects induced by six weekly injections of 1,2-dimethylhydrazine in epithelial cells of mouse distal colon. *Zeit. Krebsforsch*, **91**, 205.

Deschner, E. E. (1981). Cell proliferation as a biological marker in human colorectal neoplasia. In *Colorectal cancer: prevention, epidemiology and screening* (eds S. J. Winower, D. Schottenfield and P. Sherlock). New York: Raven Press, p. 133.

Deschner, E. E., and Lipkin, M. (1975). Proliferative patterns in colonic mucosa in familial polyposis. *Cancer*, **35**, 413.

Deschner, E. E., and Maskens, A. P. (1981). Significance of the labeling index and labeling distribution as kinetic parameters in colo-rectal mucosa of 1,2-dimethylhydrazine treated animals and cancer patients. *Proceedings of the American Association for Cancer Research*, **22**, 192.

Emmelot, P., and Scherer, E. (1980). The first relevant cell stage in rat liver carcinogenesis. A. Quantitative Approach. *Biochemica et Biophysica Acta*, **605**, 247.

Farber, E. (1973). Hyperplastic liver nodules. *Methods in Cancer Research*, **7**, 345.

Fenoglio, C. M., and Pascal, R. R. (1982). Colorectal adenomas and cancer. *Cancer*, **50**, 2601.

Fukushima, S., Arai, M., Cohen, S. M. *et al.* (1981). Scanning electron microscopy of cyclophosphamide-induced hyperplasia of rat urinary bladder. *Laboratory Investigation*, **44**, 89.

Gianelli, F., and Pawsey, S. A. (1976). DNA repair synthesis in human heteroka-
ryons. *Journal of Cell Science,* **20,** 307.

Gibson, J. B., and Chan, W. C. (1972). Primary carcinomas of the liver in Hong
Kong. Some possible aetiological factors. *Recent Results in Cancer Research,* **39,**
107.

Grinnel, R. S., and Lane, N. (1958). Benign and malignant adenomatous polyps and
papillary adenomas of colon and rectum: analysis of 1956 tumours in 1335 patients.
International Abstracts of Surgery, **106,** 519.

Haenszel, W., Correa, P., Cuello, C. *et al.* (1976). Gastric cancer in Colombia II.
Case-control epidemiologic study of precursor lesions. *Journal of National Cancer
Institute,* **57,** 1021.

Hanigan, H. M., and Pitot, H. C. (1982). Isolation of γ-glutamyl transpeptidase
positive hepatocytes during the early stages of hepatocarcinogenesis in the rat.
Carcinogenesis, **3,** 1349.

Hard, G. C. (1982). Demonstrations of the tumorigenicity of transformed rat kidney
cell-lines by intravenous allotransplantation in the neonate. *International Journal of
Cancer,* **30,** 197.

Hard, G. C., and Butler, W. H. (1970a). Cellular analysis of renal neoplasia:
Induction of renal tumours in dietary conditioned rats by dimethylnitrosamine,
with a reappraisal of morphological characteristics. *Cancer Research,* **30,** 2796.

Hard, G. C., and Butler, W. H. (1970b). Cellular analysis of renal neoplasia: Light
microscopic study of the development of interstitial lesions induced in the rat
kidney by a single carcinogenic dose of dimethylnitrosamine. *Cancer Research,* **30,**
2806.

Hard, G. C., Borland, R., and Butler, W. H. (1971). Altered morphology and
behaviour of kidney fibroblasts *in vitro,* following *in vivo* treatment of rats with a
carcinogenic dose of dimethylnitrosamine. *Experientia,* **27,** 1208.

Herd, E., and Williams, G. (1983). *Journal of Histopathology* (in press).

Hicks, R. M., and Choisaniec, J. (1978). Experimental induction, histology and
ultrastructure of hyperplasia and neoplasia of the urinary bladder epithelium.
International Review of Experimental Pathology, **18,** 199.

Hicks, R. M., and Wakefield, J. St. J. (1972). Rapid induction of bladder cancer in
rats with *N*-methyl-*N*-nitrosourea 1. Histology. *Chemico-biological Interactions,* **5,**
139.

Imai, T., Kubo, J., and Watanabe, H. (1971). Chronic gastritis in Japan with
reference to high incidence of gastric carcinoma. *Journal of the National Cancer
Institute,* **47,** 179.

Inglis, K. (1954). The relation of the renal lesions to the cerebral lesions in the
tuberous sclerosis complex. *American Journal of Pathology,* **30,** 739.

Jarrett, W. F. H. (1978). Transformation of warts to malignancy in alimentary
carcinoma in cattle. *Bulletin of Cancer,* **65,** 191.

Jensen, H. M., Rice, J. R., and Wellings, S. R. (1976). Preneoplastic lesions in the
human breast. *Science,* **191,** 295.

Judah, D. J., Legg, R. F., and Neal, S. E. (1977). Development of resistance to
cytotoxicity during aflatoxin carcinogenesis. *Nature (London),* **265,** 343.

Kennedy, A. W., and Hart, W. R. (1982). Multiple squamous-cell carcinomas in
Fanconi's anaemia. *Cancer,* **50,** 811.

Koss, L. G. (1967). A light and electron microscopic study of the effects of a single
dose of cyclophosphamide on various organs in the rat. *Laboratory Investigation,*
16, 44.

Kramer, W. (1971). Lesions of the central nervous system in multiple neurofibromatosis. *Psychiatria Neurologia Neurochirurgia,* **74,** 349.

Kunze, E., Schaner, A., Krusmann, G. (1975). Focal loss of alkaline phosphatase and increase of proliferation in preneoplastic areas of the rat urothelium after administration of N-butyl-N-(4-hydroxybutyl)-nitrosamine and N-[4-(5-nitro-2-furyl)-2-thiazolyl] formamide. *Zeitschrift für Krebsforschung und Klinische Onkologie*, **84**, 143.

Lee, F. I. (1966). Cirrhosis and hepatoma in alcoholics. *Gut*, **7**, 77.

Lipsky, M. M., Hinton, D. E., Klaunig, J. E. *et al.* (1980). Gamma glutamyl transpeptidase in safrole induced presumptive premalignant mouse hepatocytes. *Carcinogenesis*, **1**, 151.

MacMahon, B. (1982). Risk factors for cancer of the pancreas. *Cancer*, **50**, 2676.

Madara, J. L., Harte, P., Deasy, J. *et al.* (1983). Evidence for an adenoma–carcinoma sequence in dimethylhydrazine-induced neoplasms of rat intestinal epithelium. *American Journal of Pathology*, **110**, 230.

Magee, P. N., and Barnes, J. M. (1962). Induction of kidney tumours in the rat with dimethylnitrosamine (N-nitroso-dimethylamine). *Journal of Pathology and Bacteriology*, **84**, 19.

Muller, H., and Grissman, L. (1978). Mastomys natalensis papilloma virus: the causative agent of epithelial proliferation. *Journal General Virology*, **41**, 315.

Neal, G. E., Metcalfe, S. A., Legg, R. F. *et al.* (1981). Mechanism of the resistance to cytotoxicity which precedes aflatoxin B_1 hepatocarcinogenesis. *Carcinogenesis*, **2**, 457.

Newberne, P. N., Harrington, D. H., and Wogan, G. N. (1966). Effects of cirrhosis and other liver insults on induction of liver tumours by aflatoxin in rats. *Laboratory Investigation*, **15**, 962.

Obeid, D. A., Hill, F. G. H., Harnden, D. *et al.* (1980). Fanconi anaemia. Oxymethalone hepatic tumours and chromosome aberration association with leukaemic transition. *Cancer*, **46**, 1401.

Ohaki, Y., Misugi, K., Susaki, Y., and Tsunodas, A. (1983). Hepatitis B surface antigen positive hepatocellular carcinoma in children: Report of a case and review of the literature. *Cancer*, **51**, 822.

Pattern, L. M., Morris, L. E., Blot, W. J. *et al.* (1981). Oesophageal cancer among black men in Washington, DC: alcohol, tobacco and other risk factors. *Journal of the National Cancer Institute*, **67**, 777.

Peers, F. G., and Linsell, C. A. (1973). Dietary aflatoxins and liver cancer – a population based study in Kenya. *British Journal of Cancer*, **27**, 473.

Peraino, C., Fray, R. J. M., and Staffelott, E. (1971). Reduction and enhancement by phenobarbitol of hepatocarcinogenesis induced in the rat by 2-acetylaminofluorine. *Cancer Research*, **31**, 1506.

Rasmussen, C. W. (1976). A new endoscopic classification of chronic oesophagitis. *American Journal of Gastroenterology*, **65**, 409.

Reid, R., Stanhope, C. R., Herschman, B. R. *et al.* (1982). Genital warts and cervical cancer 1. Evidence of an association between subclinical papillomavirus infection and cervical malignancy. *Cancer*, **50**, 377.

Rodriguez, H. A., and Berthrong, M. (1966). Multiple primary intracranial tumours in von Recklinghausen's neurofibromatosis. *Archives of Neurology*, **14**, 467.

Rous, P., and Kidd, J. G. (1941). Conditional neoplasms and subthreshold neoplastic states. A study of the tar tumours of rabbits. *Journal of Experimental Medicine*, **73**, 365.

Simpson, H. W., Mutch, F., Halberg, F. *et al.* (1982). Bimodal age-frequency distribution of epitheliosis in cancer mastectomies. *Cancer*, **50**, 2417.

Solt, D. B., Medline, A., and Farber, E. (1977). Rapid emergence of carcinogen-induced hyperplastic lesions in a new model for the sequential analysis of liver carcinogenesis. *American Journal of Pathology*, **88**, 595.

Summers, J., O'Connell, A., Maupas, P. *et al.* (1978). Hepatic B virus DNA in primary hepatocellular carcinoma tissue. *Journal of Medical Virology*, **2**, 207.

Syverton, J. T. (1952). Mastomys natalensis papillomavirus: the causative agent of epithelial proliferation. *Journal of General Virology*, **41**, 315.

Teebor, G. W., and Becker, F. F. (1971). Regression and persistence of hyperplastic hepatic nodules induced by N-2 fluorenyl-acetamide and their relationship to hepatocarcinogenesis. *Cancer Research*, **31**, 1.

Trau, H., Scheurach-Millet, M., Fisher, B. K., and Tsur, H. (1982). Peutz–Jegher's syndrome and bilateral breast carcinomas. *Cancer*, **50**, 788.

Van Rensburg, S. J., Van der Watt, J. J., Purchase, I. F. H. *et al.* (1974). Primary liver cancer rate and aflatoxin intake in a high cancer area. *South African Medical Journal*, **48**, 1508a.

Wellings, S. R., Jensen, H. M., and Marcum, R. G. (1975). Atlas of subgross pathology of the human breast with special reference to possible precancerous lesions. *Journal of the National Cancer Institute*, **55**, 231.

Yang, C. S. (1980). Research on oesophageal cancer in China: a review. *Cancer Research*, **40**, 1633.

Yoshiharu Ohaki, Kazuaki Misugi, Yoshiro Sasaki, and Akio Tsumoda (1983). Hepatitis B surface antigen positive hepatocellular carcinoma in children. *Cancer*, **51**, 822.

Chapter

8

BRUCE K. ARMSTRONG

Variations in Pattern of Cancer Incidence

The study of variations in cancer incidence is of little value unless the observation of a significant variation leads us to ask 'why?' For example, why has mortality from cancer of the stomach fallen in developed countries? Why does the incidence of cancer of the oesophagus vary more than 40-fold between different countries? Why are women at higher risk to cancer of the thyroid gland than are men? Why does the incidence of cancer of the cervix cease to rise appreciably after the menopause? Why does mortality from melanoma in European migrants fail to rise subtantially with increasing duration of residence in Australia?

MEASUREMENT OF CANCER INCIDENCE

The incidence of cancer is measured directly by recording all new cases of cancer arising in a defined total population over a defined period of time. This can be done either by the conduct of a special incidence survey (Holman *et al.*, 1980) or by routine recording in a population-based cancer registry (MacLennan *et al.*, 1975). There are now cancer registries throughout the world (Waterhouse *et al.*, 1976; World Health Organization, 1979) but only about 15% of the total world population is covered by some form of population-based cancer registration. The longest continuously operating registry is that in Connecticut, USA, which has published incidence estimates since 1935.

These limitations on the coverage and period of operation of cancer registries have meant that extensive use has been made of cancer mortality data to estimate cancer incidence. The WHO publishes cancer mortality data from about 36% of the world's population (World Health Organization, 1979) but even in such data, there is substantial variation in population coverage by region – from 100% in Europe to 10% in Asia and Africa. Inevitably, therefore, factors other than variations in the true incidence of cancer can influence the rates estimated by cancer registration or other means. The major factors affecting the accuracy of cancer registration are summarized in Table 1, and discussed below.

The aim of a population-based cancer registry is the counting of all newly occurring cancers in its population base but this aim is probably never achieved. It may be particularly difficult to ascertain all cancers occurring in elderly or other population subgroups who may not seek medical advice, or in those who have less ready access to medical care. The problems in comparability produced by these effects can be overcome in part at least, by restricting comparisons to younger people (the age band 35 to 64 years is often chosen) in whom the degree of ascertainment should be high and more nearly uniform (Doll and Peto, 1981).

The problem of variation in the definition of cancer applies particularly to *in situ* and borderline lesions such as carcinoma *in situ* of the cervix, preinvasive melanoma, and papilloma of the bladder (Holman *et al.*, 1980; Saxen, 1982). Unless lesions are registered in a uniform manner in different populations and at different times, artificial variation in cancer incidence will result. An example was the apparent 15- to 30-fold increase in mortality from malignant neoplasms of the brain and nervous system which manifested in Australia between 1910 and 1979 (Holman and Armstrong, 1982). Most (if not all) of this change was explained by transfer of some tumours from one category of the International Classification of Diseases to another.

The degree to which diagnoses of cancer are confirmed histologically varies between cancer registries of one country and another (Muir and Waterhouse, 1976), and by age and cancer site even in the one registry. For example, in the Birmingham registry in 1968–72, histological confirmation was at the max-

Table 1   Factors producing artificial variation in cancer incidence rates (from Saxen, 1982)

1. Variation in completeness of coverage of the target populations by cancer registration
2. Variation in the definition of cancer
3. Variation in the proportion with histological confirmation of the diagnosis of cancer
4. Variation in the necropsy rate
5. Variation in diagnostic accuracy
6. The occurrence of mass screening

imum of 92% in males aged 25–29 years, and fell to the minimum of 46% in those aged 75+ years; the highest histological confirmation rate was for cancer of the testis and Hodgkin's disease (97%), and the lowest was for cancer of the pancrease (35%) (Muir and Waterhouse, 1976).

Lack of histological confirmation will affect particularly the distinction between primary and secondary tumours, and the correct attribution of lymphomas to a morphological category rather than to a site such as the small intestine (Saxen, 1982). The necropsy rate prevailing in a population will affect the estimated incidence of non-aggressive cancers which tend not to manifest in life, such as latent carcinoma of the prostate (Saxen, 1982).

In addition to the particular issues of histological confirmation and necropsy rate, there is the more general issue of diagnostic accuracy. For example, review by a panel of pathologists and haematologists of a group of lympho-haematopoietic neoplasms can produce an appreciable change in incidence rates; particularly of non-Hodgkin's lymphomas, many of which were reclassified as other neoplasms by Dougan *et al.* (1981). The existence of a special interest or special expertise in the diagnosis of a particular group of tumours may thus have an effect on recorded incidence rates.

Mass screening methods such as cervical cytology, breast examination or mammography, may temporarily increase incidence rates by bringing forward the time of diagnosis (Saxen, 1982). They may even increase incidence rates permanently if they bring to light lesions which would never have become manifest clinically as cancer (Doll and Peto, 1981).

All those factors which affect recorded cancer incidence can also affect records of cancer mortality. In addition, however, cancer mortality statistics have problems of their own and variations in cancer survival rates between countries may give false impressions regarding the underlying incidence rates. Firstly, there are considerable opportunities for error on the part of those who complete the death certificate (Davies, 1977; Percy *et al.*, 1981). Cancer mortality statistics are also limited in detail, providing only the histological information specified in the International Classification of Diseases, and rarely providing subsite information.

The above problems mean that artefact will be a component of almost all variations in cancer incidence however measured and care is needed in interpreting patterns of variation. Mortality statistics, while superficially inferior to directly collected incidence statistics, may in some situations lead to more valid inferences because of the inherent stability of the method whereby they are collected (Doll and Peto, 1981).

In the following discussion, the patterns of variation in cancer incidence will be described along three axes – time, place, and personal characteristics:

Time – refers to the study of trends over time, usually within a single, geographically defined population. Trends may be compared between different populations.

Place – refers to the study of differences between geographically defined populations, often countries, but sometimes subunits within a single country.

Person – refers to personal characteristics shared by subgroups within a geographically defined population; including sex, age, place of birth, ethnic origin, marital status, religion, socio-economic status, occupation, etc. In practice, the number of characteristics which can be studied in this way in the whole population is limited to what can be collected by cancer registries or on death certificates, and to data reported in census tables.

VARIATION IN CANCER INCIDENCE OVER TIME

This brief review will be limited to trends observed in some developed countries over the past 50 years and will draw mainly on mortality data for the reasons discussed above. Tables 2, 3, and 4 compare the main trends in cancer

Table 2 Major changes in age-standardized annual mortality from cancer in Australia between 1930–34 and 1970–74 in males and females of all ages (from Holman and Armstrong, 1982)[a]

MALES	Net change per 100,000	FEMALES	Net change per 100,000
Rises		*Rises*	
Pancreas	+ 3.9	Lung	+ 4.8
Lung	+40.9	Brain and nervous system	+ 2.9
Melanoma of skin	+ 2.5	Lymphoma (non-Hodgkin's lymphoma and myeloma; since 1950)	+ 2.3
Prostate	+ 4.9	Leukaemia	+ 3.4
Brain and nervous system	+ 4.2		
Lymphoma (non-Hodgkin's lymphoma and myeloma; since 1950)	+ 2.9		
Leukaemia	+ 6.0		
Falls		*Falls*	
Mouth	− 5.1	Stomach	−12.4
Stomach	−20.6	Liver not specified as primary (to 1967)	− 3.8
Liver, not specified as primary (to 1967)	− 3.3	Uterus	− 7.7

[a]Cancer sites with a change in mortality of >2/100,000 have been shown.

Table 3   Major changes in age-standardized annual mortality from cancer in England and Wales between 1931–35 and 1971–75 in males and females 45–64 years of age (from Doll, 1979)[a]

MALES	Net change per 100,000	FEMALES	Net change per 100,000
Rises		*Rises*	
Pancreas	+ 5.2	Lung	+32.8
Lung	+137.4	Breast	+ 6.1
Brain and nervous system	+ 5.3	Ovary	+ 9.4
Lymphoma (non-Hodgkin's lymphoma + myeloma)	+ 3.3		
Leukaemia	+ 4.6		
Falls		*Falls*	
Tongue	− 10.5	Stomach	−28.0
Mouth and tonsil	− 5.4	Large intestine (except rectum)	− 7.9
Oesophagus	− 8.9	Rectum	− 4.8
Stomach	− 34.9	Liver and gallbladder[b]	−10.8
Large intestine (except rectum)	− 9.2	Uterus (since 1950)	− 3.7
Rectum	− 14.6		
Liver and gallbladder[b]	− 9.3		
Larynx	− 7.2		

[a]Cancer sites with a change in mortality of >3/100,000 have been shown.
[b]Probably includes cancers not specified as primary.

mortality in Australia, England, and Wales, and the *white* population of the USA since the early 1930s. In each country, males showed a net rise in cancer mortality (due mainly to the rise in lung cancer beginning in the 1930s) while females showed a net fall. The patterns of change by site of cancer show some similarities and some differences between the countries.

The three populations are almost completely concordant in showing absolute rises in mortality from cancer of the lung, tumours of the brain and nervous system, and lymphoma in both sexes, and in addition from cancer of the pancreas and leukaemia in males, and cancer of the ovary in females (the rise in Australian females was not quite 2 per 100,000). They are essentially concordant also in showing falls in mortality from cancers of the stomach and liver (the latter probably mainly secondary cancers) in both sexes, mouth

Table 4   Major changes in age-standardized annual mortality from cancer in the USA between 1935 and 1973–74 in white males and females of all ages (from Devesa and Silverman, 1978)[a]

MALES	Net change per 100,000	FEMALES	Net change per 100,000
Rises		*Rises*	
Intestines (except rectum)	+ 3.9	Pancreas	+ 2.1
Pancreas	+ 5.0	Lung	+ 9.9
Lung	+50.1	Ovary	+ 3.0
Brain and nervous system	+ 3.8	Brain and nervous system	+ 2.4
Lymphoma (non-Hodgkin's lymphoma + myeloma; since 1950)	+ 3.3	Lymphoma (non-Hodgkin's lymphoma + myeloma; since 1950)	+ 2.4
Leukaemia	+ 4.2		
Falls		*Falls*	
Stomach	−23.7	Stomach	−18.0
Rectum	− 2.6	Rectum	− 3.3
		Uterus	−19.3

[a]Cancer sites with a change in mortality of >2/100,000.

cancer in males (cancers of the mouth were omitted from the US tables), and uterine cancer in females.

The disagreements with respect to rises in mortality seen in these tables are more apparent than real. Melanoma mortality rose in England and Wales, and in the USA as well as in Australia, but as the data in the former two countries extended only from 1950 the rises did not reach the threshold for tabulation. Mortality from cancer of the prostate, which rose in Australia, also rose by a small amount in the USA but fell in Britain; the detail of age-specific trends, however, differs little between England and Wales and Australia (Holman *et al.*, 1981). Mortality from cancer of the breast rose subtantially in England and Wales but not in Australia and the USA; there is evidence, however, of recent increases in both the USA and Australia (Fleming *et al.*, 1981; Stevens *et al.*, 1982).

The main discordance between mortality trends in these countries is in cancer of the large bowel. There was a rise in cancer of the colon in US males, little change in Australians of either sex, and falls in both sexes in England and Wales. Mortality from cancer of the rectum fell appreciably in both sexes in England and Wales and in the USA, but not in Australia. A detailed analysis of the Australian and British data suggests that this complex, discordant pattern can be explained by differing trends in alcohol consumption (McMichael, 1979). The falls in mortality from cancers of the oesophagus and larynx in England and Wales, but not in the other two populations, may have a similar explanation (McMichael, 1978, 1979).

For convenience, the mainly concordant trends are summarized in Table 5. This changing pattern in cancer mortality is probably shared by many other Western countries and can be seen in other more recently developed countries such as Japan (Kuroishi *et al.*, 1981).

Additional detail on trends in cancer mortality in Australia is shown in Figures 1 and 2 and rates for most of the sites cover the period 1910 to 1979. It will be noted that for some sites which show an increase in mortality, much of the increase occurred before 1930; for example colon, rectum, pancreas (in females), ovary, and prostate. These earlier changes are likely to be due to improved diagnosis. The fall in mortality from cancer of the lip, not

Table 5   Cancers showing appreciable absolute changes in age-standardized mortality in at least two countries (out of Australia, England and Wales and the United States of America) between 1930 and 1975[a]

MALES	
Rises	*Falls*
Lung	Stomach
Brain and nervous system	Mouth
Pancreas	Liver (probably mainly secondary)
Leukaemia	
Lymphoma (non-Hodgkin's lymphoma and myeloma)	

FEMALES	
Rises	*Falls*
Lung	Stomach
Ovary	Liver (probably mainly secondary)
Lymphoma (non-Hodgkin's lymphoma and myeloma)	Uterus
Brain and nervous system	

[a]Changes listed in descending order according to the size of the absolute change in mortality in England and Wales.

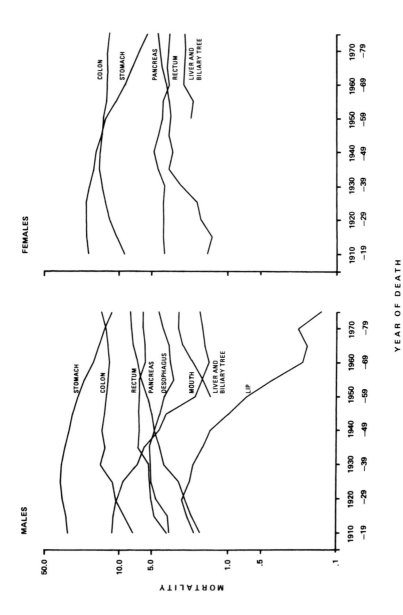

Figure 1   Trends in age-standardized annual mortality (per 100,000) from the main gastrointestinal cancers in Australia, 1910 to 1979. (Holman and Armstrong, 1982.)

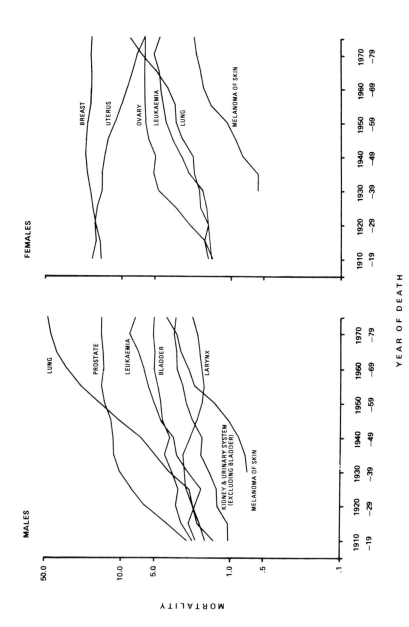

Figure 2 Trends in age-standardized annual mortality (per 100,000) from the other main cancers in Australia, 1910 to 1979. (Holman and Armstrong, 1982.)

highlighted in Table 2 because of its small absolute size, was quite dramatic. The undulating curves of mortality from cancers of the colon, rectum, and oesophagus in males indicate the complexity of the mortality trends in these cancers, as discussed above.

The extent to which these patterns of cancer mortality reflect patterns in incidence is difficult to assess because, as pointed out above, cancer registration rates may be less accurate indicators of true trends in cancer incidence over time than are mortality rates. None the less, trends in cancer incidence can be examined in the USA over the three National Cancer Surveys conducted in 1937–39, 1947–48, and 1969–71 (Devesa and Silverman, 1978). There is agreement between incidence and mortality on at least the main features (compare Tables 4 and 6) – the rise in cancer of the lung, and falls in cancer of the stomach and uterus. Buccal cavity was not included in analysis of US mortality; the fall in incidence is consistent with falls in mortality in Australia and England and Wales (Tables 2 and 3). Lymphoma and leukaemia were not tabulated for the First National Cancer Survey; they

Table 6   Major changes in age-standardized annual incidence of cancer in the USA between the First (1937–39) and Third (1969–71) National Cancer Surveys (seven common areas) in white males and females of all ages (from Devesa and Silverman, 1978)[a]

MALES	Net change per 100,000	FEMALES	Net change per 100,000
Rises		*Rises*	
Intestines (except rectum)	+ 9.2	Intestines (except rectum)	+ 3.0
Lung	+55.3	Lung	+11.8
Prostate	+13.2	Breast	+ 6.7
Kidney	+ 3.9	Melanoma of skin	+ 2.2
Bladder	+ 7.2		
Melanoma of skin	+ 2.9		
Brain	+ 2.3		
Falls		*Falls*	
Buccal cavity	−12.3	Buccal cavity	− 2.4
Stomach	−29.7	Stomach	−19.6
Liver, gallbladder, and biliary tract	− 3.8	Liver, gallbladder, and biliary tract	− 6.7
		Uterus	−26.8

[a]Cancer sites with a change in incidence of >2/100,000 have been shown.

showed appreciable increases (>2/100,000 in both sexes) between the Second and Third National Cancer Surveys.

The main inconsistencies between incidence and mortality trends lie in cancers of the colon, prostate, and urinary organs. All showed apparent large increases in incidence (in males at least), whereas only colon cancers showed an appreciable increase in mortality (in males), and then only to a smaller degree. The mortality from cancer of the colon in females fell. These divergent trends can be plausibly attributed to improving survival rates (Devesa and Silverman, 1978), but may also be due to problems in incidence measurement (Doll and Peto, 1981).

In a few instances, the factors involved in major trends in cancer incidence and mortality (in terms of changes in exposure to cancer risk factors) are fairly obvious, and this applies to the relationship between trends in lung cancer mortality and use of cigarettes (Doll and Peto, 1981). They are more often obscure, as in the falls in incidence of cancers of the stomach and uterus which still lack adequate explanations.

VARIATION IN CANCER INCIDENCE WITH GEOGRAPHY

Between countries

Table 7 provides a summary (Muir and Nectoux, 1982) of the variation in cancer incidence between countries, based on age-standardized rates measured by 60 cancer registries in 28 countries (Waterhouse *et al.*, 1976). Only the populations with the highest rates have been shown because many of the low-rate populations may have underestimated their rates and there were usually several populations at the lowest level. For the former reason some of the ratios of highest to lowest rates may overestimate the true range of variation.

The ratios in Table 7 emphasize that the incidence of cancer varies widely throughout the world and that for the cancer sites shown, the apparent variation was never less than fivefold, and was as high as 180-fold for non-melanotic cancer of the skin. Even the latter may underestimate the true variation because of the well-known difficulty in ascertaining all such cancers; its true rate in (non-Spanish) white males in El Paso, Texas may be higher than that shown. In addition, no current, accurate estimate of the incidence of this cancer in Queensland, Australia is available; it is commonly thought to be the highest in the world.

Other populations for which incidence rates of cancer are not readily available may also have higher rates than those shown in Table 7. Thus, for example, age-standardized mortality from cancer of the nasopharynx in Hong Kong males in 1975 was 17.0 per 100,000 (Aoki *et al.*, 1981), only slightly less than the incidence rate shown for this tumour in San Francisco Chinese males

Table 7 Populations showing the highest age-standardized incidence rates for particular cancers (from Waterhouse *et al.*, 1976)[a]

Cancer site	Sex	Highest incidence per 100,000	Rate	Ratio of highest to lowest rate
Lip	M	Newfoundland	27.1	90
Tongue	M	Bombay	12.6	25
Mouth	F	Singapore Indian	16.9	84
Oropharynx	M	Bombay	5.6	28
Nasopharynx	M	San Francisco Chinese	19.1	64
Hypopharynx	M	Bombay	7.7	38
Oesophagus	M	Bulawayo African	63.8	42
Stomach	M	Osaka	91.4	13
Colon	M	Connecticut	30.1	23
Rectum	M	Hawaii Chinese	20.4	17
Liver	M	Bulawayo African	64.6	81
Gallbladder, etc.	F	Warsaw City	13.8	20
Pancreas	M	Hawaii Hawaiian	15.8	10
Nose and sinuses	M	Osaka	2.6	9
Larynx	M	Sao Paulo	14.1	10
Lung	M	Liverpool	89.5	112
Bone	M	Zaragoza	3.0	5
Connective tissue	M	Hawaii Hawaiian	8.1	20
Melanoma of skin	F	New Zealand Non-Maori	11.7	58
Other skin	M	El Paso White	144.9	181
Breast	F	Hawaii Caucasian	80.3	7
Cervix uteri	F	El Paso Spanish	80.9	20
Corpus uteri	F	Alameda White	33.3	37
Ovary	F	Denmark	15.1	5
Other female genital	F	Okayama	5.6	14
Prostate	M	San Francisco Black	77.0	28
Testis	M	Denmark	4.9	24
Penis	M	Recife	6.8	17
Bladder	M	Bulawayo African	28.7	10
Other urinary organs	M	Iceland	12.2	11
Brain, etc.	M	Israel Jews	10.5	13
Thyroid	F	Hawaii Filipino	18.7	37
Lymphosarcoma, etc.	M	Ibadan	9.1	6
Hodgkin's disease	M	San Francisco White	4.7	6
Myeloma	M	San Francisco Black	8.2	16
Lymphatic leukaemia	M	Bulawayo African	7.5	12
Myeloid leukaemia	M	Alameda White	4.6	6

[a]Includes only cancers with maximum rates >2/100,000. Minimum rates were used for the calculation of ratios only if based on >10 cases.

(19.1 per 100,000). It is likely, therefore, that the incidence in Hong Kong Chinese males is higher than in San Francisco Chinese males; but probably higher again in Chinese males in parts of Guangdong Province in China itself (Armstrong, 1980).

Similarly, very high rates of cancer of the oesophagus are known to occur in central China, in Iran around the shores of the Caspian Sea, and in adjacent regions of the USSR (Armstrong, 1980). Age-standardized mortality from cancer of the oesophagus in essentially the whole of mainland China in 1973–75 was estimated at 31.7 per 100,000 in males, which is more than double the highest mortality rate (14.9 per 100,000 in males in Uruguay) listed by Aoki *et al.* (1981) for 1975. In 1973–75, Linxien County in Henan Province in China recorded a mortality from cancer of the oesophagus of 161.3 per 100,000 – more than double the incidence rate shown in Table 7 for Africans in Bulawayo, Zimbabwe.

Within countries

Variation in cancer incidence or mortality rates between different regions of single countries has also been described. These descriptions include cancer mortality by county in the USA (Mason *et al.*, 1975), an atlas of cancer mortality in China (Li *et al.*, 1981), the recently completed but not yet fully reported analysis of cancer mortality in local authority areas of England and Wales (Gardner *et al.*, 1982), and analysis of cancer mortality by prefecture in Japan (Kuroishi *et al.*, 1981).

The range of variation in cancer incidence between regions of a single country is likely to be less than that observed world-wide. The quality of the data, however, should be more uniform and, therefore, artefact is less likely to be responsible for variations observed. In the case of cancer mortality in 25 regions of the United States, observed variations exceeded threefold for cancers of the rectum, oesophagus, mouth and pharynx in white males and for cancer of the lip in white females. An additional nine sites of cancer in white males (including colon and lung) and six in white females (including rectum and oesophagus) varied more than twofold in cancer mortality (Blot and Fraumeni, 1982). Even more pronounced variation in cancer mortality by region was observed in the black population of the USA.

Interpretation of geographic variation

Variations in cancer incidence between geographic areas within and between countries can be used both to generate and explore hypotheses about cancer risk factors. For example, in the USA cancers of the colon and rectum showed similar geographic patterns, being most common in the northeast and least common in the south – a pattern at least superficially consistent with known gradients in dietary intake of fat and fibre (Blot and Fraumeni, 1982).

Cancers of the mouth and oesophagus in US males also showed high rates in the northeast, and an association with urbanization, due probably to their association with alcohol and tobacco use. In contrast, cancer of the mouth in females was highest in the rural south where it corresponded geographically to the chronic use of snuff.

In Britain, Gardner *et al.* (1982) showed that high rates of mesothelioma were found around the main ports where asbestos, particularly crocidolite, was used in shipbuilding and repairing; and also in London around an asbestos textile factory. Five local authority areas were found to have very high rates of cancer of the nose and sinuses. Three were already well known from studies of nasal cancer in the woodworking and boot and shoe industries while the other two were unsuspected.

VARIATION IN CANCER INCIDENCE ACCORDING TO PERSONAL CHARACTERISTICS

Sex

Surprisingly little attention has been paid to sex differences in cancer incidence. Table 8 shows ratios of male to female cancer incidence rates in Birmingham, England, in 1968–72 for organs common to both sexes (excluding breast). The most striking feature of this table is the preponderance of ratios greater than unity; in only 8 out of 29 cancer sites is the male/female ratio less than 1.5 and in only 4 is it less than 1.0 (Doll, 1976).

There are probably a number of factors contributing to this male excess of cancer. The largest excesses are for sites of tobacco carcinogenesis (lip, mouth, pharynx, larynx, lung, bladder, and kidneys), with or without interaction with some other factor such as occupational exposure to the sun in the case of cancer of the lip, alcohol in the case of cancers of the mouth, pharynx and larynx, and occupational exposure to chemicals for cancer of the bladder. Alcohol or occupational factors may also contribute to the male preponderance for cancers of the liver and skin and myeloid leukaemia.

The other male excesses of cancer do not have a ready environmental explanation. Is there, perhaps, an endogenous factor, such as capacity to inactivate carcinogens, which differs between males and females? There is at least some evidence for this possibility (Armstrong, 1982).

The cancers having a female excess may be of special interest – salivary gland, gallbladder and bile ducts, melanoma of the skin, and thyroid. A case can be made for the effects of endogenous hormonal factors in cancers of the gallbladder and bile ducts, cancer of the thyroid and, perhaps, melanoma (Armstrong, 1982). Melanoma excess may also be explained by differences between the sexes in their habits of sun exposure (Holman *et al.*, 1980).

Table 8   Sex ratios of age-standardized cancer incidence in Birmingham, England, 1968 to 1972 (from Doll, 1976)

Cancer site	Male/female ratio	Cancer site	Male/female ratio
Lip	18.0	Larynx	7.8
Tongue	2.7	Lung	6.8
Salivary gland	0.8	Connective tissue	1.5
Mouth	2.9	Melanoma of skin	0.6
Oropharynx	3.3	Other skin	1.6
Hypopharynx	1.4	Bladder	4.3
Oesophagus	1.9	Kidney, etc.	2.2
Stomach	2.1	Brain and nervous system	1.4
Colon	1.1	Thyroid	0.6
Rectum	1.9	Lymphosarcoma, etc.	1.6
Liver	1.8	Hodgkin's disease	1.6
Gallbladder, etc.	0.9	Myeloma	1.5
Pancreas	1.8	Lymphatic leukaemia	1.8
Nose, etc.	2.0	Myeloid leukaemia	1.2

[a]Includes only cancers for which the male or female age-standardized rate was greater than 1.0 per 100,000 per year.

Age

Variation in the incidence of cancer with age raises complex issues (Doll, 1971). Most cancers increase in incidence progressively with age and the increase generally fits a simple power function in which incidence varies approximately as the fourth power of age. This relationship may indicate an effect of ageing on susceptibility to cancer, or that age is highly correlated with duration of exposure and time since first exposure to the relevant carcinogens. For lung cancer (at least in smokers) the relevant variable is probably duration of cigarette smoking rather than age (Doll and Peto, 1978).

Figure 3 illustrates the marked complexity of the relationship of cancer incidence with age which may apply in some cases. Over all body sites, the incidence of melanoma in both males and females increases progressively with age, although there is a plateau around the age of menopause in females which has been taken by some to suggest an effect of endogenous hormones on risk of melanoma (Sadoff *et al.*, 1973). However, the age incidence curves by body sites (Figure 3) show that the overall curve is made up of several quite different components. At one extreme we have the progressively rising

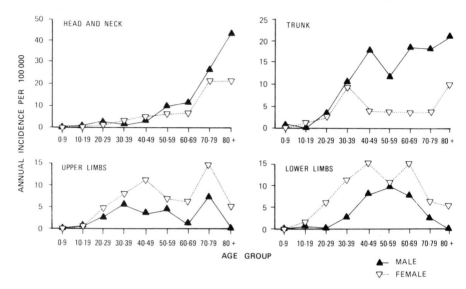

Figure 3   Annual incidence of invasive melanoma of the skin by body site in Western Australia, 1975 to 1976. (From Holman *et al.*, 1980. Published with permission of the Editor *International Journal of Cancer.*)

incidence in head and neck melanoma; at the other extreme, the rise, peak, then fall of incidence with age for melanoma on the lower limbs.

The pattern of incidence of melanoma of the head and neck is what would reasonably be expected from the fact that these sites are more or less continuously exposed to the sun throughout life. The peak followed by a fall in incidence of melanoma on the lower limbs may be the result of intense exposure of the legs to the sun during recreation in teenage and early adult life but with reduced exposure thereafter. For melanoma also, therefore, it may be that exposure to the relevant risk factors rather than age itself is the main determinant of the relationship between incidence and age.

Place of birth

Study of the variation of cancer incidence by place of birth in migrating populations has contributed to the explanation of some geographical variations in cancer incidence. If, where migration occurs along a gradient of cancer incidence, it can be shown that cancer incidence in the migrants is initially similar to that in their home country but, over time following migration, deviates towards that in their host country, it may be inferred that the observed geographical difference is due to environmental factors rather than to artefact or genetic differences between the compared populations.

Most interest in cancer epidemiology has focused on the experience of Asian populations, particularly the Japanese and Chinese, migrating to the USA (Locke and King, 1980; King and Locke, 1980). For example, in Japanese migrants, mortality from cancers of the oesophagus and stomach, initially high, has fallen while mortality from cancers of the colon, ovary and prostate and lymphoma, initially low, has risen (Locke and King, 1980). For some cancer sites, notably breast, the observed rise in mortality has been delayed until the generation born in the USA of Japanese parentage. This pattern suggests either that environment in early life is of predominant importance or that acculturation in ways relevant to breast cancer may have been delayed until the first post-migration generation.

A more detailed illustration of the effect of country of birth on cancer risk is given in Table 9 for lung cancer in male migrants to Australia. This table updates data originally published by McCall and Stenhouse (1971). The highest relative rates of lung cancer were in those born in Britain. This would be expected from the fact that male incidence rates of lung cancer in Britain are the highest in the world (Table 7). The pattern of variation by duration of residence in Australia, however, is unusual (Table 10).

Relative rates are comparatively low in recent migrants, much higher in intermediate-term migrants, and then lower again in long-term migrants. The initially low rate is suggestive of what might be called 'the healthy migrant effect'; that is, people who are sick and likely to die soon from lung cancer are unlikely to migrate. The effect of this selection on mortality becomes less with time after migration and so the intermediate-term rate in migrants is high. The later fall in mortality with long duration of residence may indicate either the operation of environmental factors in Australia to lower lung cancer mortality or the removal of adverse factors present in the British environment.

Other variables

Appreciable variation in cancer incidence can also be shown when populations are categorized by ethnic origin (Mason *et al.*, 1976), marital status (Ernster *et al.*, 1979), religion (Phillips *et al.*, 1980) or occupation (Office of Population Censuses and Surveys, 1978). In each case high and low risk populations can be identified, study of which may lead to further insights into the causes of cancer.

As an example, in 1970–72 mortality from cancer of the cervix in England and Wales varied four-fold between a low in women in social class I (classified according to their husbands' occupations) and a high in women in social class

Table 9   Ratios of age-standardized mortality from lung cancer in male migrants to Australia to that in native-born Australian males in the period 1962 to 1971[a]

Country of birth	Standardized mortality ratio	
	Point estimate	95% Confidence interval
Australia	1.00	—
New Zealand	1.18	1.02–1.36
England	1.53	1.48–1.59
Wales	2.28	1.96–2.66
Scotland	1.95	1.84–2.08
Ireland	1.43	1.27–1.61
Austria	0.76	0.53–1.09
Czechoslovakia	1.08	0.71–1.64
Germany	1.20	1.02–1.43
Greece	1.03	0.86–1.22
Hungary	1.26	0.97–1.64
Italy	1.02	0.92–1.13
Malta	1.51	1.20–1.89
Holland	1.75	1.48–2.06
Poland	1.29	1.08–1.54
Scandinavia	1.35	1.14–1.61
USSR	1.10	0.92–1.31
Yugoslavia	1.66	1.38–1.99
Elsewhere in Europe	1.06	0.89–1.25
India or Pakistan	1.26	0.96–1.66
Elsewhere in Asia	1.02	0.84–1.24
United Arab Republic	1.11	0.74–1.65
Elsewhere in Africa	1.25	0.92–1.69
USA	1.23	0.88–1.71
Elsewhere in America	1.50	1.09–2.06

[a]Confined to those aged 40+ years.

V (Office of Population Censuses and Surveys, 1978). Does it seem reasonable to attribute this to variations in sexual activity, based on present concepts of the aetiology of cancer of the cervix? If not, study of this situation may lead to identification of new risk factors for cancer of the cervix; carcinogens from the husbands' workplaces have been put forward as one possibility (Robinson, 1982).

Table 10   Mortality ratios from lung cancer in male British migrants to Australia according to duration of residence in Australia[a]

Country of birth	Duration of residence (years)	Standardized mortality ratio	
		Point estimate	95% Confidence interval
England	0– 5	1.94	1.72–2.18
	6–16	2.23	2.03–2.44
	17+	1.43	1.37–1.50
Wales	0– 5	2.66	1.45–4.90
	6–16	4.52	2.86–7.16
	17+	2.10	1.76–2.51
Scotland	0– 5	2.85	2.23–3.63
	6–16	2.42	2.00–2.93
	17+	1.88	1.74–2.02
Ireland	0– 5	1.71	1.04–2.82
	6–16	2.28	1.59–3.27
	17+	1.33	1.15–1.53

[a]Relative to rates in native-born Australian males; confined to those aged 40+ years.

REFERENCES

Aoki, K., Tominaga, S., and Kuroishi, T. (1981). Age-adjusted death rates for cancer by site (ICD 8th Revision) in 50 countries in 1975. In *Cancer mortality and morbidity statistics. Japan and the world* (eds M. Segi, S. Tominaga, K. Aoki, and I. Fujimoto). GANN Monograph on cancer research, No. 26. Tokyo: Japan Scientific Societies Press, p. 251.

Armstrong, B. (1980). The epidemiology of cancer in the People's Republic of China. *International Journal of Epidemiology,* **9,** 305.

Armstrong, B. (1982). Endocrine factors in human carcinogenesis. In *Host factors in human carcinogenesis.* (eds H. Bartsch and B. Armstrong). *IARC Scientific Publications,* No. 39. Lyon: International Agency for Research on Cancer, p. 193.

Blot, W. J., and Fraumeni, J. F. (1982). Geographic epidemiology of cancer in the United States. In *Cancer epidemiology and prevention.* (eds D. Schottenfeld and J. F. Fraumeni). Philadelphia: W. B. Saunders, p. 179.

Davies, J. M. (1977). Two aspects of the epidemiology of bladder cancer in England and Wales. *Proceedings of the Royal Society of Medicine,* **70,** 411.

Devesa, S. S., and Silverman, D. T. (1978). Cancer incidence and mortality trends in the United States: 1935–74. *Journal of the National Cancer Institute,* **60,** 545.

Doll, R. (1971). The age distribution of cancer. Implications for models of carcinogenesis. *Journal of the Royal Statistical Society, Series A,* **134,** 133.

Doll, R. (1976). Comparison between registries age-standardized rates. In *Cancer incidence in five continents*, Vol. 3. (eds J. Waterhouse, C. Muir, P. Correa, and J. Powell). IARC Scientific Publications, No. 15. Lyon: International Agency for Research on Cancer, p. 453.

Doll, R. (1979). The pattern of disease in the post-infection era: national trends. *Proceedings of the Royal Society of London, B*, **205**, 47.

Doll, R., and Peto, R. (1978). Cigarette smoking and bronchial carcinoma. Dose and time relationships among regular smokers and life-long non-smokers. *Journal of Epidemiology and Community Health*, **32**, 303.

Doll, R., and Peto, R. (1981). *The causes of cancer*. Quantitative estimates of avoidable risks of cancer in the United States today. New York: Oxford University Press.

Dougan, L. E., Matthews, M. L. V., and Armstrong, B. K. (1981). The effect of diagnostic review on the estimated incidence of lymphatic and haematopoietic neoplasms in Western Australia. *Cancer*, **48**, 866.

Ernster, W. L., Sacks, S. T., Selvin, S., and Petrakis, N. (1979). Cancer incidence by marital status: US Third national cancer survey. *Journal of the National Cancer Institute*, **63**, 567.

Fleming, N. T., Armstrong, B. K., Sheiner, H. J., and James, I. R. (1981). Occurrence of breast cancer in Australian women. *Medical Journal of Australia*, **1**, 289.

Gardner, M. J., Winter, P. D., and Acheson, E. D. (1982). Variations in cancer mortality among local authority areas in England and Wales: relations with environmental factors and search for causes. *British Medical Journal*, **284**, 784.

Holman, D., and Armstrong, B. (1982). *Cancer mortality trends in Australia 1910–1979*. Perth: Cancer Council of Western Australia.

Holman, C. D. J., James, I. R., Segal, M. R., and Armstrong, B. K. (1981). Recent trends in mortality from prostate cancer in male populations of Australia and England and Wales. *British Journal of Cancer*, **44**, 340.

Holman, C. D. J., Mulroney, C. D., and Armstrong, B. K. (1980). Epidemiology of pre-invasive and invasive malignant melanoma in Western Australia. *International Journal of Cancer*, **25**, 317.

Institute of Cancer Research (1976). *Serial mortality tables, neoplastic diseases*, Vol. 1. *England and Wales*. London: Institute of Cancer Research.

King, H., and Locke, F. B. (1980). Cancer mortality among Chinese in the United States. *Journal of the National Cancer Institute*, **5**, 1141.

Kuroishi, T., Tominaga, S., Hirose, K. *et al.* (1981). Cancer mortality in Japan. In *Cancer mortality and morbidity statistics. Japan and the world* (eds M. Segi, S. Tominaga, K. Aoki, and I. Fujimoto). GANN Monograph on cancer research, No. 26. Tokyo: Japan Scientific Societies Press, p. 1.

Li Jun-Yao, Liu Be-Qi, Li Guang-Yi *et al.* (1981). Atlas of cancer mortality in the People's Republic of China. An aid for cancer control and research. *International Journal of Epidemiology*, **10**, 127.

Locke, F. B., and King, H. (1980). Cancer mortality risk among Japanese in the United States. *Journal of the National Cancer Institute*, **65**, 1149.

MacLennan, R., Muir, C., Steinitz, R., and Winkler, A. (1975). *Cancer registration and its techniques*. IARC Scientific Publications, No. 21. Lyon: International Agency for Research on Cancer.

Mason, T. J., McKay, F. W., Hoover, R. *et al.* (1975). *Atlas of cancer mortality for US Counties 1950–1969*, Washington: US Department of Health, Education and Welfare.

Mason, T. J., McKay, F. W., Hoover, R. *et al.* (1976). *Atlas of cancer mortality among US non-whites 1950–1969.* Washington: US Department of Health, Education and Welfare.

McCall, M. G., and Stenhouse, N. S. (1971). Deaths from lung cancer in Australia. *Medical Journal of Australia*, **1**, 524.

McMichael, A. J. (1978). Increases in laryngeal cancer in Britain and Australia in relation to alcohol and tobacco consumption trends. *Lancet*, **1**, 1244.

McMichael, A. J. (1979). Alimentary tract cancer in Australia in relation to diet and alcohol. *Nutrition and Cancer*, **1**, 82.

Muir, C. S., and Nectoux, J. (1982). International patterns of cancer. In *Cancer epidemiology and prevention* (eds D. Schottenfeld and J. F. Fraumeni). Philadelphia: W. B. Saunders, p. 119.

Muir, C., and Waterhouse, J. (1976). Reliability of registration. In *Cancer incidence in five continents*, Vol. 3. (eds J. Waterhouse, C. Muir, P. Correa, and J. Powell). IARC Scientific Publications, No. 15. Lyon: International Agency for Research on Cancer, p. 45.

Office of Population Censuses and Surveys (1978). *Occupational mortality.* The Registrar General's decennial supplement for England and Wales, 1970–72. London: Her Majesty's Stationery Office.

Percy, C., Stanek, E., and Gloeckler, L. (1981). Accuracy of cancer death certificates and its effect on cancer mortality statistics. *American Journal of Public Health*, **71**, 242.

Phillips, R. L., Garfinkel, L., Kuzma, J. W. *et al.* (1980). Mortality among California Seventh-Day Adventists for selected cancer sites. *Journal of the National Cancer Institute*, **65**, 1097.

Robinson, J. (1982). Cancer of the cervix: Occupational risks of husbands and wives and possible preventive strategies. In *Pre-clinical neoplasia of the cervix* (ed. J. A. Jordan). *Proceedings of the ninth study group of the Royal College of Obstetricians and Gynaecologists, 1981.* London: Royal College of Obstetricians and Gynaecologists.

Sadoff, L., Winkley, J., and Tyson, S. (1973). Is malignant melanoma an endocrine-dependent tumor? The possible effects of estrogen. *Oncology*, **27**, 244.

Saxen, E. A. (1982). Trends: Facts or fallacy. In *Trends in cancer incidence, causes and practical implications* (ed. K. Magnus). Washington: Hemisphere Publishing, p. 5.

Segi, M., Aoki, K., and Kurihara, M. (1981). World cancer mortality. In *Cancer mortality and morbidity statistics, Japan and the world* (eds M. Segi, S. Tominaga, K. Aoki, and I. Fujimoto). GANN Monograph on Cancer Research, No. 26. Tokyo: Japan Scientific Societies Press, p. 121.

Stevens, R. G., Moolgavkar, S. H., and Lee, J. A. (1982). Temporal trends in breast cancer. *American Journal of Epidemiology*, **115**, 759.

Waterhouse, J., Muir, C., Correa, P., and Powell, J. (eds) (1976). *Cancer incidence in five continents*, Vol. 3. IARC Scientific Publication, No. 15. Lyon: International Agency for Research on Cancer.

World Health Organization (1979). *Cancer statistics.* Report of a WHO–IARC Expert Committee, Technical Report series, No. 632. Geneva: World Health Organization.

Risk Factors and Multiple Cancer
Edited by B.A. Stoll
© 1984 John Wiley and Sons Ltd.

Chapter

9   B. A. J. PONDER

Role of Genetic and Familial Factors

Cancer is not generally regarded as a disease with a major inherited component. The results of epidemiological studies (Higginson, 1969; Peto and Doll, 1981) suggest that about 80% of cancer incidence may be attributable to environmental factors. Although this has directed attention to the potential for prevention of cancer by avoiding environmental carcinogens, there is a danger that the contribution of genetic factors and their implications for clinical management and for research may be overlooked. This aspect will be discussed under the following headings:

– Inherited factors and cancer risk.
– Inherited disorders predisposing to cancer.
– Familial aggregation of cancer.
– Clinical implications.

INHERITED FACTORS AND CANCER RISK

The strongest evidence for genetically determined susceptibility to cancer in man comes from the cancers which are inherited in a pattern consistent with a single Mendelian trait. These include retinoblastoma, the multiple endocrine neoplasia syndromes, familial polyposis coli, and the recessively inherited chromosomal instability syndromes such as Bloom's syndrome. Although only a small minority, these inherited cancer syndromes are of clinical importance because of the opportunities they provide for screening and early diagnosis, and because of the need for family counselling. They can also provide vital information about the processes involved in carcinogenesis.

Apart from the inherited cancer syndromes, most of the cancers at the common sites show only a slight degree of familial aggregation. Review of some 15,000 British families in which one or more children developed cancer under the age of 15 showed that, after tumours with a known genetic basis such as retinoblastoma were excluded, the risk among siblings of affected children was about twice normal, overall and for individual types of cancer (Draper *et al.*, 1977). Many of the common adult cancers show a consistent two- to fourfold risk for relatives of patients, compared to control relatives or the general population (Anderson, 1975).

Twin studies show at the most, only a slightly greater concordance for cancer in monozygous than in dizygous twins, a comparison which helps to minimize the effects of shared environment (Holm *et al.*, 1982). The obvious inference that inherited factors are unimportant in the great majority of cancers may not, however, be correct. Peto (1980) has shown that a considerable degree of inherited predisposition may be present without giving rise to marked family clustering. Where almost all the incidence of a cancer occurs in a minority of genetically predisposed individuals, there may be almost no familial aggregation.

Interaction between environmental and genetic factors might, therefore, provide the basis for a substantial individual variation in susceptibility to cancer which is so far largely unrecognized. The best-known example is xeroderma pigmentosum (XP), in which an inherited defect in the enzyme systems for repair of ultraviolet light damage to DNA is associated with the development of multiple cancers in skin exposed to sunlight (Robbins, 1978). Better understanding of similar interactions would have major implications for cancer prevention.

Before discussing individual examples of inherited cancer risk in more detail, it may be helpful to review briefly current ideas about the process of development of a cancer. All inherited predisposition must ultimately operate by increasing the probability of one or other of the steps involved in carcinogenesis. The development of a cancer may take many years: the peak incidence of leukaemia attributable to the atomic bombings in Japan, for example, occurred eight years later; and the excess incidence of solid tumours was still rising after 20 years (Cairns, 1978). Both experimental and epidemiological evidence indicates that a number of distinct steps is involved. The experimental evidence originates with the work of Berenblum and is fully discussed in Chapter 1.

The epidemiological evidence for multiple steps in carcinogenesis derives largely from studies of age-related variation in the incidence of cancers at specific sites. The incidence of most common cancers of man and animals rises steeply with age. That time, rather than age *per se*, is the important factor is suggested by the results of experiments in which carcinogens were applied to animals of different ages (Peto *et al.*, 1975).

For many common human cancers a log/log plot of cancer incidence against age (or time of exposure to a carcinogen) yields a straight line, the slope of which is about five. In other words, for those cancers, incidence is related to approximately the fifth power of time, and a possible explanation of this relationship is that a number of separate time-dependent events must occur before a cancer is produced (Peto, 1976).

Individuals who have inherited one of the steps in the development of a cancer, or a predisposition for it to occur, will be more likely to develop multiple tumours. On average, the first of these tumours will occur at a younger age than in the general population. Examples in which such a pattern has suggested an hereditary component to various tumours will be described below.

The evidence at present favours the concept that most cancers originate from a mutation in a somatic cell. Stable changes in gene expression may of course occur without mutation. Such 'epigenetic' changes are thought to be the basis of cell differentiation during development. In mice, teratomas can be induced by explanting early embryos to an ectopic site such as the kidney capsule (Martin, 1975), and since there is no evident mutation, these tumours are thought to arise as a result of epigenetic events. There is no evidence at present to say whether or not the development of all naturally occurring human cancers involves a mutational step.

The nature of promotion, the stages which are supposed to follow the initial mutation, is still quite unclear. Experimental evidence suggests that there may be at least two components, one involving a 'resetting' of the controls of gene expression in a pattern inappropriate for the cell, and the other a stimulus to proliferation (Slaga *et al.*, 1980). Agents which induce disordered tissue organization of proliferation are found experimentally to have a promoting effect. One might speculate, therefore, that inherited abnormalities in the genes controlling cellular interactions or differentiation might have a disruptive effect on the organization of a tissue, and so provide another mechanism for inherited predisposition to cancer.

INHERITED DISORDERS PREDISPOSING TO CANCER

There are difficulties in the classification of the inherited conditions which carry an increased risk of cancer in man, but a suggested scheme which groups the conditions by possible mechanisms of predisposition is shown in Table 1.

Constitutional chromosomal abnormalities

A few conditions have been described in which a constitutional chromosome abnormality – that is, one present in every cell in the body – is associated with an increased risk of cancer. The increased cancer risk usually forms part of a

Table 1   Examples of inherited disorders associated with an increased risk of cancer

---

1. **Constitutional chromosomal abnormalities**
   Down's syndrome
   Klinefelter's syndrome

2. **Mendelian traits**[a]
   (a)   'Inherited cancer syndromes'
         Retinoblastoma
         Familial polyposis coli
         Multiple endocrine neoplasia syndromes

   (b)   Inherited preneoplastic states
         (i) DNA repair defects and chromosomal instability syndromes:
             xeroderma pigmentosum; Fanconi; Bloom's;
             ataxia telangiectasia

         (ii) Disturbances of tissue organization
             (a)   Hamartomatous syndromes: Peutz–Jegher's; Cowden;
                   neurofibromatosis
             (b)   Other conditions in which disturbance of tissue proliferation,
                   differentiation or organization is associated with increased
                   cancer risk:
                   ? Disorders of skin keratinization
                   ? Alpha-1- anti-trypsin deficiency

         (iii) Immune deficiency syndromes

         (iv) Metabolic variation:
                   Albinism
                   ? Aryl hydrocarbon hydroxylase inducibility
                   ? Variations in œstrogen metabolism

3. **Multifactorial predisposition**
   Ethnic cancer differences
   Familial cancer aggregations

---

[a] For an extended list, see Mulvihill (1977), Gorlin (1977).

syndrome of physical anomalies, and the risk is confined to cancers of one or a few types. This is in contrast to the hereditary syndromes of chromosome breakage (described later) in which there is probably a more general increase in cancer risk. The disorders fall into two groups, according to how direct the correspondence is between the presence of the chromosomal abnormality and the appearance of the cancer.

In the first group, the link seems to be less clearly direct. In Down's syndrome, trisomy 21 is associated with the features of mongolism, and also with a substantially increased incidence of leukaemia although by no means every affected individual develops leukaemia (Miller, 1970). There is no conclusive evidence of an increased risk of other malignancies, nor of increased risk of leukaemia in the families as a whole (Miller, 1970).

Klinefelter's syndrome consists of an abnormality of sexual differentiation, in which male phenotype is associated with eunuchoid habitus and dysgenesis of seminiferous tubules, and with one or more extra X chromosomes. There is gynaecomastia, and a risk of breast cancer at least 20 times that in normal males (Scheike *et al.*, 1973; Jackson *et al.*, 1965). It is uncertain whether there is also an increased risk of leukaemia and lymphoma (Miller, 1966; Sohn and Boggs, 1974).

Other constitutional chromosomal abnormalities of the sex chromosomes are associated with gonadal dysgenesis. In dysgenetic gonads in which a Y chromosome is present in a phenotypically female environment, there is a high risk of gonadal malignancy (Simpson and Photopoulos, 1976).

A variety of constitutional deletions or translocations involving autosomes has been reported, but except in the specific instances described below, there is insufficient evidence to link these to either a particular or a general increased cancer risk. A search for chromosomal abnormalities in the cultured peripheral blood lymphocytes of 3068 patients attending a radiotherapy department in Edinburgh (O'Riordan *et al.*, 1972) showed no difference in the incidence of either aneuploidy or balanced rearrangements compared with' a selected normal population. The inference is that gross constitutional chromosomal abnormalities of this kind are not an important source of increased cancer risk in the general population.

In the second group of constitutional chromosomal abnormalities, the link with the development of the cancer appears to be more direct. They include: a deletion in the long arm of chromosome 13 in some patients with retinoblastoma; a deletion in the short arm of chromosome 11 in patients with the familial Wilm's tumour – aniridia syndrome; a translocation between chromosomes 3 and 8 in a family with renal cell carcinoma; and a possible deletion in chromosome 2 in families with polyposis and colon cancer (Harnden and Herbert, 1982). As the resolution of techniques for studying chromosomes improves, it is possible that other linked abnormalities will be discovered.

The constitutional chromosomal abnormalities may reflect the operation of the same mechanisms as the rearrangement of specific chromosomal segments which are described in the cancer cells of non-hereditary cancers (Klein, 1981). Some lymphoproliferative disorders, for example, are associated with consistent rearrangements of the chromosomal segments bearing the immunoglobulin genes. Chromosomal rearrangements which predispose to cancer may do so by bringing together genes and genetic controlling sequences which are not normally associated (Sager, 1979; Ponder, 1980; Cairns, 1981).

Recent advances in molecular genetics have already led to the identification of genes involved in some of these chromosomal events. Some appear to be homologues of the transforming genes carried by the RNA tumour viruses (Cooper, 1982), which are also active in the experimental transfer of the malignant phenotype from cancer cells to other cells in culture by means of DNA fragments (Logan and Cairns, 1982). These new developments promise the most important advances in our understanding of carcinogenesis and in the case of the inherited cancer syndromes, identification of these genes may provide markers to detect family members at high risk.

The next two sections will deal with a group of inherited neoplasms or preneoplastic disorders based on uncommon Mendelian traits. They have attracted a good deal of interest because of the possibility (as for chromosomal deletions in the last section) that elucidation of the inherited defect will throw light on the processes of carcinogenesis, and possibly prevent cancer by identification of individuals at high risk.

Inherited cancer syndromes

This group includes retinoblastoma, familial polyposis coli, and the multiple endocrine neoplasia syndromes. (For detailed reviews, see Mulvihill *et al.*, 1977; Knudson *et al.*, 1973; Knudson, 1977b; Harnden and Herbert, 1982).

Retinoblastoma

About 40% of cases of retinoblastoma are hereditary, and the rest sporadic (Knudson, 1971). In inherited cases the tumours are commonly multiple and bilateral, and they develop earlier than in sporadic cases. Even in inherited cases the number of tumours is obviously very small compared to the number of retinal cells at risk, and so at least one further event appears to be necessary for the inherited defect to be manifest as a tumour. The number of tumours in hereditary cases follows a Poisson distribution about a mean of 3–4 (Knudson *et al.*, 1975), whereas the incidence of retinoblastoma in individuals without a predisposing gene is 1 in 30,000. The gene, therefore, confers about a 100,000-fold increased risk.

These observations led Knudson *et al.* (1973) to propose a general model for inherited cancers in which the hereditary form of the tumour is the result of two events: a germinal mutation affecting all the retinal cells, and a second somatic mutation affecting one or a small number. Two events are also needed for the development of the sporadic tumours, but both must occur in the same somatic cell. The evidence that the second step in retinoblastoma is mutational was based on the pattern of incidence of the tumours with time, which was thought to be that expected if their development required a single random event.

Re-examination of the data on tumour incidence suggests, however, an alternative explanation (Matsunaga, 1979). Firstly, bilateral tumours occur too closely linked in time to be consistent with the occurrence of separate random events. Secondly, the degree of expression of the gene (reflected in the occurrence of bilateral, unilateral or no tumours in gene carriers) tends to vary between families. Thirdly, the distribution of gene carriers with bilateral, unilateral, and no tumours does not fit that expected if the development of each tumour is determined separately by a second, random event.

Matsunaga, therefore, envisages the interaction of more than one gene in the expression of the retinoblastoma phenotype. The dominant susceptibility gene for retinoblastoma may act not as an inherited initiating mutation, but through influencing the probability of emergence of a tumour from already initiated cells at some specific stage in retinal development.

Familial polyposis coli

Hereditary adenomatosis of the colon and rectum (ACR) is a single-gene disorder, inherited in an autosomal dominant pattern, associated with the development in early adult life of multiple polyps of the colon and rectum. The polyps have a high malignant potential, and affected individuals almost invariably develop one or more malignant tumours by the age of 50 unless prophylactic colectomy is carried out (Alm and Licznerski, 1973). Carcinoma in polyposis coli develops through several intermediate stages of epithelial change and polyp formation (Hill *et al.*, 1978), and occurs at a much later age than the tumours in retinoblastoma so one might suppose that the number of events involved in colonic carcinogenesis is greater (Fisher, 1958; Ashley, 1969; Knudson, 1977a).

Phenotypic abnormalities have been recognized in patients with familial polyposis which may give a clue to the mechanisms of cancer development. They comprise proliferative abnormalities of the colonic epithelium preceding polyp formation and also abnormalities of cultured skin fibroblasts (Deschner and Lipkin, 1975; Pfeffer and Kopelovich, 1977; Kopelovich, 1982).

In normal colonic epithelium, the epithelial cells differentiate as they migrate to the surface of the mucosa, and their ability to proliferate, as measured by DNA synthesis, is lost. In ACR, there is failure of this mechanism, so that throughout the mucosa there are foci of epithelial cells at the surface which have retained the ability to proliferate. Subsequently, these cells accumulate and form the adenomatous polyps, some of which progress to malignancy.

The abnormalities in cultured skin fibroblasts have been described both in classical ACR and in Gardner's syndrome, a closely related condition in which colonic polyposis of the ACR type is associated with multiple benign tumours of connective tissue in other organs (Davies *et al.*, 1977). These abnormalities are said not to be present in the general population of patients with or without colon cancer. The phenotypic abnormalities in the fibroblast in culture are a subset of those associated with experimentally induced malignant transformation. In addition, the cells have increased susceptibility to transformation by certain tumour viruses, and they are abnormally sensitive to the effects of phorbol ester tumour promoters (Kopelovich, 1982).

The explanation of these abnormalities and their significance in relation to colonic carcinogenesis is not yet understood. It is hoped that they may provide phenotypic markers for the early detection of gene carriers, a possibility which is being tested at present. Even though closely linked, it is not necessary that they be implicated in the cause of the colonic cancer.

Multiple endocrine neoplasia type 2 (MEN 2: Sipple's syndrome)

A number of inherited tumour syndromes involve tissues which are derived embryologically from neural crest (reviewed by Schimke, 1977). MEN 2 consists of medullary thyroid carcinoma, which arises from the parafollicular or C-cells of the thyroid, and (in some families) phaeochromocytoma, which arises from the cells of the adrenal medulla. In a rare variant, MEN 2b, these tumours are also associated with neuromas of the oral cavity and eyelids, and a variety of other physical abnormalities including features of Marfan's syndrome. The syndrome is inherited in an autosomal dominant pattern but, as with the other tumours which form part of inherited cancer syndromes, sporadic cases also occur. Tumours in the inherited cases show the expected multiplicity and early age of onset, compared with sporadic cases.

Development of the tumours occurs through a preceding stage of hyperplasia, and it has been claimed that the presence of multiple foci of hyperplasia in thyroid or adrenal accompanying the tumours is pathognomic of the inherited form of the syndrome (Jackson *et al.*, 1979). Studies of the clonality of each of the multiple tumours in thyroid and adrenal using the X-linked glucose phosphate dehydrogenase marker have shown that while each tumour is clonal, different tumours are derived from different progenitors (Baylin *et al.*, 1978). It seems, therefore, that the inherited defect in MEN 2 cases affects cells of neural crest origin (in some families only the C-cell lineage, but in others the adrenal medullary lineage also) in such a way that they are subsequently at increased risk of undergoing an event which leads to clonal proliferation and subsequent neoplasia.

Because C-cells secrete calcitonin, and adrenal medullary cells secrete catecholamines, there are markers available for the diagnosis of the inherited syndrome at the stage of hyperplasia (Wells *et al.*, 1978). Screening of family members might seem worthwhile because surgery of both thyroid and adrenal tumours at an early stage should be curative, but in practice, the difficulty of distinguishing sporadic from familial cases and the variability of the natural history of untreated tumours raise a variety of problems. These will be discussed with other implications of genetic cancer risk in the last section of this chapter.

Inherited preneoplastic states

Separate classification of this group is based on the concept that the inherited defect facilitates the processes of carcinogenesis, rather than constituting itself one of the steps, as was suggested might be the case in the hereditary neoplasms.

Chromosomal instability syndromes and xeroderma pigmentosum

A number of rare autosomal recessive inherited syndromes have been described in which chromosomal instability, leading to an increased incidence of chromosomal rearrangements, is associated with an increased risk of malignancy. The best known of these disorders are Bloom's syndrome, Fanconi's anaemia, and ataxia telangiectasia. These have been extensively reviewed (German, 1972) and will not be described in detail here.

Often included in discussion of the chromosomal instability syndromes is xeroderma pigmentosum (XP), a genetically heterogeneous group of disorders (also inherited in an autosomal recessive fashion) which have in common impaired ability to repair ultraviolet-induced damage to DNA, and a very high incidence of cancer of exposed skin (Cleaver and Bootsma, 1975; Robbins, 1978). XP cannot strictly be described as a chromosomal instability disorder, because there is no increase in spontaneous chromosome aberrations. XP cells do, however, respond to damage induced by ultraviolet light or by a variety of chemical mutagens with an increased level of chromosome aberrations compared with normal cells (Wolff *et al.*, 1977).

The XP syndrome is of considerable scientific interest because it provides one of the most direct pieces of evidence linking damage to DNA with the development of tumours. It is also of clinical significance as an example of an inherited syndrome in which the mechanism of predisposition to cancer is known, so that rational preventive action can be applied (by avoidance of sunlight) to minimize the chances of cancer developing.

Although the same abnormalities in DNA repair are present in all tissues of affected individuals with XP, it has been suggested that the excess risk of cancer does not extend to tissues other than skin (German, 1972; Cairns, 1981). If true, this is rather surprising, since many putative carcinogens are thought to act by causing DNA damage of a type to which XP cells would be expected to be abnormally sensitive. This has led to the suggestion (Cairns, 1981) that such mutational events are not, after all, rate-limiting in carcinogenesis in the majority of human cancers.

Disturbances of tissue organization

There may be distinct varieties of disruption of tissue organization which, although not themselves neoplastic, predispose to the development of cancer.

(a) *Hamartomatous syndromes*   Hamartomas are focal benign tissue abnormalities whose hallmark is tissue malformation; there is disordered arrangement of tissue elements which are otherwise normal and indigenous to that tissue. The majority of the hamartomas show an autosomal dominant pattern of inheritance and some examples are given in Table 1. In most of these conditions there is probably a small increased risk of benign or malignant neoplastic change, but the rarity of the conditions prevents accurate determination of the excess risk.

In the gastrointestinal tract two hamartomatous syndromes are recognized: Peutz–Jegher's syndrome and juvenile polyposis (Alm and Licznerski, 1973). Both are characterized by multiple gastrointestinal polyps. A few cases of malignancy of the small intestine (which is otherwise rare) have been described in patients with Peutz–Jegher's syndrome, and in some it seems probable that the malignancy arose in a polyp. Even so, the presence of an excess risk of cancer in this condition has been a matter of debate (Morson and Dawson, 1972). The malignant propensity in juvenile polyposis seems better established, at least in one kindred (Stemper *et al.*, 1975), but here the carcinomas described were not closely related to the polyps in time or location. This suggests that the increased risk of malignancy may be related to a second action of the gene, rather than resulting directly from the tissue disorganization within the polyps.

In addition to the syndromes which fulfil the histological criteria for hamartoses, there are a large number of disorders in which benign focal abnormalities of different tissues occur in consistent associations, in some cases with an apparently increased risk of malignancy in one or more sites (Mulvihill, 1977; Warkany, 1977). For example, Cowden syndrome (Gentry *et al.*, 1974) consists of a variety of benign lesions of certain areas of the skin, which histologically have a variety of patterns; fibroadenomatosis, virginal hypertrophy, and carcinoma of the breast; adenoma and follicular carcinoma of the thyroid; soft-tissue 'neoplasms' including ovarian cysts, neuromas of the acoustic nerve, lipomas and angiomas of various tissues and polyps of the gastrointestinal tract (with in some cases adenocarcinoma). This disorder is often called 'multiple hamartoma syndrome' but it is not clear whether all of the lesions are in fact hamartomata, nor what is the link that binds them together.

A similar example is the naevoid basal cell carcinoma syndrome, in which development of multiple skin carcinomas is associated with skeletal abnorma-litics, fibromas of the ovary, mesenteric cysts, and medulloblastoma. In this case, the development of the basal cell carcinomas is markedly enhanced by radiation used to treat the associated brain tumour (Strong, 1977).

(b) *Skin cancers associated with syndromes of abnormal keratinization* The inherited syndromes of abnormal keratinization of the skin provide a series of examples within a single tissue of the apparent association of disturbances of tissue organization with an increased risk of cancer. Once again the mechan-ism of cause and effect is hard to define.

Porokeratosis (Cort and Abdel Aziz, 1972; Guss *et al.*, 1971) is a rare condition characterized by skin lesions between 2 mm and 20 mm in diameter, which consist of a peripheral zone of hyperkeratosis surrounding a central zone of atrophy. It appears usually to be familial, with autosomal dominant inheritance, although in a number of cases there has been no family history. Malignancy has developed in the skin lesions in about 7% of the 200 or so recorded cases, generally many years after the lesions have first appeared. In three cases the cancer developed after irradiation (Cort and Abdel Aziz, 1972).

Another dominantly inherited condition in which hyperkeratosis of the skin has been associated with carcinoma is hyperkeratosis lenticularis perstans (Bean, 1969). In this condition, hyperkeratoses develop in the third and fourth decades, and in one of two reported families there has been a high incidence of squamous and basal cell skin cancers. The cancers, however, did not arise from the areas of hyperkeratosis (Beveridge and Langlands, 1973) and there is no evidence to incriminate a generalized disorder of the epidermis.

Tylosis (Harper *et al.*, 1970) is an autosomal dominant condition characte-rized by localized hyperkeratosis giving rise to symmetrical thickening of the skin of the palms and the soles. There are two varieties: one with onset in the first year of life and no association with malignancy, and the other, described in two Liverpool families, with onset about 10 years of age. In the second variety, over half of those affected have developed carcinoma of the squamous epithelium at the lower end of the oesophagus at an early age. The link between tylosis and the oesophageal cancer is unclear: there seems to be no increased risk of local skin malignancy, and there is little evidence of preneoplastic lesions in the oesophageal epithelium. Genetic studies (Harper *et al.*, 1970) suggest that a single locus (or possibly two closely linked loci) are involved and possibly linked to the locus for the MNS blood group system.

In two other inherited conditions, abnormalities of the skin epithelium are associated with malignancy: epidermolysis bullosa dystrophica and dyskerato-sis congenita. Epidermolysis bullosa (Didolkar *et al.*, 1974) is characterized by recurrent skin ulceration and scarring, and here it is the constant reparative proliferation, as in scars from other causes, that probably predisposes to malignancy. Dyskeratosis congenita is a complex disorder in which a variety of dysplastic skin changes are associated with features resembling Fanconi's anaemia. There is an excess of malignancies predominantly involving squamous epithelium other than skin (Sirinavin and Trowbridge, 1975).

Disturbances in immune function

Immune deficiency, whether inherited or acquired, is associated with an increased risk of malignancy (Penn and Starzl, 1972; Kinlen *et al.*, 1979). In the case of inherited immune deficiency, the excess risk is about 100-fold (Kersey and Spector, 1975) but the excess of tumours is very largely confined to the lymphoid system (Penn and Starzl, 1972; Kersey and Spector, 1975; Stutman, 1975).

Whether immune deficiency predisposes to malignancies of other tissues, in particular the common epithelial cancers, remains contentious, but there may be special cases. For example, there seems to be a relationship between inherited immune defects and stomach cancer, and a family has been described (Creagen and Fraumeni, 1973) in which stomach cancer was associated with a genetic defect of T-lymphocyte function. There is also evidence suggesting an excess risk of stomach cancer among adults with common variable immune deficiency (Gatti and Good, 1971) and in patients with ataxia telangiectasia, in which chromosomal instability is associated with immune defects including IgA deficiency (Haerer *et al.*, 1969).

Gastric cancer is well known to be associated with atrophic gastritis, which may largely be genetically determined (Harper, 1973). In this condition epithelial changes in the stomach, including proliferation and turnover of epithelial cells, are commonly associated with the presence of autoantibodies against the gastric parietal cells. The propensity to form such autoantibodies itself seems to have a genetic basis (Chanarin, 1968). Whether there is a causal relationship between the immunological abnormalities and the epithelial proliferation is not known.

Correlation of the functional disturbances in the inherited immune deficiency syndromes with the types of tumour which develop may provide one way of understanding the interrelationships of cells in the immune system. There seems no reason to suppose at present, however, that the recognized inherited immune deficiency syndromes are of general relevance to cancer risk in other tissues.

Metabolic variation as a preneoplastic state

This category includes metabolic traits which may predispose to cancer by increasing the availability of endogenous or exogenous carcinogens. They include variations in hormonal metabolism in breast cancer (Henderson *et al.*, 1975; Schneider *et al.*, 1982) and of metabolism of carcinogens in cigarette smoke in the case of the still-controversial link between increased aryl hydrocarbon hydroxylase inducibility and lung cancer (Kellerman *et al.*, 1973; Emery *et al.*, 1978; McLemore *et al.*, 1978). Single- or multiple-gene predisposition of this type, in conjunction with environmental factors, might be responsible for much of the familial clustering of cancer to be discussed in the next section.

Ethnic differences in cancer incidence

Geographical differences in cancer incidence provide the principal evidence that much of cancer is environmentally induced. Particularly telling is the adoption of the pattern of incidence of their new country by migrant groups, such as the Japanese now living in the USA (Cairns, 1978) (see Chapter 8). There are, however, examples of ethnic differences in cancer incidence which have persisted despite migration, which suggests that they are genetically influenced. Thus, Ewing's tumour of bone is virtually absent in black populations in the USA and Africa (Fraumeni and Glass, 1970; Williams, 1975), while the incidence of other bone tumours in blacks and whites shows no such difference. The peak in mortality from testicular tumours at age 25–29 in white populations is absent in US and African blacks (Miller, 1977). These differences are unexplained. The low incidence of cutaneous melanoma in blacks, on the other hand, is reasonably explained by the protective effect against solar radiation of a genetically determined trait, skin pigmentation.

FAMILIAL AGGREGATION OF CANCER

The rather slight degree of familial aggregation of most of the common cancers has already been noted, but it was argued that even small differences are consistent with a substantial contribution of genetic factors to the frequency of the disease. The occurrence of more marked familial clustering has been described by Lynch and his co-workers (Lynch *et al.*, 1981; Lynch, 1981; Albano *et al.*, 1981). They have reported that 4% of patients referred to a university oncology clinic had a pedigree consistent with a hereditary predisposition to cancer, the most frequent site being breast. They have also reported associations between the occurrence of breast and ovarian cancer and between cancer of the colon and corpus uteri within the same family (Lynch *et al.*, 1977a). They recommend systemic attempts to identify such families in order to offer surveillance to family members from an early age.

There are two limitations to this approach to the identification of inherited cancer risk. First, in any particular family it may be difficult to be sure that the clustering is attributable to genetic, rather than to environmental or chance factors. Various statistical models have been designed to which family data can be fitted, to see whether a genetic or environmental model is the more probable; and if genetic, what is the likely mode of transmission (Elston *et al.*, 1981). It seems, however, that it is almost always possible to argue for a plausible alternative explanation of the data, whatever model is chosen. Second, even if it is established that inherited factors are involved, the genetic data are generally insufficient to enable one to assign an individual estimate of risk with confidence to any one family member.

Both of these difficulties might be overcome if it were possible to demonstrate segregation of disease susceptibility in the family with some clear-cut genetic marker. This would establish the genetic component of susceptibility and its mode of inheritance, and provide a means of identifying family members at risk. The prospects for this aproach will be discussed in the final section of this chapter.

Inferences from the study of familial aggregation

Familial aggregations of cancer are almost all confined to one or a few sites characteristic for the family and this suggests that the genes which confer susceptibility may be correspondingly limited in their expression. If this is true, there are practical consequences for the search for phenotypic markers of susceptibility (such as metabolic peculiarities), because it implies that the presence of the gene might only be assayed in the tissues in which the cancers arise. This might be difficult and it is to be noted that the examples which have been mentioned so far (skin fibroblasts in polyposis coli, aryl hydrocarbon hydroxylase inducibility in blood lymphocytes in patients with lung cancer) rely on the expression of the trait of interest in another, more convenient, tissue.

Analysis of family pedigrees suggests considerable heterogeneity in cancer at the common sites. For example, at least four dominantly inherited varieties of colonic cancer without associated polyposis have been described (Anderson, 1978, 1980). The tumours in each case tend to arise in the ascending and transverse colon rather than the descending colon, which is the common site for polyposis. Each type has a characteristic penetrance and age of onset, and in three of the four types there are characteristic associations with malignancy at other sites (in particular, stomach and endometrium). Taking these tumours together with the inherited polyposis syndromes (Erbe, 1976), it seems that colonic carcinoma may be predisposed to as a result of at least 11 different inherited traits and to what extent these are allelic is not known. The preferential involvement of different sites in the colon suggests either a role for carcinogens which are unevenly distributed within the colonic contents, or that the colonic epithelium itself is not a homogeneous tissue.

Similar heterogeneity is seen in breast cancer (Anderson, 1974, 1978; Knudson *et al.*, 1973; Lynch *et al.*, 1981). Relatives of patients with premenopausal onset and bilateral tumours are at especially high risk. Other tissues may be involved in distinct syndromes: for example, in some families breast cancer is aggregated with various sarcomas, leukaemia and brain tumours and possibly adrenocortical carcinoma (Li and Fraumeni, 1975; Blattner *et al.*, 1979). Linkage studies have been used to examine the genetic basis of familial clustering of breast cancer, and to separate distinct groups. Preliminary results suggest linkage between susceptibility to breast cancer and the glutamate–pyruvate transaminase locus on chromosome 10 in one group of families, defined by relatively young onset and associated ovarian and endometrial cancers (King *et al.*, 1980; King, 1982).

Mechanisms of familial susceptibility

Mechanisms (as distinct from genetic linkage) for familial or ethnic aggregations of cancer have been proposed in only a few instances, yet the prospects for prevention are likely to be based on the avoidance of predisposing factors. A major area of interest is the possibility of genetic–environmental interactions through metabolism or exogenous carcinogens. The existence of genetically determined differences in the metabolism of drugs between individuals (Dollery, 1972) suggests that such interactions may exist also with carcinogens (Nebert, 1980).

The most extensively studied system in man and in the mouse is the cytochrome P_{450}-dependent membrane-based mono-oxygenase system, which is required for the metabolism of many known carcinogens, in particular the polycyclic aromatic hydrocarbons (reviewed by Atlas and Nebert, 1978). Although the relationship between this system and cancer risk in man remains controversial, it provides a prototype for this mechanism of cancer predisposition, and so it will be described in some detail.

The P_{450}-dependent system exists in a variety of forms each differing in tissue distribution, in pattern of metabolites produced, and in inducibility by a variety of agents including the polycyclic hydrocarbons themselves. Studies in mice, using aryl hydrocarbon hydroxylase (AHH) activity as a marker for the P_{450}-dependent system, have defined a regulatory gene locus (the Ah locus) by which inducibility of the AHH system is governed (Atlas and Nebert, 1978). Two alleles are postulated: inducible and non-inducible. Heterozygotes show evidence of a gene dosage effect (Niwa *et al.*, 1975), and crosses between inbred inducible and non-inducible strains indicate that inducibility behaves as an autosomal dominant trait (Atlas and Nebert, 1978).

AHH inducibility has been studied in human tissues by comparing the 'basal' level of AHH activity in an unstimulated tissue with that after a period of exposure to an inducer such as 3-methyl cholanthrene. In most studies, cultured mitogen-stimulated lymphocytes have been used as test material. Possibly because of technical problems with the method, the results have been extremely variable and interpretation difficult. They do show a wide variation in inducibility within the human population, and studies of twins indicate that much of this population heterogeneity is genetically controlled. Results to date do not support (neither do they deny) the conclusion that the level of inducibility in man is determined by two alleles at a single locus.

Even if distinct subgroups for AHH inducibility cannot be defined, however, inducibility might still be of value as a quantitative indicator of cancer risk; for example, to identify those individuals at exceptional risk of cancers related to smoking. Lung cancer has been shown to aggregate in families (Tokuhata and Lilienfeld, 1963); the familial factor is independent of smoking, but interacts synergistically with it. The initial reports did indeed suggest a correlation between AHH inducibility and lung cancer risk, but subsequent reports by other groups (Emery *et al.*, 1978; McLemore *et al.*, 1978; Paigen *et al.*, 1977) have been contradictory and the matter is still in dispute. The ratio of induced to uninduced AHH activity in most series is seldom greater than 5, and until this ratio can be increased (or the background 'noise' of the technique reduced) it seems unlikely that AHH inducibility will become of practical value. The hope remains that this or a similar system will prove to be of predictive value in the future.

A quite different mechanism related to carcinogen exposure has been proposed to account for some of the excess in breast cancer among Caucasian compared to Oriental women (Petrakis, 1977). The hypothesis is based on the observation that the adult non-lactating breast secretes and resorbs fluid within the alveolar–ductal system. If exogenous carcinogens enter the secretion, as many other substances do, the level of secretory activity may influence the exposure of the breast epithelium to carcinogens. It appears that a higher proportion of Caucasian than Oriental women are breast-fluid secretors, which is consistent with the hypothesis. Moreover, secretion is correlated with the production of wet, rather than dry, cerumen (ear-wax). Cerumen type, which is inherited in a simple Mendelian fashion, might thus be expected to provide an indicator of breast cancer risk, but a correlation between wet cerumen type and breast cancer could not be substantiated (Ing *et al.*, 1973).

The cancer family pedigrees which have been studied generally are consistent with an autosomal dominant mode of inheritance. By contrast, most of the inherited non-neoplastic diseases for which a mechanism has been established are recessively inherited simple enzyme defects. In familial hyperbetalipoproteinaemia, which is autosomal dominant, a cell surface receptor is at fault (Brown and Goldstein, 1976). One might speculate, therefore, that the majority of familial cancer syndromes (unlike the inborn errors of metabolism or the disorders of DNA repair such as xeroderma pigmentosum) will not turn out to be the straightforward consequence of a systemic enzyme defect. The mechanisms are likely to be harder to elucidate and tissue-specific, possible involving regulatory genes or cell-surface components, as the above examples suggest.

It has been proposed nevertheless in that the recessive genes of Fanconi's anaemia, ataxia telangiectasia, Bloom's syndrome, and similar disorders might contribute to familial aggregations of cancer when they are present in the heterozygous state (Swift, 1976). The proposal was based on the finding of an increased incidence of cancer among families of homozygous probands, relative to the incidence expected from population statistics. If correct, this hypothesis would have considerable implications: it can be calculated, for example, that as many as 10% of patients under 55 years of age with ovarian cancer would be carriers of an AT gene. A more recent analysis of a large group of families by the same authors has, however, cast doubt on the validity of the original conclusions (Swift *et al.*, 1980).

CLINICAL IMPLICATIONS

The possibility that a component of inherited predisposition exists in a patient with cancer (or his relatives) presents the clinician with two problems: (1) What should be done for the patient and his family? (2) Can this be investigated further, either to confirm the operation of genetic factors, or to elucidate the mechanism of predisposition?

Identification of an inherited component

To decide whether an inherited component of risk is present in the cancer patient, the most important information is from the family history. Features which may indicate an inherited component are, firstly, the aggregation in the family of cancers of particular types, especially of uncommon cancers, for example, in the families with breast cancer, a history of leukaemia, sarcoma, and brain tumours (Blattner *et al.*, 1979); secondly, evidence of multiple primary tumours in the same individual (Forrest *et al.*, 1981; Lynch *et al.*, 1977a; Anderson, 1980; Albano *et al.*, 1981); thirdly, unusually early age of onset; fourthly, the presence of associated malformations, benign tumours or hamartomatous lesions (e.g. Cowden syndrome or naevoid basal cell carcinoma syndrome (Mulvihill, 1977; Lutzner, 1977)). The history should be supplemented by clinical examination of family members with these points in mind.

Even when this has been done, there may still be doubt whether a familial cluster has a genetic basis. The tumours which occur in the inherited cancer syndromes also occur in sporadic form. If these individuals could be distinguished, their families could be spared the anxiety of screening. There may be too few family members at risk from whom information is available, or the patient may represent a new mutation to the inherited form, whose parents and siblings will be unaffected, but whose children will be at risk. If the tumour is one of an aggregation of cancers within a family but not part of a well-defined syndrome with a known pattern of inheritance, it may again be a problem to establish that the aggregation has a genetic rather than a chance or environmental basis.

How are these difficulties to be overcome? In each case, what is needed is a marker which will indicate the presence of an inherited predisposition to the cancer. This might be a particular phenotypic trait, due either to the susceptibility gene itself or perhaps to altered activity of adjacent genes (involved, for example in a translocation). Alternatively, we need a genetic marker, in practice, at present, a visible chromosomal abnormality which can be consistently associated with susceptibility to the tumour.

Several phenotypic traits which can be used as markers have already been mentioned. In polyposis coli, there are the polyps themselves and possibly the abnormalities of *in vitro* behaviour of skin fibroblasts. In MEN 2, the presence of multifocal hyperplasia in the C-cells or adrenal medullary cells adjacent to the tumours is reported to be characteristic of the inherited syndrome, possibly reflecting the effects of the inherited mutation (Jackson *et al.*, 1979). In some of the cancer family syndromes, characteristic associations with other tumours, malformations or hamartomas may provide strong evidence of the operation of genetic factors.

In many cases, however, including most examples of familial clustering, such phenotypic markers are not available. Constitutional chromosomal abnormalities may identify some hereditary cases in some of the inherited cancer syndromes (such as renal cell carcinoma and familial Wilms's tumour described earlier) but they have not so far been described in family aggregations where the operation of genetic factors has been in doubt. A marker of inherited susceptibility would be a valuable tool in the management of these families. Its presence would not only confirm that inherited factors were involved; the use of different markers might resolve a heterogeneous group of similar families into truly homogeneous groups, with benefits both for clinical management and for studies of aetiology.

How, then, should markers of susceptibility be sought? The usual approach until recently has been to test for phenotypic abnormalities, basing the search on current ideas of cancer development. Thus, for example, Forrest *et al.* (1981) tested a patient with nine primary cancers for deficiency in various aspects of DNA repair and immune function.

In general, in the absence of some clue, such as sensitivity to sunlight in patients with xeroderma pigmentosum, such searches for phenotypic traits are laborious and have been unproductive. Systematic screening for genetically determined differences in metabolism of potential carcinogens may ultimately prove to be a successful example of this approach, but it is hampered by our lack of knowledge of what exogenous or endogenous materials are likely to be relevant. In the medium term, attempts to establish linkage of the cancer susceptibility with a genetic marker seem likely to provide the most powerful approach.

Management of the patient and his family

These patients provide opportunities for prevention, early diagnosis, prophylactic treatment, and genetic counselling to reduce the morbidity and mortality of the disease in the index patient and his family. As emphasized in several recent reviews (Fraumeni, 1975; Mulvihill *et al.*, 1977; Mulvihill, 1981), there is a balance to be struck between costs and benefits in each individual case.

Against the potential benefits outlined above must be set the costs of the anxiety and uncertainty induced in the family by the suggestion that they may have a gene for cancer risk; the cost in time and money and perhaps in physical discomfort of screening or surveillance procedures; the costs of possible false-positive diagnosis and consequent 'unnecessary' treatments; and the costs of 'necessary' treatments such as prophylactic surgery in MEN 2 or polyposis coli. The potential costs and potential benefits will vary from family to family, and between individuals in a single family. In general, the greater the potential total costs, the more accurately must the clinician be able to estimate both them and the benefits for an individual patient before recommending a policy of management.

In polyposis coli, for example, there is the discomfort and cost of regular surveillance by sigmoidoscopy (see Chapter 18). Major prophylactic surgery may be advised on the basis that the risk of cancer approaches 100% if no action is taken, and that the treatment is highly effective. If the skin fibroblast studies (Kopelovich, 1982) can be confirmed to be accurate indicators of individuals at risk, up to half the family members may eventually be spared the preliminary surveillance.

In MEN 2 cases, the equation is not so easy. There is the problem of distinguishing hereditary from sporadic cases, so that if an aggressive approach to screening is taken, many families will be included in whom there is in fact a rather low risk that the index case has the inherited form – although at present one cannot tell them what that risk is. Even within known MEN 2 families, only half the family members being screened at yearly intervals from early childhood will in fact be carriers of the gene. Because there is no way of recognizing them, screening of all family members must go on until some, as yet ill-defined, age (probably 35–40 years) when the risk that the syndrome is still undiagnosed is slight.

Perhaps most important, the natural history of the tumours in MEN 2 cases is not clearly defined, and may vary from one individual to another: quite commonly patients seem to coexist with their tumours for many years without evident ill-effects of tumour progression. It is, therefore, not clear whether operation is always of benefit to a patient with proven tumour, nor whether it is always important to diagnose the thyroid tumours at the earliest stage of multifocal C-cell hyperplasia (Wells *et al.*, 1978). The earlier one tries to make the diagnosis, the more frequent and more sensitive the screening must be, and the greater the risk of false positive results.

As the costs and benefits become more difficult to estimate exactly, it becomes correspondingly more difficult for the clinician to be sure in his advice to the families. At this point, emotional factors in the response to screening become more important, in two ways. First, uncertainty in the clinician may communicate itself to the family, with possibly damaging results. Second, the enthusiasm (or lack of it) for screening shown by the family is likely to be a larger factor in the formulation of screening policy.

In the cancer family syndromes and familial aggregations, estimates of risk are likely to be even less precise because the numbers of families studied are generally smaller, the patterns of inheritance of susceptibility (if indeed inheritance has been established) may not be clear-cut, and the extent of the differences between families with apparently similar clusterings of cancers is not yet known. There is, in addition, some data to suggest that the cancers in these families may have a more benign behaviour than their sporadic equivalents, so that the extent of risk cannot necessarily be extrapolated from the common cancers of similar type (Forrest *et al.*, 1981; Anderson, 1980).

In general, members of these families have been offered surveillance for early detection of cancers at sites known to be affected in that family, especially colon and uterine cancer (Lynch *et al.*, 1977b). This policy is reported to have led to the diagnosis of cancers in several family members at a stage curable by surgery. Provided the resources are available and the families wish to avail themselves of the service, it seems sensible because the 'costs' are relatively low.

More difficult problems arise if prophylactic surgery is contemplated – for example, mastectomy in a young woman in a 'breast cancer family' or prophylactic oophorectomy in a family with a high incidence of ovarian cancer (Lynch *et al.*, 1977b). Such a potentially 'high cost' decision should be based on as accurate an estimate as possible of the future risk of cancer in that individual. Since the data to make such an estimate may not be available, the decision becomes a matter of judgement, taking into account the perception of the disease by the individual concerned.

In summary, our aim is to understand the mechanism of predisposition sufficiently to be able to identify individuals at risk and adopt preventive measures, rather than rely on surveillance and prophylactic surgery. Prevention is the only reasonable approach to the postulated high-risk individuals in the general population. The studies of AHH inducibility discussed earlier were aimed at this. With the exception of xeroderma pigmentosum, where prevention is possible by avoidance of sunlight (Lynch *et al.*, 1977b), this ideal has not yet been achieved.

Prospects for the future: genetic markers

The availability of genetic markers for linkage studies will greatly extend our knowledge of inherited predisposition to cancer. In the inherited cancer syndromes, markers will be used to identify individuals who have inherited the susceptibility gene, and who therefore require surveillance. In family clusters, demonstration of linkage of the cancers to a genetic locus will provide concrete evidence of an inherited component and, once again, the marker locus may be used to indicate the family members at risk. If family groups are found with predisposition to the same cancers but linkage to different genetic loci, this will provide evidence of the heterogeneity of cancers at a single site. More accurate definition of subtypes in this way may be important both for management and for studies of aetiology.

Finally, the postulated existence of genetic susceptibility without evident family clustering can be tested by examining the distribution of a genetic marker among siblings, in cases where two or more siblings are affected by a particular cancer. If the affected siblings share the same marker significantly more often than randomly chosen pairs of siblings, it may be inferred that there is an inherited component of susceptibility linked to that marker (Bodmer, 1982).

Linkage has already been demonstrated to HL-A haplotypes for Hodgkin's disease in siblings in 15 families, and possibly for some other cancers (Dausset *et al.*, 1982); and to the glutamate–pyruvate transaminase locus on chromosome 10 for a group of families with breast cancer (King *et al.*, 1980). In general, however, linkage studies to date have been unsuccessful, probably because of the paucity of genetic markers. Only about 30 suitable loci are available, and it is a fortunate coincidence if the susceptibility gene for the cancer in question lies close enough to one of these for linkage to be demonstrated.

This problem is now being overcome by the use of markers generated by the many slight differences in DNA nucleotide sequences between individuals. A class of enzymes, the 'restriction enzymes', recognize specific nucleotide sequences at which they cut the DNA strand. A difference in sequence between individuals can thus be revealed as the presence or absence of cutting of the strand, which will produce DNA fragments of different sizes which can easily be recognized by the pattern they produce upon electrophoresis in a gel. A very large number of such polymorphic genetic markers can in theory be identified (White, 1980). It has been estimated that a set of around 200 (depending upon the size of pedigree available), evenly spaced along the chromosomes, would be sufficient to allow the detection of linkage of a susceptibility gene, whatever its location (Bishop and Skolnick, 1980).

This type of analysis has already been successfully developed in the X-linked inherited Duchenne muscular dystrophy (Murray *et al.*, 1982), and is entering routine application in the management of these families. The problems of covering all the other chromosomes as well, and of assembling suitable pedigrees or sibling pairs for analysis of cancer susceptibility, are clearly far greater, but may possibly be accomplished in the next 10 years.

CONCLUSION

Inherited susceptibility to cancer has been shown unequivocally in only a few, rather uncommon, inherited cancer syndromes. Substantial inherited predisposition to cancer at the common sites may, however, be present with only a small degree of familial clustering. The role of inherited factors should soon be clarified by the development of genetic markers which can be used in linkage studies.

Recognition of inherited predisposition to cancer is important because of the possibilities for early diagnosis and prevention in individuals at high risk, and because insight into the mechanism of predisposition may tell us something about the processes of carcinogenesis. In syndromes such as polyposis coli, where the risks are well defined, effective prevention by surgery is possible without understanding the mechanism of predisposition. But if cancer prevention is to be extended to high-risk individuals in the general population, the kinds of intervention that can be contemplated are likely to require that the mechanism of the predisposition is at least partly understood.

Acknowledgements

B. A. J. Ponder holds a Career Development Award from the Cancer Research Campaign. Manuscript submitted February 1983.

REFERENCES

Albano, W. A., Lynch, H. T., Recabaren, J. A. *et al.* (1981). Familial cancer in an oncology clinic. *Cancer, 47,* 2113.

Alm, T., and Licznerski, G. (1973). The intestinal polyposes. *Clinics in Gastroenterology, 2,* 577. Philadelphia: Saunders.

Anderson, D. E. (1974). Genetic study of breast cancer. Identification of a high risk group. *Cancer, 34,* 1090.

Anderson, D. E. (1975). Familial susceptibility. In *Persons at high risk of cancer. An approach to cancer etiology and control* (ed. J. F. Fraumeni). New York: Academic Press, p. 39.

Anderson, D. E. (1978). Familial cancer and cancer families. *Seminars in Oncology,* **5,** 11.

Anderson, D. E. (1980). An inherited form of large bowel cancer. *Cancer,* **45,** 1103.

Ashley, D. J. B. (1969). Colonic cancer arising in polyposis coli. *Journal of Medical Genetics,* **6,** 376.

Atlas, S. A., and Nebert, D. W. (1978). Pharmacogenetics: a possible pragmatic perspective in neoplasm predictability. *Seminars in Oncology,* **5,** 89.

Baylin, S. B., Hsu, S. H., Gann, D. S. *et al.* (1978). Inherited medullary thyroid carcinoma: A final monoclonal mutation in one of multiple clones of susceptible cells. *Science,* **199,** 429.

Bean, S. F. (1969). Hyperkeratosis lenticularis perstans. *Archives of Dermatology,* **99,** 705.

Beveridge, G. W., and Langlands, A. O. (1973). Familial hyperkeratosis lenticularis perstans associated with tumours of the skin. *British Journal of Dermatology,* **88,** 453.

Bishop, D. T., and Skolnick, M. H. (1980). Linkage and polymorphic DNA markers. In *Cancer incidence in defined populations,* Banbury Report, No. 4 (eds J. Cairns, J. L. Lyon, and M. H. Skolnick). New York: Cold Spring Harbor Laboratory, p. 421.

Blattner, W. A., McGuire, D. B., Mulvihill, J. J. *et al.* (1979). Genealogy of cancer in a family. *Journal of the American Medical Association,* **241,** 259.

Bodmer, W. F. (ed.) (1982). *Cancer surveys,* Vol. 1. *Inheritance of susceptibility to cancer in man.* Oxford University Press.

Brown, M. S., and Goldstein, J. L. (1976). Receptor-mediated control of cholesterol metabolism. *Science,* **191,** 150.

Cairns, J. (1978). *Cancer, science and society.* San Francisco: W. H. Freeman.

Cairns, J. (1981). The origin of human cancers. *Nature,* **289,** 353.

Chanarin, I. (1968). In *Clinical aspects of immunology,* 2nd edn (eds P. G. H. Gell, and R. R. A. Coombes). Oxford: Blackwell, p. 1020.

Cleaver, J. E., and Bootsma, D. (1975). Xeroderma pigmentosum – biochemical and genetic characteristics. *Annual Review Genetics,* **9,** 19.

Cooper, G. M. (1982). Cellular transforming genes. *Science,* **218,** 801.

Cort, D. F., and Abdel Aziz, A.-H. M. (1972). Epithelioma arising in porokeratosis of mibelli. *British Journal of Plastic Surgery,* **25,** 318.

Creagen, E. T., and Fraumeni, J. F. (1973). Familial gastric cancer and immunological abnormalities. *Cancer,* **32,** 1325.

Dausset, J., Colombani, J., and Hors, J. (1982). Major histocompatibility complex and cancer, with special reference to human familial tumours (Hodgkin's disease and other malignancies). In *Cancer surveys,* Vol. 1. Oxford University Press, p. 119.

Davies, B. S., Krush, A. J., and Gardner, E. J. (1977). Is Gardner syndrome a distinct genetic disorder? *Lancet,* **2,** 925.

Deschner, E. E., and Lipkin, M. (1975). Proliferative patterns in colonic mucosa in familial polyposis. *Cancer,* **35,** 413.

Didolkar, M. S., Gerner, R. E., and Moore, G. E. (1974). Epidermolysis bullosa dystrophica and epithelium of the skin. *Cancer,* **32,** 198.

Dollery, C. T. (1972). Individual differences in response to drugs in man. *Eighth symposium on advanced medicine* (ed. G. Neale). London: Pitman Medical.

Draper, G. J., Heaf, M. M., and Kinnier-Wilson, L. M. (1977). Occurrence of childhood cancers among sibs and estimation of familial risks. *Journal of Medical Genetics,* **14,** 81.

Elston, R. C., Go, R. C. P., King, M. C., and Lynch, H. T. (1981). A statistical model for the study of familial breast cancer. In *Genetics and breast cancer* (ed. H. T. Lynch). New York: Van Nostrand Reinhold.

Emery, A. E. H., Anand, R., Danford, N. *et al.* (1978). Aryl-hydrocarbon-hydroxylase inducibility in patients with cancer. *Lancet*, **1**, 470.

Erbe, R. W. (1976). Inherited gastrointestinal-polyposis syndromes. *New England Journal of Medicine*, **294**, 1101.

Fisher, J. C. (1958). Multiple-mutation theory of carcinogenesis. *Nature*, **181**, 651.

Forrest, J., Slaney, G., Crocker, J. *et al.* (1981). Multiple malignancy with a familial tendency. *Clinical Oncology*, **7**, 357.

Fraumeni, J. F. (ed.) (1975). *Persons at high risk of cancer*. New York: Academic Press.

Fraumeni, J. F., and Glass, A. G. (1970). Rarity of Ewing's sarcoma among US negro children. *Lancet*, **1**, 366.

Gatti, R. A., and Good, R. A. (1971). Occurrence of malignancy in immunodeficiency diseases. *Cancer*, **28**, 89.

Gentry, W. C., Eskritt, N. R., and Gorlin, R. J. (1974). Multiple hamartoma syndrome (Cowden's disease). *Archives of Dermatology*, **109**, 521.

German, J. (1972). Genes which increase chromosomal instability in somatic cells and predispose to cancer. In *Progress in medical genetics*, Vol. III. New York: John Wiley, p. 61.

Gorlin, R. J. (1977). Monogenic disorders associated with neoplasia. In *Genetics of human cancer. Progress in cancer research and therapy*, Vol. 3. (eds J. J. Mulvihill, R. W. Miller, and J. F. Fraumeni), New York: Raven Press, p. 169.

Guss, S. B., Osbourn, R. A., and Lutzner, M. A. (1971). Porokeratosis Plantaris, Pulmaris et Disseminata. *Archives of Dermatology*, **104**, 366.

Haerer, A. F., Jackson, J. F., and Evers, C. G. (1969). Ataxia-telangiectasia with gastric adenocarcinoma. *Journal of the American Medical Association*, **210**, 1884.

Harnden, D. G., and Herbert, A. (1982). Association of constitutional chromosomal rearrangements with neoplasia. In *Cancer Surveys* Vol. 1. Inheritance of susceptibility to cancer in man. (ed. W. F. Bodmer) Oxford University Press, p. 150.

Harper, P. S. (1973). Hereditary and gastrointestinal tumours. *Clinics in Gastroenterology*, **2**, 675.

Harper, P. S., Harper, P. M. J., and Howel-Evans, A. W. (1970). Carcinoma of the oesophagus with tylosis. *Quarterly Journal of Medicine (NS)*, **39**, 317.

Henderson, B. E., Gerkins, V., Rosario, I. *et al.* (1975). Elevated levels of estrogen and prolactin in daughters of patients with breast cancer. *New England Journal of Medicine*, **293**, 790.

Higginson, J. (1969). Present trends in cancer epidemiology. *Canadian Cancer Conference*, **8**, 40.

Hill, M. J., Morson, B. C., and Bussey, H. J. R. (1978). Aetiology of adenoma–carcinoma sequence in large bowel. *Lancet*, **1**, 245.

Holm, N. V., Hauge, M., and Jensen, O. M. (1982). Studies of cancer aetiology in a complete twin population. In *Cancer surveys*, Vol. 1. (ed. W. F. Bodmer). Oxford University Press, p. 18.

Ing, R., Petrakis, N. L., and Ho, H. C. (1973). Evidence against association between wet cerumen and breast cancer. *Lancet*, **1**, 41.

Jackson, A. W., Muldal, S., Ockey, C. H., and O'Connor, P. J. (1965). Carcinoma of male breast in association with the Klinefelter syndrome. *British Medical Journal*, **1**, 223.

Jackson, C. E., Block, M. A., Greenawald, K. A., and Tashjian, A. H. (1979). The two-mutational event theory in medullary thyroid cancer. *American Journal of Human Genetics*, **31**, 704.

Kellerman, G., Shaw, C. R., and Lutycn-Kellerman, M. (1973). Aryl hydrocarbon hydroxylase inducibility and bronchogenic carcinoma. *New England Journal of Medicine*, **289**, 934.

Kersey, J. H., and Spector, B. D. (1975). Immune deficiency diseases. In *Persons at high risk of cancer* (ed. J. F. Fraumeni). New York: Academic Press, p. 55.

King, M.-C. (1982). Genetic and epidemiological analysis of cancer in families: Breast cancer as an example. In *Cancer surveys*, Vol. 1. *Inheritance of susceptibility to cancer in man.* (ed. W. F. Bodmer). Oxford University Press, p. 33.

King, M.-C., Go, R. C. P., Elston, R. C. *et al.* (1980). Allele increasing susceptibility to human breast cancer may be linked to the glutamate-pyruvate transamine locus. *Science*, **208**, 406.

Kinlen, L. J., Sheil, A. G. R., Peto, J., and Doll, R. (1979). Collaborative United Kingdom–Australasian study of cancer in patients treated with immunosuppressive drugs. *British Medical Journal*, **2**, 1461.

Klein, G. (1981). The role of gene dosage and genetic transposition in carcinogenesis. *Nature*, **294**, 313.

Knudson, A. G. (1971). Mutation and cancer: Statistical study of retinoblastoma. *Proceedings of the National Academy of Science USA*, **68**, 820.

Knudson, A. G. (1977a). Genetic and environmental interactions in the origin of human cancer. In *Genetics of human cancer. Progress in cancer research and therapy*, Vol. 3. (eds J. J. Mulvihill, R. W. Miller, and J. F. Fraumeni). New York: Raven Press, p. 391.

Knudson, A. G. (1977b). Genetics and the aetiology of human cancer. *Advances in Human Genetics*, **8**, 1.

Knudson, A. G., Hethcote, H. W., and Brown, B. W. (1975). Mutation and childhood cancer: A probabilistic model for the incidence of retinoblastoma. *Proceedings of the National Academy of Science USA*, **72**, 5116.

Knudson, A. G., Strong, L. C., and Anderson, D. E. (1973). Heredity and cancer in man. *Progress in Medical Genetics*, **3**, 113.

Kopelovich, L. (1982). Adenomatosis of the colon and rectum. In *Cancer surveys*, Vol. 1. *Inheritance of susceptibility to cancer in man.* (ed. W. F. Bodmer). Oxford University Press, p. 71.

Li, F. P., and Fraumeni, J. F. (1975). Familial breast cancer, soft-tissue sarcomas, and other neoplasms. *Annals of Internal Medicine*, **83**, 833.

Logan, J., and Cairns, J. (1982). The secrets of cancer. *Nature*, **300**, 104.

Lutzner, M. A. (1977). Nosology among the neoplastic genodermatoses. In *Genetics of human cancer. Progress in cancer research and therapy*, Vol. 3. (eds J. J. Mulvihill, R. W. Miller, and J. F. Fraumeni). New York: Raven Press, p. 145.

Lynch, H. T. (ed.) (1981). *Genetics in breast cancer.* New York: Van Nostrand Reinhold.

Lynch, H. T., Fain, P. C., Golgar, D. *et al.* (1981). Familial breast cancer and its recognition in an oncology clinic. *Cancer*, **47**, 2730.

Lynch, H. T., Guirgis, H. A., Lynch, P. M. *et al.* (1977a). Familial cancer syndromes: a survey. *Cancer*, **39**, 1867.

Lynch, H. T., Lynch, J., and Lynch, P. (1977b). Management and control of familial cancer. In *Genetics of human cancer. Progress in cancer research and therapy*, Vol. 3. (eds J. J. Mulvihill, R. W. Miller, and J. F. Fraumeni). New York: Raven Press, p. 235.

Martin, G. R. (1975). Teratocarcinomas as a model system for the study of embryogenesis and neoplasia. *Cell*, **5**, 229.

Matsunaga, E. (1979). Hereditary retinoblastoma: host resistance and age at onset. *Journal of the National Cancer Institute*, **63**, 933.

McLemore, T. L., Martin, R. C., Wray, N. P. *et al.* (1978). Dissociation between aryl hydrocarbon hydroxylase activity in cultured pulmonary macrophages and blood lymphocytes from cancer patients. *Cancer Research*, **38**, 3805.

Miller, R. W. (1966). Relation between cancer and congenital defects in man. *New England Journal of Medicine*, **275**, 87.

Miller, R. W. (1970). Neoplasia and Down's syndrome. *Annals of the New York Academy of Sciences*, **171**, 637.

Miller, R. W. (1977). Ethnic differences. In *Genetics of human cancer. Progress in cancer research and therapy*, Vol. 3. (eds J. J. Mulvihill, R. W. Miller, and J. F. Fraumeni). New York: Raven Press, p. 1.

Morson, B. C., and Dawson, I. M. P. (1972). *Gastrointestinal pathology*. Oxford: Blackwell.

Mulvihill, J. J. (1977). Genetic repertory of human neoplasia. In *Genetics of human cancer. Progress in cancer research and therapy*, Vol. 3. (eds J. J. Mulvihill, R. W. Miller, and J. F. Fraumeni). New York: Raven Press, p. 137.

Mulvihill, J. J. (1981). Cancer control through genetics. In *Genes, chromosomes and neoplasia* (eds F. E. Arrighi, P. N. Rao, and E. Stubblefield). New York: Raven Press, p. 501.

Mulvihill, J. J., Miller, R. W., and Fraumeni, J. F. (eds) (1977). *Genetics of human cancer. Progress in cancer research and therapy*, Vol. 3. New York: Raven Press.

Murray, J. M., Davies, K. E., Harper, P. S. *et al.* (1982). Linkage relationship of a cloned DNA sequence on the short arm of the X chromosome to Duchenne muscular dystrophy. *Nature*, **300**, 69.

Nebert, D. W. (1980). Pharmacogenetics: an approach to understanding chemical and biological aspects of cancer. *Journal of the National Cancer Institute*, **64**, 1279.

Niwa, A., Kumaki, K., Nebert, D. W., and Poland, A. P. (1975). Genetic expression of aryl hydrocarbon hydroxylase activity in the mouse. *Archives of Biochemistry and Biophysics*, **166**, 559.

O'Riordan, M. L., Langlands, A. O., and Harnden, D. G. (1972). Further studies on the frequency of constitutional chromosome aberrations in patients with malignant disease. *European Journal of Cancer*, **8**, 373.

Paigen, B., Gurtoo, H. L., Minowada, J. *et al.* (1977). Questionable relation of aryl hydrocarbon hydroxylase to lung-cancer risk. *New England Journal of Medicine*, **297**, 346.

Penn, I., and Starzl, T. E. (1972). Malignant tumours arising *de novo* in immunosuppressed organ transplant recipients. *Transplantation*, **14**, 407.

Peto, J. (1980). Genetic predisposition to cancer. In *Cancer incidence in defined populations*. Banbury Report, No. 4. (eds J. Cairns, J. L. Lyon, and M. H. Skolnick). New York: Cold Spring Harbor Laboratory, p. 203.

Peto, R. (1976). Epidemiology, multistage models and short-term mutagenicity tests. *Cold Spring Harbor Conferences in Cell Proliferation*, **4**, 1403.

Peto, R., and Doll, R. (1981). The causes of cancer: quantitative estimates of avoidable risks of cancer in the United States today. *Journal of the National Cancer Institute*, **66**, 1192.

Peto, R., Roe, F. J. C., Lee, P. N. *et al.* (1975). Cancer and ageing in mice and men. *British Journal of Cancer*, **32**, 411.

Petrakis, N. L. (1977). Genetic cerumen type, breast secretory activity and breast cancer epidemiology. In *Genetics of human cancer. Progress in cancer research and therapy*, Vol. 3. (eds J. J. Mulvihill, R. W. Miller, and J. F. Fraumeni). New York: Raven Press, p. 297.

Pfeffer, L. M., and Kopelovich, L. (1977). Differential genetic susceptibility of cultured human skin fibroblasts to transformation by Kirsten murine sarcoma virus. *Cell*, **10**, 313.

Ponder, B. A. J. (1980). Genetics and cancer. *Biochimica et Biophysica*, **605**, 369.

Robbins, J. H. (1978). Significance of repair of human DNA: evidence from studies of xeroderma pigmentosum. *Journal of the National Cancer Institute*, **61**, 645.

Sager, R. (1979). Transposable elements and chromosomal rearrangements in cancer – a possible link. *Nature*, **289**, 447.

Scheike, O., Visfeldt, J., and Petersen, B. (1973). Male breast cancer. *Acta Pathologica Microbiologica Scandinavica*, **81**, 352.

Schimke, R. N. (1977). Tumours of the neural crest system. In *Genetics of human cancer. Progress in cancer research and therapy*, Vol. 3. (eds J. J. Mulvihill, R. W. Miller, and J. F. Fraumeni). New York: Raven Press, p. 179.

Schneider, J., Kinne, D., Fracchia, A. *et al.* (1982). Abnormal oxidative metabolism of estradiol in women with breast cancer. *Proceedings of the National Academy of Sciences USA*, **79**, 3047.

Simpson, J. L., and Photopoulos, G. (1976). The relationship of neoplasia to disorders of abnormal sexual differentiation. In *Cancer and genetics: Original article series*, Vol. 12. New York: March of Dimes Birth Defects Foundation. p. 15.

Sirinavin, C., and Trowbridge, A. A. (1975). Dyskeratosis congenita: Clinical features and genetic aspects. *Journal of Medical Genetics*, **12**, 339.

Slaga, T. J., Klein-Szanto, A. J. P., Fischer, S. M. *et al.* (1980). Studies on mechanism of action of anti-tumour-promoting agents: their specificity in two-stage promotion. *Proceedings of the National Academy of Sciences*, **77**, 2251.

Sohn, K. Y., and Boggs, D. R. (1974). Klinefelter's syndrome, LSD usage and acute lymphoblastic leukaemia. *Clinical Genetics*, **6**, 20.

Stemper, T. J., Kent, T. H., and Summers, R. W. (1975). Juvenile Polyposis and gastrointestinal carcinoma: a study of a kindred. *Annals of Internal Medicine*, **83**, 639.

Strong, L. C. (1977). Theories of pathogenesis: mutation and cancer. In *Genetics of human cancer. Progress in cancer research and therapy*. Vol. 3. (eds J. J. Mulvihill, R. W. Miller, and J. F. Fraumeni). New York: Raven Press, p. 401.

Stutman, O. (1975). Immunodepression and malignancy. *Advances in Cancer Research*, **22**, 261.

Swift, M. (1976). Malignant disease in heterozygous carriers. In *Cancer and genetics : birth defects: Original article series*, Vol. 12, No. 1. New York: March of Dimes Birth Defects Foundation, p. 133.

Swift, M., Caldwell, R. J., and Chase, C. (1980). Reassessment of cancer predisposition of Fanconi anaemia heterozygotes. *Journal of the National Cancer Institute*, **65**, 863.

Tokuhata, G. K., and Lilienfeld, A. M. (1963). Familial aggregation of lung cancer in humans. *Journal of the National Cancer Institute*, **30**, 289.

Warkany, J. (1977). Phacomatoses, hamartoses, neurocristopathies. In *Genetics of human cancer. Progress in cancer research and therapy*, Vol. 3. (eds J. J. Mulvihill, R. W. Miller, and J. F. Fraumeni). New York: Raven Press, p. 199.

Wells, S. A., Baylin, S. B., Gann, D. S. *et al.* (1978). Medullary thyroid carcinoma : relationship of method of diagnosis to pathologic staging. *Annals of Surgery*, **188**, 377.

White, R. (1980). In search of DNA polymorphism in humans. In *Cancer incidence in defined populations.* Banbury Report, No. 4. (eds J. Cairns, J. L. Lyon, and M. H. Skolnick). New York: Cold Spring Harbor Laboratory, p. 409.

Williams, A. O. (1975). Tumours of childhood in Ibadan, Nigeria. *Cancer,* **36,** 370.

Wolff, S., Rodin, B., and Cleaver, J. C. (1977). Sister chromatid exchanges induced by mutagenic carcinogenesis in normal and xeroderma pigmentosum cells. *Nature,* **265,** 347.

Risk Factors and Multiple Cancer
Edited by B.A. Stoll
© 1984 John Wiley and Sons Ltd.

Chapter

10 HENRY M. LEMON

Sex Hormones and Multiple Cancers

Early reports of the incidence of multiple primary cancers indicated a predilection for females (Greenberg, 1963). While some associations of multiple primary tumours in endometrium, breast, and colon may have a genetic basis in the Cancer Family Syndrome (Lynch *et al.*, 1981), it is probable that most sporadic multiple cancers arising in the female involve the carcinogenic potential inherent in oestrogenic hormones derived from the ovaries.

Hormone production from the adrenal cortex may also be important in affecting the risk of multiple cancer in the female. Throughout life, but especially following the menopause, an increasing fraction of adrenal-secreted androstenedione is converted to oestrone by adipose and muscle tissue. There is a high correlation between this conversion rate and body weight, so that the most obese women would be at highest risk of multiple cancers.

This chapter summarizes the more important aspects of endocrine pathophysiology predisposing to multiple primary cancers in either sex, or contributing to their protection from such neoplasms. They are discussed under the following headings:

– Sex hormones as carcinogens.
– Oestrogen metabolism and carcinogenesis.
– Association of colorectal, breast, and genital cancers.
– Malignant melanoma; oestrogen-related pathogenesis?
– Receptor proteins and hormonal interactions.
– Endocrine pathophysiology affecting cancer-risk.

SEX HORMONES AS CARCINOGENS

Increasing epidemiologic evidence has confirmed an increased risk of carcinomas of the breast, endometrium or ovary in adult women following prolonged oestrogenic supplementation (Hoover *et al.*, 1976; Ross *et al.*, 1980; Hoover *et al.*, 1981; Gusberg, 1980; Weiss *et al.*, 1982). The principal oestrogen chronically administered to castrate or postmenopausal women has been conjugated oestrogens of equine origin.

While most investigations have not as yet indicated any clear increase in breast cancer risk from oral contraceptive usage, a French case-control study has concluded that a significantly increased risk of 1.6-fold did exist (Clavel *et al.*, 1981). Women with biopsy-proven proliferative benign breast tumors who utilized contraceptives for more than five years had an 11-fold increase in breast cancers (Fasal and Paffenbarger, 1975).

Diethylstilbestrol administered to pregnant women for threatened abortion resulted in a small epidemic 10–25 years later of vaginal and cervical carcinomas in girls and young women (Herbst and Bern, 1981). Among the mothers so treated, a 50% increase has been noted so far in the incidence of breast cancer, compared to retrospectively selected control women who did not receive hormonal therapy ($p = 0.16$). Treated women developed breast cancers at an earlier median age than the controls. Ovarian but not endometrial cancers were increased in the treated women 25 years later (Bibbo *et al.*, 1978; Clark and Portier, 1979). Endometrial carcinoma developing at a median age of 31 years has also been reported after more than five years' diethylstilbestrol therapy for gonodal dysgenesis (Cutler *et al.*, 1972).

Endometrial carcinomas have been infrequently reported in young women on sequential oral contraceptives, containing long-acting high potency oestrogens such as ethinyl oestradiol (Lyon, 1975; Silverberg and Makowski, 1975). Malignant tumors in other organs do not appear to increase in women following either oestrogen or contraceptive therapy. Although reported, hepatocellular carcinomas are extremely rare following oral contraceptive usage (Lingemam, 1979).

Unlike cancer of the endometrium, cancer of the cervix does not seem to have its pathogenesis influenced by an endocrine stimulus, although cancers of the vagina and cervix are inducible with high dose, prolonged oestrogen therapy in rodents (Lingeman, 1979).

Progesterone therapy has not so far been reported to enhance risk of cancer in human epidemiologic investigations. In fact, cyclic progesterone administration to menopausal women reduces the risk of endometrial carcinoma (Thom *et al.*, 1979; Gambrell *et al.*, 1980). Methylated derivatives, or anabolic steroids modelled after testosterone have not been proven to have any significant human carcinogenicity, except for rare malignant tumors of the liver (Lingeman, 1979).

Ovarian carcinomas have been induced in dogs by diethylstilbestrol administration (Johnson *et al.*, 1972; Lingeman, 1979). The epidemiologic setting for ovarian carcinoma is similar to that of endometrial and breast carcinomas, including increased cancer risk in women previously receiving estrogens (Hoover *et al.*, 1977; Rosenberg *et al.*, 1982). About 50–75% of ovarian carcinomas have been shown to possess oestrogen, androgen or progesterone receptors (Holt *et al.*, 1979; Berggvist *et al.*, 1981; Naftolin and Eisenfeld, 1982; Hähnel *et al.*, 1982).

Furthermore, advanced ovarian carcinomas may respond objectively clinically to therapy with androgens, anti-oestrogens (Schwartz *et al.*, 1982b) and progestins, suggesting that these receptors are functional in terms of tumor promotion, as in the case of breast and endometrial carcinoma (Schwartz *et al.*, 1982a; Hamilton *et al.*, 1981). Ovarian carcinomas have also been induced by unilateral oophorectomy, with transplantation of the remaining ovary into the spleen.

Occult or overt prostatic carcinoma coexists frequently with the common malignant neoplasms of the aging male. In its early stages, prostatic carcinoma, like breast carcinoma, may be multicentric (Wellings *et al.*, 1975; McNeal, 1970). Unlike the considerable decrease in oestrogen secretion from the ovaries following menopause in women, there is a slower and more gradual decrease in testosterone secretion by the testes of the male with aging. Persistent androgenic stimulation of the prostatic epithelium of the posterior lobes of the prostate gland appears consistent with the earliest manifestations of carcinomatous transformation in this area (McNeal, 1970).

Many investigators have now confirmed the increased ratio of intranuclear dihydrotestosterone present bound to receptor proteins in the majority of moderate to well-differentiated prostate carcinomas (Geller *et al.*, 1978; Gustafson *et al.*, 1978; Ekman *et al.*, 1979; Lehoux *et al.*, 1980; Trachtenberg and Walsh, 1982). The concentration of intranuclear dihydrotestosterone (believed to be the most active reduced form of testosterone) correlates closely with the chances of regression of Stage D prostate carcinoma after diethylstilbestrol therapy, or castration.

In addition to androgen receptors, prostatic cancers often possess oestrogen or progesterone receptors, and Stage D prostate carcinomas may respond clinically to progestational therapy with oral Megestrol acetate in cases relapsing after castration or diethylstilbestrol treatment. Megestrol acetate may function as an anti-androgen (blocking the binding of dihydrotestosterone to cytosol receptor) and it also decreases plasma testosterone concentrations, presumably as a result of pituitary inhibition of gonadotropin release (Geller *et al.*, 1981).

The presence of oestrogen receptors in the prostate indicates the possibility of oestrogen-induced carcinogenesis with increasing age. Recent investigations have emphasized the increased plasma oestrogen and decreased plasma testosterone levels in aging males, with increased disparity in these hormonal parameters in prostate cancer (Hill *et al.*, 1982). It is believed that an increased oestrogen : androgen ratio may lead to ductal hyperplasia as a precancerous change.

OESTROGEN METABOLISM AND CARCINOGENESIS

Oestradiol 17β is the principal oestrogen secreted by the human ovary and binds to rodent uterine cytosol receptor proteins with an affinity second only to that of diethylstilbestrol (Korenman, 1969). Oestrone and oestradiol are readily interconverted *in vivo* in human metabolism, and oestradiol is the principal oestrogen transferred into the human endometrial nuclei in the receptor–protein complex, even when oestrone is the oestrogen infused pre-operatively prior to hysterectomy (Thijssen *et al.*, 1978).

Human metabolism of oestrone and oestradiol follows either of two major pathways which are mutually exclusive. Additional oxidation of the steroid nucleus takes place on Ring A at C-2 or C-4 forming catechol oestrogens, which are the largest group of degradative metabolites, or at Ring D at C-16 to produce oestriol and its epimers. There are numerous other hydroxylations carried out at C-6 and C-15 which represent a minority of compounds finally excreted in faeces or urine.

During the past decade, the urinary excretion ratio of oestriol/oestrone + oestradiol 17β has been extensively investigated throughout the world in relation to mammary carcinogenesis, as a result of the 'oestriol hypothesis' (Lemon *et al.*, 1966; Cole and MacMahon, 1969). The oestriol ratio was found to be *inversely* correlated with breast cancer risk according to economic status in young nulliparous women (Trichopoulos *et al.*, 1980), with cancer risk of premenopausal women in Africa, Asia, North America, and Western Europe (Briggs, 1972; Dickinson *et al.*, 1974; MacMahon *et al.*, 1974; MacMahon *et al.*, 1980) and with cancer risk of postmenopausal women in Israeli women from many parts of the world (Gross *et al.*, 1977).

Nulliparity was associated with low oestriol ratios, compared to parous women, in whom elevated oestriol excretion persisted for several years after parturition (Cole *et al.*, 1976; Trichopoulos *et al.*, 1980). Precancerous breast disease (fibrocystic disease) has been associated with low oestriol ratios (Lemon *et al.*, 1966; Bacigalupo and Shubert, 1966). However, patients with cancer of the breast have not been consistently different from age-matched non-cancer control healthy women in their oestriol excretion ratios (Lemon *et al.*, 1966; Bacigalupo and Shubert, 1966; Cole *et al.*, 1978; Morreal *et al.*, 1979). Significantly increased excretion of oestrone, oestradiol, and oestriol compared to controls was observed pre-operatively in postmenopausal cancer patients using gas–liquid chromatography (Morreal *et al.*, 1979).

Newer studies of urinary oestrogen fractions have failed to confirm earlier findings of a significant difference in urinary oestriol ratios between nulliparous and parous women (Yu *et al.*, 1981). Diet plays a major role in modifying plasma oestradiol and oestriol concentrations as a result of altered metabolism and absorption of oestrogens in the enterohepatic cycle. At present, therefore, it seems unlikely that any readily measurable parameter of oestrogen metabolism (and especially those that rely on urinary excretion) can be equated with cancer risk without serious exceptions or qualifications (see Tables 1 and 2).

Table 1   Significance of oestriol ratio as a possible indicator of catechol oestrogen production in relation to multi-organ carcinogenesis

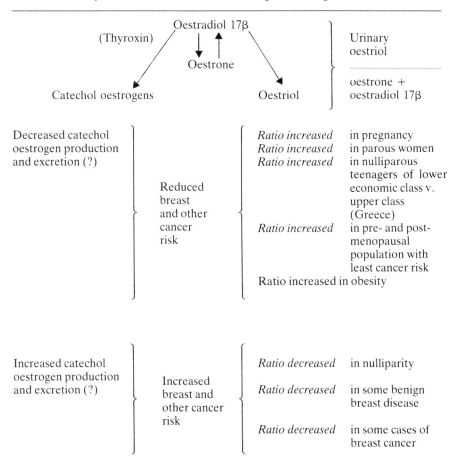

Table 2   Indications of sex hormonal carcinogenesis at multiple sites

Epidemiology	ORGAN SITE					
	Breast	Endometrium	Ovary	Prostate	Colon	Melanoma
Predispose	Oestrogen therapy Nulliparity Infertility Obesity High fat diet Genetic	Oestrogen therapy Nulliparity Infertility Obesity High fat diet Genetic	Oestrogen therapy Nulliparity Infertility — High fat diet Genetic	— — —	— Nulliparity — High fat diet Genetic	— — — US radiation. fair skin —
Protect	Castration Vegetarian diet Early pregnancy	Castration Vegetarian diet Early pregnancy Progestin therapy	Castration — —	Castration Vegetarian diet —	Vegetarian diet —	—
Exp. induction by hormones	Oestrogen therapy	Oestrogen therapy	Oestrogen therapy Chronic LH, FSH increase	None	None	None
Exp. prevention	Oestriol therapy Anti-oestrogen therapy Castration Low fat diet			—	Increased diet fiber, reduction diet fat, cholesterol	
Hormone receptors in tumours	A, E, P, G	E, P	A, E, P	A, E, P	A, E, P, G	E
Hormonal therapy of tumours	Oestrogens Anti-oestrogens Androgens Glucocorticoids Castration	Anti-oestrogens Progestins	Anti-oestrogens Progestins Androgens	Oestrogens Anti-oestrogens Progestins	—	Anti-oestrogens

A = androgen, E = oestrogen, G = growth hormone, P = progesterone, G = glucocorticoid

ASSOCIATION OF COLORECTAL, BREAST, AND GENITAL CANCERS

Malignant neoplasms of the colon and rectum occur with almost equal frequency in both sexes, and age at their clinical appearance is similar to that for breast, endometrial, and ovarian carcinomas. Recent investigations have indicated that nulliparity doubles the risk of colon cancer compared to multiparous women (Dales *et al.*, 1979; Weiss *et al.*, 1981), and in the case of rats, dimethylhydrazine-induced large bowel cancer incidence is increased in nulliparous compared to multiparous and breeding females (Sjogren, 1977). A recent study has indicated no variation in the mortality from breast, ovarian or colorectal cancer in nulliparous women in relation to dietary fat intake (Kinlen, 1982).

About two-thirds of small groups of human colon cancers have been found to contain one or more hormone receptors of various types – oestrogens, progesterone, dihydrotestosterone or glucocorticoid (Alford *et al.*, 1979; Sica *et al.*, 1981). Androgen receptors have been identified in dimethylhydrazine-induced colorectal carcinomas (Mehta *et al.*, 1980). As yet, there have been no reports of objective responses of advanced colorectal cancers to anti-sex-hormone synthetic agents.

Epidemiologically, the incidence rates of colorectal cancer reflect closely the average annual dietary fat intake, as is seen also in the case of breast, endometrial, and prostatic cancers (Carroll and Khor, 1975) (Table 3). Japan has been notably low in the incidence of colorectal, prostate, and breast cancer in the past, compared to other highly industrialized nations. Bile salts and/or their metabolites may be cocarcinogenic for colorectal carcinoma (Carroll and Khor, 1975) and the rate of bile salt excretion will depend upon the amount of dietary fat ingested (Reddy, 1981).

Table 3   Correction coefficients between mortality rates and *per capita* annual fat consumption in endocrine-related neoplasms (40 countries) (Adapted from Carroll and Khor, 1975; Armstrong and Doll, 1975)

Neoplasms	Correlation coefficients	
	Males	Females
Breast carcinoma	...	+0.89, +0.94
Endometrial carcinoma	...	+0.85
Ovary, fallopian tube, and broad ligament	...	+0.73
Intestine (except rectum)	+0.85, +0.93	+0.81, +0.91
Rectal carcinoma	+0.74, +0.83	+0.64, +0.79
Prostate carcinoma	+0.74, +0.89	...

Since a large fraction of plasma oestrogens is excreted in the biliary tract ($\pm50\%$), re-absorption in the enterohepatic cycle in the small intestine will be influenced by the absolute amount of bile salts present, and perhaps also by the amount of dietary fiber (or other components such as lignans) which might serve to sequester oestrogens (Adlercreutz *et al.*, 1982). Dietary fiber is believed to play an important role in modifying the risk of colorectal cancer, through modifying fecal transit time. Higher dietary fiber intake in underdeveloped countries is associated with low rates of colorectal carcinoma, and a threefold increase in the rate of transit of enteric contents through the gastrointestinal tract.

Low fat (vegetarian) diets reduce plasma oestradiol and oestrone concentrations (Armstrong *et al.*, 1981; Adlercreutz *et al.*, 1981), possibly reducing the risk of induction of cancers of the female reproductive system. Low fat diets also may reduce the exposure of the colorectal mucosa to enteric carcinogens and cocarcinogens through the reduced bile salt excretion and a more rapid transit time, if there is an accompanying increase in fiber intake and excretion (Kay, 1981).

At the present time, it seems most likely that the connection between reproductive tract cancer in women and colorectal cancer is through the physiologic linkages between bile salt production and excretion, and oestrogen re-absorption in the enterohepatic cycle (see Chapter 6). A strong genetic linkage to these aspects of human physiology could explain in part the cancer family syndrome when it includes this spectrum of multiple cancers (Lynch *et al.*, 1981).

MALIGNANT MELANOMA: OESTROGEN-RELATED PATHOGENESIS?

Malignant melanoma is not frequently encountered as a component of multiple malignant neoplasms, but has been reported as a subgroup of the cancer family syndrome, mainly in association with cancers of the breast, colon, lung, and stomach (Lynch *et al.*, 1975). Chronic ultraviolet skin exposure is the major known pathogenetic factor in Caucasians, with increasing incidence with decrease in latitude. In spite of its nearly equal distribution between the two sexes, many papers have been published about its possible endocrine dependence and the fact that women have a considerably better prognosis than men.

Benign nevi usually lack detectable oestrogen or other receptors but nearly one-half of benign nevi resected from patients from whom a malignant melanoma had been previously removed were shown to possess cytosol receptor proteins for oestrogens (Chandhuri *et al.*, 1980). About 50% of malignant melanomas or their metastases contain oestrogen or progesterone cytosol receptor proteins (Fisher *et al.*, 1976; Masiel *et al.*, 1980). Partial objective remissions of metastatic melanoma have been induced by the anti-oestrogen Tamoxifen, mostly in women to date (Nesbit *et al.*, 1979; Masiel *et al.*, 1980; Mirimanoff *et al.*, 1981). The response rate is only about 20% however, and there has been no report to our knowledge of correlation between receptor content and responsiveness to therapy.

RECEPTOR PROTEIN AND HORMONAL INTERACTIONS

The most striking and important feature of hormone–receptor interaction is the rapid transfer of the complex to the cell nucleus, in close chemical relationship with chromatin-containing DNA. The following observations are related to the possible role of receptor protein in the induction of cancer at different target sites:

1. The duration of nuclear binding to acceptor sites is directly related to oestrogenic activity. Oestriol receptor complexes remain bound for only 4 hours to rat nuclear sites, while part of the oestradiol bound persists in excess of 24 hours.
2. A minimum number of nuclear acceptor sites need to be filled with receptor–oestrogen complexes for maximum functional activity. Progesterone, whose receptor mechanism is induced following oestrogenic stimulus, interacts during nuclear binding to reduce the number of available oestrogen receptor sites, thereby limiting the oestrogenic response (Okulicz *et al.*, 1981). This modulation of oestrogenic activity by progesterone is probably of major importance in the reduction of carcinogenic risk for the uterus and breast. Anovulatory cycles (resulting in decreased progesterone biosynthesis) have been implicated in the etiology of benign and malignant breast disease and of endometrial carcinoma (Sitruk-Ware *et al.*, 1977; Bulbrook *et al.*, 1978).
3. Regeneration of cytosol receptor proteins must occur for continued oestrogenic activity. Synthetic oestradiol antagonists such as Tamoxifen translocate most of the receptor protein into the nucleus, without regeneration of cytosol receptors. This results in over 90% of receptor proteins remaining bound to nuclear acceptors for up to 48 hours (Jordan *et al.*, 1977). It is not yet known whether the lack of regeneration of unfilled cytosol receptors results in unresponsiveness to further oestrogenic stimuli under these circumstances, or whether there is another metabolic block in the expression of genome activity by such oestrogen antagonists (Sutherland *et al.*, 1980).
4. Unfilled cytosol oestrogen receptor proteins in significant titre (>3–5 fmol/mg) are present in only about 20% of premenopausal breast cancers, compared to more than one-half of cancers from postmenopausal woemn. Part of this difference may result from endogenous oestrogen binding to receptors, but it is also possible that the better retention of unfilled cytosol oestrogen receptors in postmenopausal breast cancer tissues may reflect a

different endocrine pathogenesis of breast cancer in the two age-groups. Thus, it has been observed that mammary cancers induced in intact female rats by 350–400 r whole body radiation retain most of their oestrogen receptor function, the majority being inhibited by treatment with Tamoxifen (Welsch *et al.*, 1981; Lemon and Kumar, 1983). These radiation-induced tumors closely resemble *postmenopausal* breast cancers in their high degree of inhibition by Tamoxifen, whereas chemically induced breast cancers in rats appear to resemble *premenopausal* human breast cancer, in the low amount or absence of unfilled oestrogen receptors and minimal suppression of neoplasia by anti-oestrogens.

5. Prolactin appears more important in the pathogenesis of rodent than human breast cancers, but is said to promote oestrogen receptor biosynthesis syngergistically with oestrogens in neoplastic mammary tissues and not in the uterus (Asselin and Labrie, 1978). Nulliparous women have a 35% higher morning serum prolactin than parous women, independent of age, weight or age at menarche (Yu *et al.*, 1981). Vegetarian diets reduce nocturnal prolactin secretion (Weisburger *et al.*, 1977). Breast cancers which occur bilaterally in 5–10% of women may reflect a combined oestrogenic and prolactin stimulus in postmenopausal women, tending to preserve oestrogenic and progestational receptors in the transformed cells.

Testosterone has the ability to translocate 'empty' oestrogen receptors to the nucleus (Rochefort *et al.*, 1972; Ruh *et al.*, 1975), resulting in minimal biologic activity (Zava and McGuire, 1978). Glucocorticoid binding receptors in human breast cancer cells when filled and transferred to the nucleus, antagonize the action of oestrogens, by inhibiting DNA synthesis and causing a cessation of mitotic activity (Lippman *et al.*, 1976). These observations illustrate other aspects of hormonal interaction which can have modifying influences *in vivo* upon the effect of oestrogens, possibly even in carcinogenesis.

ENDOCRINE PATHOPHYSIOLOGY AFFECTING CANCER RISK

The incidence of cancer in the breast, uterus, ovary, prostate, and gastrointestinal tract varies considerably between populations with different diets, lifestyles, and environments. Some progress has been made in understanding nutritional and other factors that alter endocrine physiology and affect cancer risk, since the close correlation between average annual dietary fat intake and mortality from these cancers was recognized (Table 3).

Effects of diet

Ovo-lacto-vegetarians in highly developed countries such as the United States are 30–40% less likely to develop cancers of the breast. Non-vegetarians such as the Mormons in Utah also have a reduced risk of breast and endometrial cancer, but their incidence rates for prostatic cancer are significantly increased (Lyon *et al.*, 1976). From dietary comparisons in Hawaii and Canada, reduction of both fat and protein intake reduce endometrial and breast cancer risk (Miller *et al.*, 1978; Kolonel *et al.*, 1981). Mixed function oxidase activity in the liver and gastrointestinal tract is influenced by protein intake (Kappas *et al.*, 1976; Mucklow *et al.*, 1979), fat consumption (Mucklow *et al.*, 1980), and the flavone content of the diet (Wattenburg *et al.*, 1968). Vegetarians consuming only 30% of their total calories as fat, consumed more than twice as much fiber as omnivores with a 40% fraction of caloric intake as fats.

Vegetarians excreted more oestrogen in their stools, with a 15–19% reduction in plasma oestrone and oestradiol 17β. Plasma levels of androstenedione and testosterone remained constant or increased slightly. However, none of the observed differences was significant owing to the small number of tested subjects (Goldin *et al.*, 1982). Urinary equol, derived from a phyto-oestrogen with anti-oestrogenic potentialities, was excreted in similar amounts in both omnivores and vegetarians (Adlercreutz *et al.*, 1982). Some vegetarians excreted 20–70-fold more equol than endogenous oestrogens, so that an anti-oestrogenic dietary effect could not be ruled out.

Changes in serum protein binding of sex hormones

Over 95% of plasma oestrone, oestradiol, and testosterone are bound to sex hormone binding globulin (SHBG) and to serum albumin, which reduces the physiologically active dialysable free oestrogens and androgens to a very small fraction of the total. Since so much plasma testosterone and oestradiol is bound to SHBG, variations in the plasma concentration of this protein produced in the liver may be critical in determining the ratio of bound to free circulating sex hormone, which will regulate the local tissue availability for end organ activation.

Hepatic cirrhosis impairs SHBG production, decreasing plasma concentrations, and reducing the available protein high affinity binding sites for sex hormones in plasma. Since testosterone has a higher affinity for SHBG than has oestradiol, transport of the latter in an inactive form will be more impaired, resulting in a chronic net oestrogenic effect in either sex (Vigersky *et al.*, 1979). In males this can lead to testicular atrophy and gynecomastia. In females this can lead to amenorrhea, with a sustained chronic oestrogenic stimulation, but has not so far led to a significant increase in cancers in target organs, probably because of the limited life expectancy of the cirrhotic patient.

Both obese men and women may have reduced sex hormone binding proteins in their plasma (O'Dea *et al.*, 1979; Davidson *et al.*, 1981). In the latter study in cancerous and non-cancerous women, body size was positively correlated with total plasma oestradiol, non-SHBG bound oestradiol and absolute free oestradiol. Body size was inversely correlated with the concentration of SHBG in blood.

The greater biologically active diffusible oestradiol in obese older women compared to leaner women was confirmed by analysing the penetration of human plasma samples tagged with tritiated oestradiol across the blood–brain barrier of anesthetized rats (Gambone *et al.*, 1982). The oestradiol fraction capable of diffusing across the blood–brain barrier represented the sum of albumin-bound oestradiol + free (dialysable) oestradiol. Correlation coefficients of −0.86 to 0.98 were established in cancer and control subjects between per cent SHBG and the brain uptake index. Although the 20% mean increase in brain uptake index of endometrial cancer patients was not significantly different from the control mean, positive correlation coefficients were noted between this index and the per cent of ideal weight in the cancer patients (0.65) and in the controls (0.21). These studies confirm clinical observations many years ago, that obese women with endometrial cancer retained 44% of an administered oestradiol dose in their tissues, compared to only 32% retention in non-obese women (Twombley *et al.*, 1961).

These investigations emphasize the increased risk that chronic obesity may confer for carcinogenesis in mammary, endometrial, and ovarian epithelia, even though not all investigators agree as to the degree of this risk (De Waard and Baanders-Halewijn, 1974; Choi *et al.*, 1978). Weight reduction has been shown to decrease plasma oestrone, oestradiol, and free testosterone in obese males, without much change in SHBG concentration (Stanik *et al.*, 1981). Postmenopausal vegetarian women were noted to have lower urinary levels of oestriol, total oestrogen, lower plasma prolactins, and higher concentrations of SHBG (Armstrong *et al.*, 1981). Plasma SHBG levels were highly correlated with plasma high density lipoprotein cholesterol. Neither body weight nor obesity was a confounding factor.

Therefore, weight reduction and low-fat, high-fiber (vegetarian) diets may both offer an approach to multiple cancer prevention in women, affecting about one-half of their total risk of cancer. The mortality rates for breast, endometrial and ovarian cancers, as well as for prostatic and colorectal cancer, are linearly correlated with the average consumption of meat protein, fat and total calories per person in many countries of the world (Lea, 1966; Doll *et al.*, 1970; Armstrong and Doll, 1975) (Table 3).

Chronic drug therapy stimulating mixed function tissue oxidases

Diphenylhydantoin (Dilantin) and phenobarbital are noteworthy inducers of mixed function oxidases in animals and man. In some women, Dilantin therapy has induced a marked anti-oestrogenic syndrome, with reduced serum oestrone and oestradiol levels, increased pituitary gonadotropin release, elevated SHBG, and failure of oral contraceptives to prevent conception (Notelovitz *et al.*, 1981). Prospective investigations of Dilantin therapy in both sexes have confirmed a 30–40% increase in SHBG for the duration of treatment, thereby reducing the biologically active free fraction of testosterone and oestradiol (Victor *et al.*, 1977; Barragry *et al.*, 1978; Toone *et al.*, 1980).

A Danish investigation of the carcinogenicity of anti-epileptic drugs (which included phenobarbital, Dilantin, and primidone) reported a 29% *reduction* in the incidence of breast and reproductive tract neoplasms (compared to the age-corrected expected risk) in epileptics treated for over 10 years, but not for a lesser time, out of a population of 3810 women (Clemmeson *et al.*, 1974; Clemmeson and Hjalgrim-Jensen, 1978). A British investigation of cancer mortality rates in severe epileptics, however, observed a 1.6-fold to 2.2-fold *increase* in breast and reproductive tract cancer deaths compared to the expected mortality rates, in a smaller patient series whose duration of treatment was not given (White *et al.*, 1979).

Feeding of 1% Dilantin in drinking water to intact female rats beginning two weeks before induction of mammary carcinogenesis by 7,12-dimethylbenz[*a*]anthracene has reduced by 50% the incidence of breast carcinomas compared to the DMBA-treated controls not given Dilantin, during the first four months of observation. Initiating Dilantin feeding at the same time as the carcinogen gave no protection whatsoever against breast cancer (Lemon *et al.*, 1983). These investigations emphasize the important role that chronic therapy with xenobiotic drugs may play in modifying risk of multiple carcinogenesis, and offer a possible approach to cancer prevention.

Influence of somatotype on cancer risk

Women who develop endometrial cancers without exogenous hormonal supplementation have a characteristic somatotype marked by obesity, hypertension, mild hirsutism, and diabetes mellitus (MacMahon, 1974; Koss *et al.*, 1980). These women have abundant adrenocortical secretion of dehydroepiandrosterone and Δ-4 androstenedione, the latter providing a precursor for testosterone and oestrone biosynthesis after the menopause (Siiteri *et al.*, 1972). They tend to develop minimal postmenopausal osteoporosis, while on the other hand, slender women who may show osteoporosis have much smaller muscles and fat depots for aromatization of androstenedione to oestrone (Longcope *et al.*, 1978). Reduced androstenedione and oestrone plasma concentrations have been described in postmenopausal osteoporosis, which may well have an aetiologic relationship to the more rapid skeletal demineralization and loss of bone matrix, that occurs in the 25% of elderly women crippled by this disease (Crilly *et al.*, 1978).

In our experience, osteoporotic women very seldom develop breast, endometrial or ovarian cancers, and in these women, postmenopausal administration of oestrogens is advisable for years to inhibit bone resorption and prevent fractures. The incidence of breast or genital tract malignancies has been very low in this population of oestrogen-treated osteoporotics, according to those clinicians with the greatest treatment experience (Wallach and Henneman, 1959; Gordan and Greenberg, 1976). We believe it is likely that the somatotype of osteoporotic women, with its underlying reduction in endogenous androstenedione and oestrone production, renders them less susceptible to the potential cancer-inducing effects of low dose oestrogen therapy late in life.

In a prospective investigation of breast cancer development in over 7000 Dutch women, both obesity and tallness increased cancer risk in postmenopausal women while high parity counteracted the influence of obesity on breast cancer risk (De Waard and Baanders-van Halewijn, 1974).

CONCLUSION

The significant correlation of ovarian, endometrial, and mammary cancers in women is likely to be a demonstration of the potency of oestrogenic hormones in inducing multiple carcinomas. Most of these cancers develop after the end of reproductive activity, and thus are not susceptible to being screened out through gradual elimination of the genetically predisposed carriers for the phenotype. These cancers also illustrate the modifying influence that nutrition can have on disease incidence, with the higher cancer risks most apparent in the obese.

The future control of these cancers may be influenced by current investigations of dietary modification, and of weight reduction in relation to sex hormone metabolism in women. Other investigations have resulted in a diminution of multiple cancer risk.

Since the relationship of chronic postmenopausal oestrogen supplementation to increased endometrial cancer risk was publicized in 1975–76, an impressive decrease was recorded in US sales of oestrogens, and a decrease in the incidence of endometrial and possibly of breast cancer (Greenwald, 1981; Lawson *et al.*, 1981). Following banning of diethylstilbestrol therapy to pregnant women, there has been a decrease in reports of new cases of vaginal and cervical carcinoma in girls and young women.

Whether prostatic carcinoma in males may be fitted into the pattern of sex-hormone induced cancers still remains a question. Prostatic carcinoma appears significantly associated with 50–60 years of normal male endocrine function and is marked by an increasing intranuclear concentration of dihydrotestosterone in prostatic tissue as one proceeds from normal to benign hyperplasia and finally to well-differentiated cancer. On the other hand the aging male shows an increase in circulating plasma oestrogens, inducing an increase in SHBG, and a reduction in plasma total and free testosterone, which may provide an increased oestrogenic stimulus to some portion of the prostatic gland (Griffiths *et al.*, 1981).

At present, the association between carcinomas of the lower gastrointestinal tract and those in the reproductive system of females seems most likely to be indirect, through dietary factors which influence bile acid production and excretion, and the influence of these cocarcinogens upon the recycling of oestrogens in the enterohepatic circulation. The possibility of risk reduction for both types of cancer by adoption of diets low in fat and high in fiber needs investigation.

Receptors for sex hormones have now been described in a variety of normal tissues such as gingival mucosa, endothelium, liver, and heart; also in a variety of malignant tumors such as melanoma, renal cell carcinoma, meningioma, and colorectal carcinoma, not usually considered to be hormonally induced or promoted. These latter may offer an example of derepression of genetic functions during cell transformation. They do not necessarily indicate a role for oestrogens or androgens in the induction or promotion of cancers in non-reproductive tract neoplasms. Sex hormones are unlikely to have a substantial role in treating these neoplasms, because of either very limited amounts of intracellular accumulation in normal differentiated tissues, lack of mono-oxygenases in the microsomes capable of epoxide generation, or lack of a significant proliferative response to sex hormone stimulation.

REFERENCES

Adlercreutz, H., Fotsis, T., Heikkinen, R. *et al.* (1982). Excretion of the lignans enterolactone and enterodiol and of equol in omnivorous and vegetarian post-menopausal women and in women with breast cancer. *Lancet*, **2**, 1295.

Adlercreutz, H., Goldin, B. R., Dwyer, J. T. *et al.* (1981). Effect of diet on estrogen metabolism in women. *Excerpta Medica International Congress Series*, **515**, 5.

Alford, T. C., Do, H. M., Geelhoed, G. M. *et al.* (1979). Steroid hormone receptors in human colon cancers. *Cancer*, **43**, 980.

Armstrong, B., and Doll, R. (1975). Environmental factors and cancer incidence and mortality in different countries, with special reference to dietary practices. *International Journal of Cancer*, **15**, 617.

Armstrong, B. K., Brown, J. B., Clarke, H. T. *et al.* (1981). Diet and reproductive hormones; a study of vegetarian and non-vegetarian post-menopausal women. *Journal of the National Cancer Institute*, **67**, 761.

Asselin, J., and Labrie, F. (1978). Effects of estradiol and prolactin on steroid receptor levels in 7,12-dimethylbenz(*a*)anthracene-induced mammary tumors and uterus in the rat. *Journal of Steroid Biochemistry*, **9**, 1079.

Bacigalupo, G., and Shubert, K. (1966). Some aspects of oestrogen metabolism in cases of human mammary neoplasia. *European Journal of Cancer*, **2**, 75.

Barragry, M., Makin, H. L. J., Trafford, D. J. H., and Scott, D. F. (1978). Effect of anti-convulsants on plasma testosterone and sex hormone binding globulin levels. *Journal of Neurology, Neurosurgery and Psychiatry*, **41**, 913.

Berggvist, A., Kullander, S., and Thorell, J. (1981). A study of estrogen and progesterone cytosol receptor concentration in benign and malignant ovarian tumors and a review of malignant ovarian tumors treated with medroxy-progesterone acetate. *Acta Obstetrica Gynecologica Scandinavia, Suppl.*, **101**, 75.

Bibbo, M., Haenzel, W. M., Wied, G. L. *et al.* (1978). A twenty-five year follow-up of women exposed to diethylstilbestrol during pregnancy. *New England Journal of Medicine*, **298**, 763.

Briggs, M. (1972). Ethnic differences in urinary oestrogens. *Lancet*, **1**, 324.

Bulbrook, R. D., Moore, J. W., Clark, G. M. G. *et al.* (1978). Plasma oestradiol and progesterone levels in women with varying degrees of risk of breast cancer. *European Journal of Cancer*, **14**, 1369.

Carroll, K. K., and Khor, H. T. (1975). Dietary fat in relation to tumorigenesis. *Progress Biochemical Pharmacology*, **10**, 308.

Chandhuri, P. K., Walter, M. J., Briele, H. A. *et al.* (1980). Incidence of estrogen receptors in benign nevi and human malignant melanoma. *Journal of the American Medical Association*, **244**, 791.

Choi, N. N., Howe, G. R., Miller, A. B. *et al.* (1978). An epidemiologic study of breast cancer. *American Journal of Epidemiology*, **107**, 510.

Clark, L. G., Portier, K. (1979). Diethylstilbestrol and risk of breast cancer (Letter). *New England Journal of Medicine*, **300**, 263.

Clavel, F., Le, M., and Laplanche, A. (1981). Breast cancer and use of anti-hypertensive drugs and oral contraceptives; results of a case-control study (Translation). *Bulletin Cancer*, **68**, 449.

Clemmeson, J., Fuglsang-Frederickson, V., and Plum, C. M. (1974). Are anti-convulsants carcinogenic? *Lancet*, **1**, 705.

Clemmeson, J., Hjalgrim-Jensen, S. (1978). Is phenobarbital carcinogenic? A follow-up of 8078 epileptics. *Ecotoxicology and Environmental Safety*, **1**, 457.

Cole, P., and MacMahon, B. (1969). Oestrogen fractions during early reproductive life in the aetiology of breast cancer. *Lancet*, **1**, 604.

Cole, P., Brown, J. B., and MacMahon, B. (1976). Oestrogen profiles of parous and nulliparous women. *Lancet*, **2**, 596.

Cole, P., Cramer, D., Yen, S. *et al.* (1978). Estrogen profiles of premenopausal women with breast cancer. *Cancer Research*, **38**, 745.

Crilly, R. G., Horsman, A., Marshall, D. H., Nordin, B. E. C. (1978). Postmeno-pausal and corticosteroid-induced osteoporosis. *Frontiers Hormone Research*, **5**, 53. Basel: Karger.

Cutler, B. S., Forbes, A. P., Ingersoll, F. M., and Scully, R. E. (1972). Endometrial carcinoma after stilbestrol therapy in gonadal dysgenesis. *New England Journal of Medicine*, **276**, 628.

Dales, L. G., Friedman, D. G., Ury, H. K. *et al.* (1979). A case-control study of relationship of diet and other traits to colorectal cancer in American blacks. *American Journal of Epidemiology*, **109**, 132.

Davidson, B. J., Gambone, J. C., LaGasse, L. D. *et al.* (1981). Free estradiol in post-menopausal women with and without endometrial cancer. *Journal of Clinical Endocrinology and Metabolism*, **52**, 404.

De Waard, F., and Baanders-van Halewijn, E. A. (1974). A prospective study in general practice on breast cancer risk in postmenopausal women. *International Journal of Cancer*, **14**, 153.

Dickinson, L., MacMahon, B., Cole, P., Brown, J. B. (1974). Estrogen profiles of Oriental and Caucasian women in Hawaii. *New England Journal of Medicine*, **91**, 1211.

Doll, R., Payne, R., and Waterhouse (eds) (1970). *Cancer incidence in five continents II*. Berlin: Springer Verlag.

Ekman, P., Snowchowski, M., Zetterberg, A. *et al.* (1979). Steroid receptor content in human prostatic carcinoma and response to endocrine therapy. *Cancer*, **44**, 1173.

Fasal, E., and Paffenbarger, R. (1975). Oral contraceptives as related to cancer and benign lesions of the breast. *Journal of the National Cancer Institute*, **55**, 767.

Fisher, R. I., Neifeld, J. P., and Lippman, M. E. (1976). Oestrogen receptors in malignant melanoma. *Lancet*, **2**, 337.

Gambone, J. C., Pardridge, W. M., Lagasse, L. D., Judd, H. L. (1982). *In vivo* availability of circulating estradiol in postmenopausal women with and without endometrial cancer. *Obstetrics and Gynecology*, **59**, 416.

Gambrell, R. D., Massey, F. M., Castaneda, T. A. *et al.* (1980). Use of the progestogen challenge test to reduce the risk of endometrial cancer. *Obstetrics and Gynecology*, **55**, 732.

Geller, J., Albert, J., de la Vega, D. *et al.* (1978). Dihydrotestosterone concentration in prostate cancer tissue as a predictor of tumor differentiation and hormonal dependency. *Cancer Research*, **38**, 4349.

Geller, J., Albert, J., Yen, S. S. C. *et al.* (1981). Medical castration of males with megestrol acetate and small doses of diethylstilbestrol. *Journal of Clinical Endocrinology and Metabolism*, **52**, 576.

Goldin, B. R., Adlercreutz, H., Gorbach, S. L. *et al.* (1982). Estrogen excretion patterns and plasma levels in vegetarian and omnivorous women. *New England Journal of Medicine*, **307**, 1542.

Gordan, G. S., and Greenburg, B. G. (1976). Exogenous estrogens and endometrial cancer. *Postgraduate Medicine*, **59**, 66.

Greenberg, R. A. (1963). The occurrence of multiple primary cancers in Connecticut, 1935–1954. *Connecticut Health Bulletin*, **77**, 257.

Greenwald, P. (1981). Cancer and the environment. *Current Concepts in Clinical Oncology*, **3**, 3.

Griffiths, K., Peeling, W. B., Harper, M. E. *et al.* (1981). In *Hormonal management of endocrine-related cancer*. (ed. B. A. Stoll). London: Lloyd-Luke (Medical Books), p. 131.

Gross, J., Moden, B., Bertini, B. *et al.* (1977). Relationship between steroid excretion patterns and breast cancer incidence in Israeli women of various origins. *Journal of the National Cancer Institute*, **59**, 7.

Gusberg, S. B. (1980). The changing nature of endometrial cancer. *New England Journal of Medicine*, **302**, 729.

Gustafson, J. A., Ekman, P., Snowchowski, M. *et al.* (1978). Correlation between clinical response to hormone therapy and steroid receptor content in prostatic cancer. *Cancer Research*, **38**, 4345.

Hähnel, R., Nat, R., Kelsall, G. R. *et al.* (1982). Estrogen and progesterone receptors in tumors of the human ovary. *Gynecologic Oncology*, **13**, 145.

Hamilton, T. C., Davies, P., Griffiths, K. (1981). Androgen and oestrogen binding in cytosols of human ovarian tumours. *Journal of Endocrinology*, **90**, 421.

Herbst, A. L., and Bern, H. A. (1981). Developmental effects of diethylstilbestrol (DES) in pregnancy. New York: Thieme-Stratton.

Hill, P., Wynder, E. L., Garbaczewski, L., Walker, A. R. P. (1982). Effect of diet on plasma and urinary hormones in South African black men with prostatic cancer. *Cancer Research*, **42**, 3864.

Holt, J. A., Caputo, T. A., Kelly, K. M. *et al.* (1979). Estrogen and progestin binding in cytosols of ovarian adenocarcinomas. *Obstetrics and Gynecology*, **53**, 50.

Hoover, R., Gray, L. A., Cole, P., and MacMahon, B. (1976). Menopausal estrogens and breast cancer. *New England Journal of Medicine*, **295**, 401.

Hoover, R., Gray, L. A., and Fraumeni, J. F. (1977). Stilboestrol (diethylstilboestrol) and the risk of ovarian cancer. *Lancet*, **2**, 533.

Hoover, R., Glass, L., Finkle, W. D. *et al.* (1981). Conjugated estrogens and risk of breast cancer. *Journal of the National Cancer Institute*, **67**, 815.

Johnson, F. L., Feagler, J. R., Lerner, K. G. *et al.* (1972). Association of androgenic–anabolic steroid therapy with development of hepatocellular carcinoma. *Lancet*, **2**, 1273.

Jordan, V. C., Dix, C. J., Rowsley, L., and Prestwick, G. (1977). Studies on the mechanism of action of the non-steroidal antioestrogen Tamoxifen (ICI 46474). *Molecular and Cellular Endocrinology*, **7**, 177.

Kappas, A., Andersson, K. E., Conney, A. H., and Alvares A. P. (1976). Influence of dietary protein and carbohydrate on antipyrine and theophyllin metabolism in man. *Clinical Pharmacology and Therapy*, **20**, 643.

Kay, R. M. (1981). Effects of diet on the fecal excretion and bacterial modification of acidic and neutral steroids, and implications for colon carcinogenesis. *Cancer Research*, **41**, 3774.

Kinlen, L. J. (1982). Meat and fat consumption and cancer mortality; a study of strict religious orders in Britain. *Lancet*, **1**, 946.

Kolonel, I. N., Hanku, J. H., Lea, J. *et al.* (1981). Nutrient intake in relation to cancer incidence in Hawaii. *British Journal of Cancer*, **44**, 332.

Korenman, S. (1969). Comparative binding affinity of estrogens and its relation to estrogenic potency. *Steroids*, **13**, 163.

Koss, L. G., Cramer, D., Ferenczy, A. *et al.* (1980). Recent advances in endometrial neoplasia. *Acta Cytologica*, **24**, 478.

Lawson, D. H., Jick, H., Hunter, J. R., and Madsen, S. (1981). Exogenous estrogens and breast cancer. *American Journal of Epidemiology*, **114**, 710.

Lea, A. J. (1966). Dietary factors associated with death rates from certain neoplasms in man. *Lancet*, **2**, 332.

Lehoux, J. G., Benard, B., and Elhilali, M. (1980). Dihydrotestosterone receptors in the human prostate. 1. Nuclear concentration in normal, benign and malignant tissues. *Archives of Andrology*, **5**, 237.

Lemon, H. M., and Kumar, P. (1983). Influence of method of mammary cancer induction upon Tamoxifen modification of hormone promotion. *Proceedings of the American Association for Cancer Research*, **24**, 171.

Lemon, H. M., Stohs, S. J., Pfeiffer R. A., and Campbell, J. (1984). Proceedings of the American Association for Cancer Research (in press).

Lemon, H. M., Wotiz, H. H., Parsons, L., and Mozden, P. J. (1966). Reduced estriol excretion in patients with breast cancer prior to endocrine therapy. *Journal of the American Medical Association*, **196**, 1128.

Lingeman, C. H. (1979). Hormones and hormonomimetic compounds in the etiology of cancer. In *Carcinogenic hormones*. *Recent Results in Cancer Research*, **66**, 1.

Lippman, M., Bolan, G., and Huff, K. (1976). The effect of glucocorticoids and progesterone on hormone responsive breast cancer in long term tissue culture. *Cancer Research*, **36**, 4602.

Longcope, C., Pratt, J. H., Schneider, S. H., and Fineberg, S. E. (1978) Aromatization of androgens by muscle and adipose tissue *in vivo*. *Journal of Clinical Endocrinology and Metabolism*, **46**, 146.

Lynch, H. T., Frichot, B. C., Lynch, P. *et al.* (1975). Family studies of malignant melanoma and associated cancer. *Surgery, Gynecology, Obstetrics*, **141**, 517.

Lynch, H. T., Lynch, P. M., Albano, W. A., and Lynch, J. F. (1981). The cancer syndrome, a status report. *Disease of the Colon and Rectum*, **24**, 311.

Lyon, F. A. (1975). Development of adenocarcinoma of the endometrium in young women receiving long-term sequential oral contraceptives. *American Journal of Obstetrics and Gynecology*, **123**, 299.

Lyon, J. H., Klauber, M. R., Gardner, J. W., and Smart, C. R. (1976). Cancer incidence in Mormons and non-Mormons in Utah, 1966–1970. *New England Journal of Medicine*, **294**, 129.

MacMahon, B. (1974). Risk factors for endometrial cancer. *Gynecologic Oncology*, **2**, 122.

McMahon, B., Andersen, A. P., Brown, J. *et al.* (1980). Urine estrogen profiles in European countries with high or low breast cancer rates. *European Journal of Cancer*, **16**, 1627.

MacMahon, B., Cole, P., Brown, J. B. *et al.* (1974). Urine oestrogen profiles of Asian and North American women. *International Journal of Cancer*, **14**, 161.

Masiel, A., Buttrick, P., and Bitran, J. (1980). Tamoxifen in the treatment of malignant melanoma. *Cancer Treatment Reports*, **64**, 531.

McNeal, J. E. (1970). Age-related changes in prostatic epithelium associated with carcinoma. In *Some aspects of the aetiology and biochemistry of prostatic cancer* (eds K. Griffiths and C. G. Pierrepoint). Third Tenovus Workshop, Alpha Omega Alpha, Cardiff, pp. 23–32.

Mehta, R. G., Fricks, C. M., and Noon, R. C. (1980). Androgen receptors in chemically-induced colon carcinogenesis. *Cancer*, **45**, 1085.

Miller, A. B., Kelly, A., Choi, N. W. *et al.* (1978). A study of diet and breast cancer. *American Journal of Epidemiology*, **107**, 499.

Mirimanoff, R. O., Wagenknecht, L., and Hunzicker, N. (1981). Long-term complete remission of malignant melanoma with Tamoxifen. *Lancet*, **1**, 1368.

Morreal, C. E., Dao, T. L., Nemoto, T., and Lonergan, P. A. (1979). Urinary excretion of estrone, estradiol and estriol in post-menopausal women with primary breast cancer. *Journal of the National Cancer Institute*, **63**, 1171.

Mucklow, J. C., Caraher, M. T., Henderson, D. B., and Rawlins, M. D. (1979). The effect of individual dietary constituents on antipyrine clearance in Asian immigrants. *British Journal Clinical Pharmacology*, **7**, 416.

Mucklow, J. C., Caraher, M. T., Idle, J. R. *et al.* (1980). The influence of changes in dietary fat on the clearance of antipyrine and 4-hydroxylation of debrisoquine. *British Journal Clinical Pharmacology*, **9**, 283.

Naftolin, F., and Eisenfeld, H. J. (1982). Estrogen receptors in ovarian epithelial carcinoma. *Obstetrics and Gynecology*, **59**, 229.

Nesbit, R. A., Woods, R. I., Tattersall, M. N. H. *et al.* (1979). Tamoxifen in malignant melanoma. *New England Journal of Medicine*, **301**, 1241.

Notelovitz, M., Tjapkes, J., and Ware, M. (1981). Interaction between estrogen and Dilantin in a menopausal woman. *New England Journal of Medicine*, **304**, 788.

O'Dea, J. P. K., Weiland, R. G., Hallberg, M. C. *et al.* (1979). Effect of dietary weight loss on sex steroid binding proteins and gonadotropins in obese post-menopausal women. *Journal of Laboratory and Clinical Medicine*, **93**, 1004.

Okulicz, W. C., Evans, R. W., and Leavitt, W. W. (1981). Progesterone regulation of the occupied form of the nuclear estrogen receptor. *Science*, **213**, 1503.

Reddy, B. S. (1981). Diet and excretion of bile acids. *Cancer Research*, **41**, 3766.

Rochefort, H., Lignon, F., and Capony, F. (1972). Formation of estrogen nuclear receptor in uterus; effect of androgens, estrone and nafoxidine. *Biochemical and Biophysical Research Communications*, **47**, 662.

Rosenberg, L., Shapiro, S., Slone, D. *et al.* (1982). Epithelial ovarian cancer and combination oral contraceptives. *Journal of the American Medical Association*, **247**, 3210.

Ross, R. K., Paganini-Hill, A., Gerkins, V. R. *et al.* (1980). A case-control study of menopausal estrogen therapy and breast cancer. *Journal of the American Medical Association*, **243**, 1635.

Ruh, T. S., Wassilak, S. G., and Ruh, M. F. (1975). Androgen-induced nuclear accumulation of the estrogen receptor. *Steroids*, **25**, 257.

Schwarz, P. E., Keating, G., MacLusky, N. *et al.* (1982b). Tamoxifen therapy for advanced ovarian cancer. *Obstetrics and Gynecology*, **59**, 583.

Schwarz, P. E., LiVoisi, V. A., Hildreth, N. *et al.* (1982a). Estrogen receptors in epithelial ovarian carcinoma. *Obstetrics and Gynecology*, **59**, 229.

Sica, V., Contieri, E., Nola, E. *et al.* (1981). Estrogen and progesterone binding proteins in human colorectal cancer. A preliminary characterization of estradiol receptor. *Tumori*, **67**, 307.

Siiteri, P. K., Hemsell, D. L., Edwards, C. L., and MacDonald, P. C. (1972). Estrogen and endometrial carcinoma. *Endocrinology; Procedings Fourth International Congress of Endocrinology*, Washington, DC, 18–24 June, 1972; *Excerpta Medica*, Amsterdam, pp. 1237–1242.

Silverberg, S. G., and Makowski, E. L. (1975). Endometrial carcinoma in young women taking oral contraceptive agents. *Obstetrics and Gynecology*, **46**, 503.

Sitruk-Ware, L. R., Sterkers, N., Mowszowicz, I., and Mauvais-Jarvis, P. (1977). Inadequate corpus luteum function in women with benign breast disease. *Journal of Clinical Endocrinology and Metabolism*, **44**, 771.

Sjogren, H. O. (1977). The application of immunology to the development of immunotherapeutic programs for patients with large bowel cancer. *Cancer*, **40**, 2710.

Stanik, S., Dornfeld, L. P., Maxwell, M. H. *et al.* (1981). The effect of weight loss on reproductive hormones in obese men. *Journal of Clinical Endocrinology and Metabolism*, **53**, 828.

Sutherland, R. L., Murphy, L. C., Foo, S. M. *et al.* (1980). High affinity anti-estrogen binding sites distinct from the oestrogen receptor. *Nature*, **288**, 273.

Thijssen, J. H. H., Wiegerinck, M. A. H. M., Mulder, G., and Poortman, J. (1978). On the biologic activity of estrone *in vivo*. *Frontiers Hormone Research*, **5**, 220.

Thom, M. H., White, P. J., Williams, R. M. *et al.* (1979). Prevention and treatment of endometrial disease in climacteric women receiving oestrogen therapy. *Lancet*, **2**, 455.

Toone, B. K., Wheeler, M., and Fenwick, P. B. C. (1980). Sex hormone changes in male epileptics *Clinical Endocrinology*, **12**, 391.

Trachtenberg, J., and Walsh, P. C. (1982). Correlation of prostatic nuclear androgen receptor content with duration of response and survival following hormonal therapy in advanced prostate cancer. *Journal of Urology*, **127**, 466.

Trichopoulos, D., Cole, P., Brown, J. B. *et al.* (1980). Estrogen profiles of primiparous and nulliparous. *Journal of the National Cancer Institute*. **65**, 43.

Twombley, G. H., Scheimer, S., and Levitz, M. (1961). Endometrial cancer, obesity and estrogen excretion in women. *American Journal of Obstetrics and Gynecology*, **82**, 424.

Victor, A., Lundberg, P. O., and Johansson, E. D. B. (1977). Induction of sex hormone binding globulin by phenytoin. *British Medical Journal*, **2**, 934.

Vigersky, R. A., Kono, S., Sauer, M. *et al.* (1979). Relative binding of testosterone and estradiol to testosterone estradiol-binding globulin. *Journal of Clinical Endocrinology and Metabolism*, **49**, 899.

Wallach, S., and Henneman, P. H. (1959). Prolonged estrogen therapy in post-menopausal women. *Journal of the American Medical Association,* **171,** 1637.

Wattenburg, L. W., Page, M. A., and Leong, J. L. (1968). Induction of increased benzpyrene hydroxylase activity by flavones and related compounds. *Cancer Research,* **28,** 934.

Weisburger, J. H., Cohen, L. H., Wynder, E. L. (1977). On the etiology and metabolic epidemiology of the main human cancers. In *Incidence of cancer in humans* (eds H. H. Hiatt, J. D. Watson, and J. A. Winsten). Cold Spring Harbor Conferences on Cell Proliferation, Vol. 4, Cold Spring Harbor, pp. 567–602.

Weiss, N. S., Daling, J. R., and Chow, W. H. (1981). Incidence of cancer of the large bowel in women in relation to reproductive and hormonal factors. *Journal of the National Cancer Institute,* **67,** 57.

Weiss, N. S., Lyon, J. L., Krishnamurthy, S. *et al.* (1982). Noncontraceptive estrogen use and the occurrence of ovarian cancer. *Journal of the National Cancer Institute,* **68,** 95.

Wellings, S. R., Jensen, H. M., and Marcum, R. G. (1975). An atlas of sub-gross pathology of the human breast with special reference to possible pre-cancerous lesions. *Journal of the National Cancer Institute,* **55,** 231.

Welsch, C. W., Goodrich-Smith, M., Brown, C. K. *et al.* (1981). Effect of an estrogen antagonist (Tamoxifen) on the initiation and progression of gamma-irradiation-induced mammary tumours in female Sprague–Dawley rats. *European Journal of Cancer and Clinical Oncology,* **17,** 1255.

White, S. J., McLean, A. E. M., and Howland, C. (1979). Anti-convulsant drugs and cancer, a cohort study in patients with severe epilepsy. *Lancet,* **2,** 458.

Yu, M. C., Gerkins, V. R., Henderson, B. E. *et al.* (1981). Elevated levels of prolactin in nulliparous women. *British Journal of Cancer,* **43,** 826.

Zava, D. T., and McGuire, W. L. (1978). Human breast cancers; androgen action mediated by estrogen receptor. *Science,* **199,** 787.

Risk Factors and Multiple Cancer
Edited by B.A. Stoll
© 1984 John Wiley and Sons Ltd.

Chapter

11 T. KRAUSZ, J. G. AZZOPARDI, and N. A. WRIGHT

Criteria for Diagnosis of Second Cancer

INTRODUCTION

There are numerous case reports and several detailed reviews of multiple malignant neoplasms in the literature. However, the most crucial point, the criteria used to establish the diagnosis of a second cancer have not received sufficient attention, since Warren and Gates (1932) established the following criteria: (1) each tumour must have definite features of malignancy (2) each tumour must be anatomically distinct (3) the probability of one being a metastasis from the other must be excluded as far as possible. These are the basic criteria which are essential and almost implicit in the concept of multiple cancers.

The majority of later workers have agreed that the general criteria of Warren and Gates are practical and realistic ones and they were adopted by Moertel *et al.* (1961, 1966), whose work on multiple cancers remains the most comprehensive to date. In this critical survey, we discuss *special* criteria of diagnosis, using a modification of Moertel's classification of multiple cancer:

– Multiple primary malignant neoplasms of the same tissue or organ.
  Multicentric lesions of the same organ.
  Multicentric lesions of a paired organ.
  Multicentric lesions of the same tissue in contiguous organs.
– Multiple primary malignant neoplasms of different tissues or organs.
– Multiple primary malignant neoplasms in a given organ (tissue) system plus a lesion of an unrelated organ.

Apart from this 'topographic' classification, multiple malignant neoplasms can be classified 'chronologically' as *synchronous* (simultaneous) where two or more cancers are present at the same time, or *metachronous* (interval) where the first cancer is followed by a second at a later date. This clinically useful, though arbitrary, distinction is not always easy to make when the interval between detection of the first and second tumour is short, since it is possible that the second cancer was already present although not clinically manifest, at the time of removal of the first.

SECOND CANCER OF THE SKIN

Squamous carcinoma and basal cell carcinoma

These malignant neoplasms of the skin may present as synchronous or metachronous multiple growths. Most major reviews examining the incidence of multiple cancers exclude these lesions, to avoid an unrealistic high incidence rate of multiple malignancies, but this exclusion is justifiable only in the sense that most skin cancers have a biologically low aggressiveness.

The independent primary nature of any simultaneous or interval tumour is obvious if one of them is a squamous carcinoma while the other is a basal cell carcinoma, because the two types of tumour have distinct pathways of development and the two types are generally considered to be distinct entities. Since most cutaneous squamous carcinomas have a low aggressiveness, the possibility that an anatomically distinct squamous carcinoma of the skin is metastatic from another is remote. Metastases from small (less than 1.5 cm diameter), superficially invasive squamous carcinomas are rare, if they occur at all (Lund, 1965). Even with tumours larger than 2 cm, with invasion of the reticular dermis, the incidence of regional lymph node metastases is less than 5%. Bowenoid or actinic changes in the epidermis adjacent to the tumour can provide additional evidence for the primary site of origin.

A small percentage of squamous carcinomas are histologically so poorly differentiated that the real nature of the tumour cannot be determined by routine histological investigations, and their differentiation from amelanotic melanoma or sarcomas of diverse types can be very difficult. In these cases electronmicroscopic investigation can reveal either melanosomes or tonofilaments and desmosomes, which are of diagnostic value. Immunohistochemical techniques are also helpful: staining with antibodies (a) to keratin would reveal the squamous type, (b) to vimentin the mesenchymal (sarcomatous) type, and (c) to neuron-specific enolase or S-100 protein the melanocytic nature of the tumour cells. Skin metastasis from squamous carcinomas of viscera, particularly of lung, must be excluded.

Basal cell carcinomas are locally invasive and rarely metastasize, so that anatomically distinct, even histologically identical tumours can confidently be regarded as independent primaries. The full excision of each tumour can be confirmed by histological examination.

Malignant melanoma

Patients with multiple primary melanomas are medical curiosities, not only because of their relative rarity, but also because the very aggressive biological behaviour of many melanomas makes any new lesion more likely to be metastatic rather than primary. In cases of widely disseminated melanoma, cutaneous blood-borne metastases are frequent. 'Outcrop' nodules often appear around the primary and, less frequently, even around secondary melanomas of the skin.

The crucial point is the distinction between metastatic malignant melanoma and a primary lesion, especially if the former shows invasion of the epidermis (epidermotropism). Although on gross examination primary melanomas often have an irregular margin and variable colour, while metastatic lesions have a smooth surface with a single colour, only careful histological examination can determine the real nature of these tumours (Moseley *et al.*, 1979). The presence of atypical melanocytes within the epidermis is usually considered to be the most important feature for histological diagnosis of primary malignant melanomas (Allen and Spitz, 1953), while the absence of atypical melanocytes within the epidermis and presence of tumour only in the dermis or the subcutis is characteristic of malignant melanoma metastatic to skin.

The validity of these criteria has been challenged by Kornberg *et al.* (1978) who described four cases of epidermotropic metastatic malignant melanoma; the microscopic features that favoured epidermotropic metastatic malignant melanoma, rather than primary cutaneous malignant melanoma were: (1) thinning of the epidermis by aggregates of atypical melanocytes within the dermis, often associated with widening of dermal papillae and elongation of inward turning rete ridges at the periphery of the specimen (2) atypical melanocytes within intradermal endothelial-lined spaces and (3) a zone of atypical melanocytes within the dermis equal to or broader than that within the epidermis.

Unger *et al.* (1981) added the additional criteria of a normal dermis between the epidermis and the bulk of the tumour, and a single cell population, as suggestive of a metastasis. On the other hand, extensive junctional activity and variability of the malignant cell types indicate a primary lesion. The presence of a benign naevus at the base of the tumour also supports a primary origin.

Apart from the different histological features of primary and metastatic melanomas, there are established prognostic criteria in clinical Stage I melanoma patients which can provide useful information about the probability of developing metastases in an individual patient. The two most important microscopic features which correlate with the prognosis are the *type* of the melanoma and the *thickness* of the tumour.

There are four distinctive types of primary cutaneous melanoma (Clark *et al.*, 1969): lentigo maligna melanoma, superficial spreading melanoma, nodular melanoma, acral lentiginous melanoma (melanoma on palms, soles and nail beds). Clark *et al.* (1969) demonstrated that lentigo maligna melanoma was the least malignant and nodular melanoma was the most aggressive. Wayte and Helwig (1968) studied 85 cases of lentigo maligna, 45 of which showed invasion. Only three patients died of tumour while a fourth, who developed metastases in lymph nodes, remained well after resection of the involved nodes. Clark *et al.* (1969) found that 31.5% of patients with superficial spreading melanoma died as a result of tumour spread, compared with 56.1% of patients with nodular melanoma. The three-year survival rate of acral lentiginous melanoma, only recently identified separately, was found by Coleman *et al.* (1980) to be only 11%.

The depth invasion is determined by using the level system of Clark *et al.* (1969) who divided malignant melanomas into five levels of invasion:

Level I	Intra-epidermal (*in situ* melanoma).
Level II	Invasion into the papillary dermis.
Level III	Tumour filling the papillary dermis and stopping at the interphase between the papillary and reticular dermis.
Level IV	Tumour in the reticular dermis.
Level V	Tumour in the subcutaneous fat.

They found that the prognosis was related to the level of invasion. Holmes *et al.* (1976) showed that regional nodal metastases were present in 32% of patients with level III invasion, 67% with level IV, and 66% with level V. Patients with level I and level II tumours did not undergo lymph node dissection, but none of them had clinical evidence of metastases.

The microstage system described by Breslow (1975) which measures tumour thickness was found to be a reliable index of prognosis; melanomas can be subdivided into low (<0.76 mm), intermediate (0.76 to 1.5 mm), and high risk categories (>1.5 mm). Balch *et al.* (1978) found that the three-year incidence of regional metastases in patients initially treated by wide local excision of the melanoma was 0% for tumours less than 0.76 mm, 25% for 0.76–1.5 mm lesions, 51% for 1.5–3.99 mm lesions, and 62% for lesions 4 mm in thickness or over.

In the series of Kerl *et al.* (1982), early invasive melanomas (<0.76 mm thick) had a 100% 10-year survival, while with lesions 0.76–1.5 mm in thickness the 10-year survival was only 76%. However, even melanomas thinner than 0.76 mm can metastasize, and in a series of 585 cases with Stage I cutaneous malignant melanomas, 72 cases were thin (<0.76 mm), and 10 of these (13.9%) metastasized (Schmoeckel *et al.*, 1982). In cases of thin primary malignant melanomas with histological features of regression, it may be impossible to evaluate prognosis because the tumour, at some time in the past, may have been of sufficient thickness for more aggressive biological behaviour prior to its partial involution (Gromet *et al.*, 1978). It is, therefore, probably appropriate to differentiate between thin melanomas with and without regressive phenomena (Kerl *et al.*, 1982).

In view of the varying aggressiveness with different types of melanomas, with different levels of invasion and different degrees of thickness, attention to these features in a given melanoma is important in assessing realistically the possibility of metastases in an individual case. Additional prognostic information can be gained from the mitotic activity, ulceration and vascular invasion, all of which increase the risk of developing metastases (Schmoeckel *et al.*, 1982).

In cases with multiple nodules of malignant melanoma, in which any of the tumours is in an advanced clinical stage (more than Stage I), the probability of cutaneous metastases is very high and careful evaluation of all the factors mentioned is necessary before accepting the diagnosis of an independent primary malignant melanoma.

SECOND CANCER OF UPPER AERODIGESTIVE TRACT

The squamous epithelium of the upper aerodigestive tract (lip, oral cavity, pharynx, oesophagus, larynx) is considered as a single unit in terms of their common epidemiological, aetiological, and pathogenetic factors (Monnier *et al.*, 1982). The frequent occurrence of multiple synchronous and metachronous cancers in this region is, therefore, not unexpected. McGuirt *et al.* (1982) using a panendoscopic method, also supported the belief that cancer of the upper aerodigestive tract is a panmucosal disease and emphasized that if a patient has one carcinoma in this region the chances of developing another are increased. The concept of 'field cancerization' described by Slaughter *et al.* (1953) for oral carcinomas seems to be valid for the whole upper aerodigestive tract. The common occurrence of carcinoma *in situ* contiguous with invasive carcinoma of the oesophagus is well known (Suckow *et al.*, 1962). Ushigome *et al.* (1967) observed several foci of dysplasia and carcinoma *in situ* of the oesphageal epithelium, and suggested that oesophageal squamous carcinoma is multicentric in origin.

Most of the reported multiple malignant tumours of the upper aerodigestive tract are of the same histological type; they are squamous carcinomas, although very rarely combinations of tumours of different histological type can be found. The diagnosis of a second primary cancer of a different histological type presents few problems but the diagnosis of an independent primary belonging to the same histological type is more difficult. As always, in cases of tumours of the same histological type, the possibility of tumour spread from the other has to be ruled out. Generally speaking, an epidermoid carcinoma can be regarded as primary at any particular site when it shows histological evidence of origin from the overlying squamous epithelium or, in cases of advanced and ulcerated carcinomas, the adjacent surface epithelium shows dysplasia or carcinoma *in situ*. This criterion is the most important for establishing the diagnosis of a second squamous carcinoma.

Multiple epidermoid carcinomas occurring in different anatomical regions of the upper aerodigestive tract at a relatively large distance from each other (e.g. lip and oesophagus, larynx and oesophagus, lip and tongue, tongue and oesophagus), either synchronously or metachronously, can be regarded as independent primaries, because inter-regional metastases simulating primaries are unusual. However, the independent nature of macroscopically multiple epidermoid carcinomas developing in close juxtaposition to each other can only be accepted if careful histological study (step sectioning of the tumour) shows tumour-free tissue between the two lesions. Two foci of invasive carcinoma which are linked by carcinoma *in situ* should be regarded as a single primary with multifocal invasion.

In cases of metachronous cancers occurring in the same anatomic region, it is important to have histological evidence that the first cancer was completely excised and that the second cancer is well away from the previous excision scar. Squamous carcinomas of the lip usually occur on the lower lip, but rarely there is a similar tumour at a corresponding position on the upper lip. The latter is unlikely to be due to implantation of malignant cells into the mucosa of the upper lip; it should be regarded as a separate primary carcinoma.

These criteria can be applied easily in cases of well differentiated or moderately differentiated squamous carcinomas which grow slowly and metastasize relatively late through lymphatics, or for verrucous carcinomas which very rarely metastasize. The degree of malignancy increases from the lip, posteriorly to the base of the tongue and pharyngeal wall so that squamous carcinomas in the latter locations are often poorly differentiated, quickly invade and spread widely into surrounding tissues. An attempt to prove multiplicity in such cases is probably only possible in 'early' microinvasive carcinomas, in which distant tumour spread is rare. A good prognosis, with lack of distant tumour spread, has been demonstrated for microinvasive carcinomas of the oral cavity and vocal cord (depth of invasion 5 mm and 3 mm respectively) by Platz *et al.* (1982) and Kleinsasser and Glanz (1982). In diagnosing multiple cancers in the oesophagus special care should be taken, since submucosal extension of the tumour to several centimetres above or below the gross limits can often be found and this can occasionally erupt to the epithelial surface at a distance from the main tumour mass.

Rarely, epidermoid carcinomas show a spindle cell pattern which has to be distinguished from sarcomas or amelanotic melanomas. In difficult cases, the use of immunohistochemical methods (i.e. keratin antibodies) or electron-microscopic investigation (demonstration of desmosomes and tonofilaments) can reveal the epidermoid nature of a spindle cell tumour, or the presence of melanosomes shows that the tumour is a melanoma. The type of carcinoma of the pharynx, which used to be called a lymphoepithelioma, is now recognized to be a carcinoma of pharyngeal squamous epithelium. It has to be distinguished from malignant lymphoma, a distinction which can be aided by ultrastructural and immunocytochemical methods. These tumours have a more aggressive behaviour than ordinary squamous carcinomas.

When adenocarcinoma involves the lower third of the oesophagus, the question arises whether the tumour is primary in the oesophagus or in the stomach. It is known that primary adenocarcinoma of the oesophagus can arise from the oesophageal glands or from ectopic gastric mucosa (Barrett's oesophagus). The only unquestionable cases of primary adenocarcinoma of the oesophagus, apart from those arising in Barrett's oesophagus, are those in which there is squamous epithelium on both resection margins. This criterion excludes the majority of cardiac tumours, where the lower margin is continuous with gastric mucosa, although it is conceivable that a few of these tumours arise from an oesophagus showing glandular metaplasia.

With adenocarcinoma arising in a Barrett's oesophagus, glandular epithelium is found proximal to the tumour. For practical purposes, it is best to consider all adenocarcinomas involving both sides of the cardia as primary gastric tumours with oesophageal spread, and all epidermoid carcinomas in the same location as primary oesophageal cancers with secondary gastric involvement. A small proportion of carcinomas involving the gastro-oesophageal junction have a mixed histological pattern showing both squamous and glandular differentiation (adenosquamous carcinomas) or resembling tumours of the salivary glands (mucoepidermoid carcinomas). In cases of coincident squamous carcinoma of the oesophagus and adenocarcinoma of the stomach, the separate primary nature of these tumours may be accepted if they are separated from each other by normal mucosa (Golby and Codling, 1969).

Cases of epidermoid carcinoma of the oesophagus colliding with gastric adenocarcinoma have been described. Dodge (1961) emphasized that before dual histogenesis is suggested in cases of mixed glandular and squamous carcinomas in this region, three criteria should be fulfilled: (1) the two structural components (squamous and glandular) should show at least a partial topographical separation (2) the areas of squamous differentiation should lie on the oesophageal side of the tumour, and the areas of glandular differentiation on the gastric (3) there should be little or no evidence of an intermediate histological structure.

Primary carcinomas of the oesophagus must be distinguished from carcinomas involving it secondarily: contiguous spread of tumour from the hypopharynx, larynx or lung or stomach into the oesophagus may produce a lesion resembling primary cancer of the oesophagus. Oat cell carcinoma of the oesophagus is now a well established entity occurring, as it does, in the total absence of a tumour in the respiratory tract (Cook *et al.*, 1976).

Primary malignant melanoma of the oral cavity is well known (Chaudhry *et al.*, 1958), while a few cases of primary malignant melanoma of the oesophagus have also been described (Boyd *et al.*, 1954; Piccone *et al.*, 1970). Junctional activity at the periphery of the tumour should be present in order to exclude a metastatic malignant melanoma.

SECOND CANCER IN THE LUNG

Criteria for the diagnosis of a second bronchial carcinoma

In the comprehensive reports on multiple cancers of Moertel *et al.* (1961, 1966), multiple bronchial cancers were not included because of the problem encountered in establishing, beyond reasonable doubt, that multiple lesions were not metastatic. There is, however, no doubt that independent primary cancers in the lung do exist. Mobley and Martinez (1968) stated that in order to meet the third criterion of Warren and Gates (1932), the histopathological features of the two tumours must be entirely different, a rule which excludes multiple primary squamous carcinomas although the commonest multiple cancers of the lung. Others, however, accept tumours of the same histopathological type if they show convincing evidence of separate origin from the bronchial mucosa (Smith, 1966).

It is now well recognized that the majority of squamous carcinomas of the bronchi arise in an area of carcinoma *in situ*. Eggleston *et al.* (1982), studying 20 cases of *in situ* and microinvasive squamous carcinoma, found that all microinvasive squamous carcinomas were closely associated with an *in situ* component, and that invasion was demonstrable both from the surface mucosa and from mucosal glands. It must be stressed, however, that it has not been shown that *all* cases of squamous carcinoma develop in this fashion, although it is probably reasonable to assume that the majority of clinically detected squamous carcinomas have evolved through similar *in situ* and microinvasive stages.

The presence of carcinoma *in situ* adjacent to invasive cancer can be used as morphological evidence for the origin of the invasive tumour at that site, and to exclude metastatic tumour with secondary involvement of the bronchial wall. The problem of using the *in situ* component as a hallmark for the site of origin is that, while it can be used for centrally located squamous carcinomas, it cannot be used for peripheral squamous carcinomas (where the site of origin usually cannot be found) or for lung cancers of other histological types. *In situ* phases of adenocarcinoma and oat cell carcinoma of the lung are yet to be identified.

Generally speaking, the independent primary nature of separate microinvasive squamous carcinomas can be accepted as long as they are not linked by a continuous field of *in situ* carcinoma, even if they occur in the same lobe; the possibility that a lesion of this type represents spread from the other is negligible. In cases of advanced multiple squamous carcinomas occurring bilaterally or in different lobes, their independent nature is suggested by an adjacent *in situ* component. This does not mean that tumours without an *in situ* component cannot have originated at that site, but only that is is impossible to prove this in the absence of *in situ* tumour.

In addition to these pathomorphological features, Schwartz (1961) suggested a biomathematical approach to evaluate growth rates for primary and metastatic neoplasms; separate primary tumours are, in principle, distinguishable from multiple metastases or from satellite lesions by the equivalence or non-equivalence of the corresponding doubling time.

Obviously, when separate tumours have an entirely different histological picture, the diagnosis of a second cancer is much easier, but one should remember that lung cancers sometimes show a variety of cell types in different structural arrangements; both adenocarcinoma and epidermoid carcinoma may be present in the same tumour (McGrath *et al.*, 1952). Previous radiotherapy or cytotoxic treatment can alter the morphology of any cancer, leading to an error in labelling a metastasis as an independent primary.

Fidler *et al.* (1978) emphasized the heterogeneity of malignant neoplasms, which often show a variety of subpopulations of cells with different biological behaviour. This heterogeneity does not contradict the theory of unicellular origin of malignant neoplasms, but reflects the instability of tumour cell populations and represents a type of progression in neoplastic development (Foulds, 1969, 1975). In spite of these considerations, the vast majority of bronchial carcinomas can be classified according to the WHO tumour classification, provided adequate sampling of each tumour is undertaken (Kreyberg *et al.*, 1967). Bronchoscopic biopsy material is, therefore, sometimes insufficient for correct classification. The pleomorphic histology of some bronchial carcinomas can lead to significant interobserver differences (Rohwedder and Wheatherbee, 1974). While interobserver consistency is high in cases of well-differentiated adenocarcinomas (98%) and well-differentiated squamous carcinomas (95%), there is less agreement with oat cell carcinomas (75%) and poorly differentiated carcinomas (60%) (Yesner *et al.*, 1965).

Electronmicroscopic and immunocytochemical investigations can be helpful in cases where light microscopic procedures provide insufficient information about the differentiation of a tumour. Oat cell carcinomas and carcinoid tumours show dense core granules at the ultrastructural level, and generally give positive immunocytochemical reactions using antibody against neuron-specific enolase. The presence of tonofilaments and desmosomes is consistent with squamous differentiation. But it should be noted that antibodies against keratin and prekeratin often give a positive reaction also with adenocarcinomas. The presence of osmiophilic lamellar bodies, normal constituents of

Type II pneumocytes, is important in the diagnosis of bronchioloalveolar cell carcinoma and in distinguishing it from metastatic adenocarcinoma (Bonikos *et al.*, 1977).

In spite of the frequent occurrence of dysplasia and carcinoma *in situ* of the bronchial mucosa among cigarette smokers, uranium miners, and patients with invasive lung cancer (Auerbach *et al.*, 1957), there are relatively few reported cases of multiple bronchial carcinoma. This is usually attributed to the short survival of most patients with invasive bronchial carcinoma leading to insufficient time for the appearance of a second, clinically apparent, bronchial carcnoma (Coffman *et al.*, 1983). LeGal and Bauer (1961) found that 6.4% of 63 patients who survived at least 30 months following excision of a bronchial carcinoma developed a second primary lung cancer.

Apart from this time factor and the difficulties in diagnosing a second bronchial carcinoma, inadequate histological sampling of the bronchial tree in both surgical and necropsy specimens can also be responsible for the lower frequency of reported multiple tumours compared with the expected incidence. Separate foci of microinvasive carcinomas can easily be missed because the average histological sampling (apart from that of the main lesion and the resection margin) usually includes only a few additional blocks. When Auerbach *et al.* (1967) studied between 50 and 208 blocks of the tracheobronchial tree of 255 patients dying of bronchial carcinoma, they found 3.5% of independent primary invasive cancers when strict criteria were used, and as many as 14.5% using less strict criteria.

An indication of a higher frequency of multiple bronchial cancers than hitherto recognized can be found in the work of Eggleston *et al.* (1982). Of 59 patients in three series with *in situ* or minimally invasive squamous carcinoma, only seven patients died of lung cancer or were alive with unresectable lung cancer: at least four and possibly six of these had developed a second lung cancer.

Criteria for diagnosis of a primary lung carcinoma coexisting with a primary malignant neoplasm of another organ

The lung is one of the most common sites for a wide variety of metastatic lesions, which makes for difficulty in establishing a pulmonary tumour as a true second primary cancer. Although metastases most often present as multiple pulmonary lesions, it is known that single metastases also occur, causing differential diagnostic problems between primary and secondary cancer. While the age, sex, race, symptoms, roentgenographic diagnosis, occupation, history of tobacco smoking, and time interval between the two tumours may help to make a clinical distinction between primary and metastatic disease, the real nature of the lesion can only be determined by histological examination (Cahan, 1977).

This distinction can be made easily when the tumours have entirely different histological characteristics: for example when there is a squamous carcinoma in the upper aerodigestive tract and an adenocarcinoma is present in the lung. However, if the two lesions have the same histological pattern, the distinction may be almost impossible; nevertheless, even in these cases, microscopic examination can be helpful. If the lung tumour is in contact with the bronchial mucosa and the adjacent bronchial epithelium shows *in situ* carcinoma, it most likely arises at that site, a feature which is very helpful when squamous carcinomas are found both in the lung and elsewhere.

It is difficult to establish the diagnosis of an independent primary adenocarcinoma of the lung, when associated with a known case of adenocarcinoma in the gut, pancreas, thyroid, breast or ovaries. As already mentioned, ultrastructural investigation is essential in the diagnosis of primary alveolar cell carcinoma which is often simulated by pulmonary metastases (Rossmann and Vortel, 1961). Histochemical stains, revealing different types of mucin in separate adenocarcinomas, are also helpful.

An increasing range of polyclonal and monoclonal antibodies is being produced against a variety of normal tissue components and tumours and, while the results are promising, at present very few antibodies can be used to distinguish with absolute certainty between adenocarcinomas arising at different sites. Antibody against acid phosphatase can identify the prostatic origin of a metastatic adenocarcinoma, while antibody against thyroglobulin can detect metastatic thyroid carcinoma. CEA antibody can be used to distinguish between malignant mesothelioma and adenocarcinoma arising either in the lung or at other sites.

Giant cell carcinoma of the lung should be distinguished from metastatic pleomorphic rhabdomyosarcoma, malignant fibrous histiocytoma, and adrenal cortical carcinoma. Detection of myoglobin by immunocytochemical methods or the demonstration of myofilaments on ultrastructural examination, indicates differentiation towards muscle.

Clear cell carcinoma of the lung (Morgan and Mackenzie, 1964) is very rare and must be distinguished from metastatic renal carcinoma. Katzenstein *et al.* (1980) found clear cell changes both in epidermoid carcinoma and adenocarcinoma, which suggests that the clear cell carcinoma is not a specific type of lung cancer. In renal carcinomas abundant fat is often present in the cytoplasm of the cells and this can be helpful in differential diagnosis. Clear cell carcinoma of the lung should also be distinguished from the benign clear cell (sugar) tumour of the lung (Liebow and Castleman, 1971). The cells of the benign clear cell tumour are crowded with glycogen, and fat is absent. This tumour, in contrast to carcinomas, does not show mitotic activity.

Bronchial carcinoid tumour has been reported in association with multiple endocrine adenomatosis (Williams and Celestin, 1962). The primary or metastatic nature of an endocrine tumour in cases of multiple endocrine tumours can be difficult and require immunocytochemical investigation. Cooney *et al.* (1980) studied a patient with a carcinoid tumour of the lung and pancreatic islet cell tumour. This patient also had a metastatic neoplasm of endocrine appearance in the liver, and presented with Cushing's syndrome and hyperglycaemia. Immunocytochemical investigation showed ACTH in the carcinoid tumour as well as in the hepatic metastasis, but not in the pancreatic islet cell tumour. This showed that the pancreatic and the lung tumours were independent primaries, and that the lung tumour was the source both of ACTH production and of the liver metastasis.

SECOND CANCER OF GASTROINTESTINAL TRACT

Adenocarcinoma

To establish a diagnosis of multiple synchronous or metachronous cancers of the gastrointestinal tract requires careful pathological study. The distinction between synchronous and metachronous tumours is useful though arbitrary, and it is not always easy to make when the time interval between detection of the first and second tumours is short, since it is possible that the second growth was present at the same time as the first without being clinically manifest (Bussey *et al.*, 1967).

Multiple cancers of the gastrointestinal tract can easily be distinguished from one another if they are of different histological types (e.g. adenocarcinoma, lymphoma, leiomyosarcoma or carcinoid). If they belong to the same histological category care has to be taken to ensure that the second carcinoma is not a recurrence or metastasis from the initial tumour. Bussey *et al.* (1967) found that the macroscopic appearance of the lesion is a good guide, since a recurrence growing in from the peritoneum differs in appearance from that of a new primary arising in the mucosa. Histological differences are not always conclusive, but can be helpful when taken in conjunction with the known type of spread of the first cancer.

A metastasis from a site outside of the gastrointestinal tract (breast, lung, pancreas, ovary, uterus, bile duct) also has to be excluded. This distinction is sometimes possible even if both tumours are adenocarcinomas, because recognizable histological differences exist, for example, between well-differentiated intestinal adenocarcinoma and an adenocarcinoma of the breast. Metastatic lesions are usually small and only occasionally form large polypoid nodules in the mucosa. They are usually located in the submucosa and when they infiltrate the mucosa, the gastric or intestinal glands are displaced without evidence of cellular atypia.

To fulfil the first criterion of Warren and Gates (1932) most authors have excluded cases of tubular adenomas with severe dysplasia or *in situ* carcinoma, and accepted only those cases which showed evidence of invasion, while others accepted the former cases as well. If the adenoma–carcinoma sequence is valid, a study of multiple cancers which includes cases of tubular adenomas with severe dysplasia is probably more justifiable than a study which excludes them.

To prove the independent nature of two neoplasms of the same histological type, it is essential to examine histologically the intervening gastric or intestinal wall in tumours which are closely situated. Tumours thought to be multiple on gross examination can be found microscopically to be continuous through extensive submucosal communication. In studying cases of multiple adenocarcinoma of the gastrointestinal tract, and in excluding metastasis from a site outside the gut, the finding of an adjacent precancerous lesion is extremely helpful and virtually proves the primary nature of the tumour.

Collins and Gall (1952), studying large sections of 117 cases of gastric carcinoma, found that in 22 specimens carcinoma *in situ* was in continuity with the margin of the presenting neoplasm. They also detected independent neoplastic lesions in 26 stomachs: four of these were grossly visible while the remainder were *in situ* carcinomas. Since their study was limited to single histological blocks (and thus reflected the putative multiple phenomena in only one plane) this raises the possibility that the foci considered to be independent might show a connection in three dimensions. To exclude this, step-sectioning of multiple histological blocks is required.

Lauren (1965) divided gastric carcinomas into two main histological types: intestinal and diffuse. Nakamura *et al.* (1968) demonstrated that, although advanced gastric cancers can show a variety of histological patterns, at their margins where only the mucosa is involved, only the differentiated (intestinal) or undifferentiated (diffuse) type is seen. He concluded that the additional histologic type seen in advanced gastric carcinoma is a secondary modification of the basic type. It is generally accepted that the intestinal type arises in intestinal metaplasia (Ming *et al.*, 1967) and several workers have noted heterogeneity within intestinal metaplasia (Iida *et al.*, 1978). Intestinal metaplasia can be divided into two types: complete and incomplete and Jass (1983) demonstrated that the incomplete variety of intestinal metaplasia is strongly related to gastric carcinoma.

In many organs, the presence of epithelial dysplasia adjacent to an invasive carcinoma is one of the most useful criteria for the diagnosis of a second cancer. In the stomach the degree of risk associated with epithelial dysplasia has yet to be established. Generally speaking, epithelial dysplasia is a precancerous lesion, a *histopathological* abnormality in which cancer is more likely to occur than in its normal counterpart. Epithelial dysplasia should be distinguished from a precancerous *clinical* condition which is associated statistically with an increased cancer risk (Morson *et al.*, 1980). For a long time atrophic gastritis, gastric ulcer, pernicious anaemia, gastric stumps, tubular adenomas, and Menetrier's disease were considered to be precancerous conditions, but now only atrophic gastritis, pernicious anaemia, gastric stumps, and tubular adenomas are regarded as having significant malignant potential. In these conditions epithelial dysplasia may develop and can be graded as mild, moderate or severe.

Epithelial dysplasia can occur with or without preceding intestinal metaplasia (Morson *et al.*, 1980). Jass (1983) claimed a link between incomplete intestinal metaplasia, epithelial dysplasia, and gastric adenocarcinoma of intestinal type. The demonstration of an incomplete type of intestinal metaplasia with epithelial dysplasia or of epithelial dysplasia alone at the periphery of an apparently second gastric carcinoma strongly supports its primary origin.

It is important to remember that linitis plastica, caused by gastric adenocarcinoma of diffuse type, can be simulated by metastatic lobular carcinoma of the breast. Cormier *et al.* (1980) described 31 cases of linitis plastica caused by metastatic breast carcinoma, and review of the literature revealed 33 additional cases. A small proportion of gastric carcinomas takes origin from tubular adenomas which might still be present at the edge of the infiltrative carcinoma, identifying the site of origin of the invasive cancer.

Adenocarcinoma of the small intestine is much less common than its counterpart in the large bowel; it is more common in the upper part of the small intestine. Most cases of duodenal adenocarcinoma arise from the mucosa in the region of the ampulla. Tumours of this area can arise from the common bile duct, from the true ampulla, from the lining epithelium of the intestinal mucosa or from Brunner's glands, which can cause differential diagnostic problems. Adenocarcinomas of the ampulla and duodenal mucosa often arise on the basis of a villous adenoma (Rosai, 1981). Bridge and Perzin (1975) also found that adenocarcinomas of the small intestine arose from pre-existing tubular or villous adenomas. Adenocarcinomas of the small intestine are associated with a high incidence of primary malignant neoplasms in other sites (Barclay and Schapira, 1983).

Adenocarcinoma of the colon and rectum is thought by most workers to arise usually from pre-existing tubular or villous adenomas and the presence of adenoma adjacent to infiltrative adenocarcinoma excludes, with reasonable certainty, the metastatic nature of the invasive tumour. Heald and Bussey (1975), studying multiple synchronous cancers of the colon and rectum, found that 27% of the 157 carcinomas arose in tubular or villous adenomas. In addition, they found that 70% of synchronous and 60% of metachronous adenocarcinomas were associated with separate tubular or villous adenomas, three times the incidence of such lesions in resection specimens for single cancers, and more than ten times that found in the general population. They concluded that this is strong circumstantial evidence to link colorectal cancer, particularly if multiple, with pre-existing adenomatous tumours (see Chapter 18). Agrez *et al.* (1982) studying metachronous colorectal malignancies reached the same conclusion.

Morson and Konishi (1980) pointed out that epithelial dysplasia is the main precursor lesion for colorectal cancer. The concept of dysplasia as the precursor lesion for adenocarcinoma, in cases of chronic ulcerative colitis, is already well documented. Epithelial dysplasia in ulcerative colitis is similar to the dysplasia seen in adenomas and differs only in that it occurs in a flat as well as a polypoid mucosa.

Epithelial dysplasias are graded as mild, moderate and severe, with the malignant potential increasing with increasing degrees of dysplasia. It is suggested that adenomas pass through stages of increasing grades of epithelial dysplasia before invasive cancer occurs. Except for cases of ulcerative colitis, the different grades of epithelial dysplasia of the colon and rectum are seen virtually only in adenomas, which supports the theory of the adenoma–carcinoma sequence. Morson and Konishi (1980) emphasized that the dysplasia–carcinoma sequence is a new histological concept, and reflects more appropriately the risk of cancer in patients with precancerous conditions (familial polyposis, colorectal cancer families, patients who have had a colorectal cancer removed, chronic ulcerative colitis).

Tumours other than adenocarcinoma

The most common malignant tumours (other than adenocarcinomas) of the gastrointestinal tract are carcinoids, leiomyosarcomas, and non-Hodgkin's lymphomas. These can present as multiple cancers of the same type, or in association with each other or with adenocarcinomas.

Carcinoid tumours can occur in any part of the gastrointestinal tract, but in the small intestine about one-third of all neoplasms are carcinoid tumours (Godwin, 1975). Pearse (1974) suggested that these tumours represent a group of neoplasms rather than a single pathological entity, and it is expected that ultrastructural and immunocytochemical investigation of these tumours and their parent cell will lead to a more accurate histogenetic classification. The small intestinal carcinoids are frequently multiple (16–34%) and can be associated with malignant gastrointestinal tumours of other microscopic types (Kuiper *et al.*, 1970). Barclay and Schapira (1983) found that 17% of carcinoid tumours of the small intestine were associated with primary malignant neoplasms in other sites (colon, breast, pancreas, kidney, lip, vulva, cervix, larynx, lymphoma).

The carcinoid tumours have characteristic histological, ultrastructural, and biochemical features, which show some variation according to site of origin (Soga and Tazawa, 1971). Apart from serotonin and 5-hydroxytryptophan, immunocytochemical investigations show that a variety of biogenic amines and peptides (ACTH, β-MSH, noradrenaline, gastrin, somatostatin, substance P) can be produced by these tumours. The recognition of such peptides using immunocytochemical methods is helpful in distinguishing between different endocrine tumours and identifying the source of metastasis in cases of endocrine tumours producing different hormones (Cooney *et al.*, 1980).

It is difficult to fulfil the first criterion of Warren and Gates (1932) (each lesion must be of pathologically proven malignancy) in cases of *smooth muscle tumours* of the gastrointestinal tract. Although the size, cellularity, atypia, and necrosis correlate to some extent with malignant behaviour, none is accurate in predicting metastasis (Ranchod and Kempson, 1977). The mitotic activity is the most important criterion for distinguishing a leiomyoma from a leiomyosarcoma in the uterus but the correlation between mitotic count and behaviour is not as good for smooth muscle tumours of the gastrointestinal tract. Five mitoses per ten high power fields indicate definite potential aggressive behaviour, though Ranchod and Kempson (1977) found that 40% of the gastrointestinal leiomyosarcomas had fewer than five mitoses per ten high power fields.

A distinctive variety of smooth muscle tumour is the epithelioid variety (leiomyoblastoma) which is characterized by round or polygonal cells with varying amounts of cytoplasm. According to Appleman and Helwig (1976), any epitheliod smooth muscle tumour having more than 5 mitoses per 50 high power fields should be considered malignant. If an epithelioid muscle tumour is larger than 6 cm it should also be regarded as probably malignant, since virtually all the benign cases reported by Appleman and Helwig (1976) were smaller than 6 cm. However, the small size does not necessarily indicate benignity, because about one-quarter of all epithelioid leiomyosarcomas were smaller than 6 cm.

Following the report of Tisell *et al.* (1978) on gastric epithelioid leiomyosarcoma associated with pulmonary chondroma, Carney (1979) described an unusual triad occurring exclusively in young females, and consisting of gastric epithelioid leiomyosarcomas, functioning extra-adrenal paraganglioma and pulmonary chondroma. Although the 15 reported cases suggest an unusual developmental defect, the condition is not familial. Until this syndrome was described, a lung lesion associated with the malignant gastric tumour in question would have been considered to be metastatic.

The diagnosis of *primary malignant lymphoma* of the gastrointestinal tract can also cause considerable difficulties: it has to be distinguished from benign lymphoid proliferations (pseudolymphoma of the stomach, lymphoid hyperplasia of the ileum, nodular lymphoid hyperplasia, benign lymphoid polyps and plasma cell granulomas) and from lymphomas with secondary gut involvement.

The gastrointestinal tract is the commonest site of primary extranodal lymphoma (Freeman *et al.*, 1972); however, about 10% of patients with nodal non-Hodgkin's lymphoma have involvement of some part of the gastrointestinal tract (Lewin *et al.*, 1978). The diagnosis of primary gastrointestinal lymphoma, therefore, requires a thorough clinicopathological investigation.

Dawson *et al.* (1961) used the following criteria for acceptance of a primary lymphoma of the gut: no palpable superficial lymphadenopathy at presentation; no radiological enlargement of mediastinal nodes; normal white blood cell count (total and differential); at laparotomy the bowel lesion predominates, the only obviously affected lymph nodes, if any, being those immediately related; the liver and spleen appear free of tumour.

These criteria have been almost universally adopted. With the new investigative techniques (lymphangiography of retroperitoneal nodes, and computerized axial tomography) as well as bone marrow aspiration, it is possible to detect more subtle evidence of disease in other sites, raising the question of whether the criteria laid down by Dawson *et al.* (1961) require modification. Blackshaw (1980) suggested the adoption of these criteria as those minimally essential for the diagnosis of primary gastrointestinal lymphoma, and that additional information from more sophisticated techniques could be used for the further exclusion of cases which are not genuinely primary.

The benign lymphoid lesions of the gut are characterized histologically by the presence of lymphoid follicles with germinal centres, a feature which is not seen in malignant lymphomas. Immunocytochemical staining for immunoglobulins can be helpful in distinguishing between benign (polyclonal) and malignant (monoclonal) lymphoid tumours; this is particularly useful in cases of plasma cell granulomas, plasmacytomas, and plasmacytoid lymphomas. Immunoperoxidase staining for α_1-antitrypsin can be used for the diagnosis of histiocytic intestinal lymphomas. Chloroacetate esterase (an enzyme present in mast cells and in the granulated myeloid series except for eosinophils) is useful in the histological diagnosis of granulocytic sarcoma.

The primary nature of lymphoma involving the gut is further supported by the fact that cases of heavy chain disease, coeliac disease, ulcerative colitis, and chronic gastritis, all show a higher association with lymphoma of the gut. In cases of Mediterranean lymphoma developing in patients suffering from heavy chain disease, the mucosa away from the tumour shows a heavy infiltration by mature plasma cells (Rappaport *et al.*, 1972), the cytoplasm of which contains monoclonal heavy chains of immunoglobulin (Isaacson, 1979). Pangalis and Rappaport (1977) demonstrated a similar immunohistochemical staining, in heavy chain disease, of both the overt tumour cells and the mature plasma cell infiltration.

Van den Heule *et al.* (1979) demonstrated that some lymphomas of the stomach were associated with follicular gastritis, and noted apparent zones of transition between the lymphomatous areas and the adjacent benign lymphoid infiltrates, suggesting that the former developed from the latter. Dutz (1978) consistently found an associated perifoveolar plasma cell gastritis when examining the adjacent non-lymphomatous mucosa of primary lymphomas. This was absent in cases of secondary lymphomatous involvement. He believed this type of 'gastritis' represented a precursor lesion of lymphoma rather than a reaction to it.

SECOND CANCER OF THE UROTHELIUM

The renal pelves, ureters, urinary bladder, and proximal urethra have a continuous lining of urothelium which is exposed to the same carcinogenic agents. The frequent occurrence of multiple cancers at these sites supports the theory of the unity of the urothelium as a target organ for neoplastic events. As in other organs, in attempting to establish criteria for diagnosis of a second cancer, it is essential to understand the morphogenesis of the tumours. Studies of urothelium adjacent to or intervening between grossly visible tumours and mapping studies of cystectomy and nephroureterectomy specimens showed that invasive carcinoma is not merely a local disease but a focal manifestation of a diffuse abnormality of the urothelium (Melicow, 1952).

There are two distinct forms of cancer development in the urinary tract: papillary and the non-papillary tumours, which probably represent different pathogenetic pathways with some degree of overlap (Koss, 1979). It is generally agreed that invasive urothelial cancer arises from non-invasive carcinomas which can be of either the papillary or the flat variety. The flat variety of non-invasive carcinoma is called carcinoma *in situ*, while a papillary carcinoma confined to the epithelial surface is classified as a non-invasive papillary carcinoma rather than as papillary carcinoma *in situ* (Friedell *et al.*, 1980).

Koss (1979) emphasized that although papillary tumours can invade the lamina propria, they usually do not invade the muscularis and they have a 'pushing border': metastasis, therefore, is unlikely. Nevertheless, patients with papillary carcinoma can develop metastatic disease and, in these cases (and also in those without papillary disease) the metastasizing urothelial cancer originates from non-papillary lesions of the urothelium, viz. carcinoma *in situ*. Invasion from a flat lesion, as opposed to the 'pushing border' of invasive papillary carcinoma, proceeds in pinpoint fashion, with penetration not only of the lamina propria but also of the muscularis.

For a long time, the multiplicity of urothelial cancers and their frequent recurrences were explained on the basis of implantation metastasis. Although there are some data supporting the possibility of implantation (McDonald and Thorson, 1956), most workers agree that implantation requires traumatized, denuded mucosa and does not explain the vast majority of cases of multicentricity. On the other hand, mapping studies clearly show that extensive and multiple precancerous lesions (dysplasia, carcinoma *in situ*) are present in most cases of invasive carcinoma. Accepting the theory that most invasive carcinomas of the urothelium develop from precancerous lesions (dysplasia, carcinoma *in situ*), one can conclude that implantation metastasis as a source of multiplicity or recurrence is a rare phenomenon and does not challenge the presently widely held theory of a carcinoma *in situ*–invasive carcinoma sequence.

Based on these data, the independent origin of a papillary transitional cell carcinoma (even when invasive) can be accepted if a given lesion is separated from another one by tumour-free tissue covered by normal urothelium. The possibility of metastatic spread in pure papillary carcinomas with superficial invasion and a 'pushing border' is negligible.

By contrast, proof of the independent origin of non-papillary invasive transitional cell carcinomas, arising from 'flat' carcinoma *in situ*, is very much more difficult to obtain, because these tumours often infiltrate extensively and readily metastasize. To exclude the metastatic origin of a second cancer, contiguous carcinoma *in situ* must be present in both lesions. Furthermore, the two lesions must not be linked by *in situ* carcinoma.

SECOND CANCER OF THE BREAST

The relatively frequent multicentric and bilateral presentation of breast carcinoma has led to the concept of breast carcinoma as a diffuse neoplastic process originating in the epithelium of mammary ducts, ductules and lobules. Gallager and Martin (1969) found that epithelial hyperplasia, atypia, and non-invasive carcinoma were almost universally present in breasts containing invasive carcinoma.

It should be pointed out that the objective criteria for the separation of benign epithelial hyperplasia and *in situ* carcinoma in the breast are not as well appreciated as in some other organs. The illustrations and descriptions of some workers lead one to believe that epitheliosis is sometimes diagnosed as carcinoma *in situ* and this is a major obstacle to a realistic assessment of the frequency of multicentric cancers in the breast. Since most mammary cancers have a preinvasive, *in situ* phase, the presence of *in situ* carcinoma can be used as morphological evidence for the primary site of origin of an adjacent invasive carcinoma.

Multicentric carcinoma in the same breast

The wide range (13–75%) of reported frequencies of multicentric breast carcinomas is attributed to differences of definition and specimen preparation techniquès (Qualheim and Gall, 1957; Tellem *et al.*, 1962; Fisher *et al.*, 1975; Gallager and Martin, 1969). Lagios (1977) and Egan (1982) both cite Gallager and Martin (1969) as finding an incidence of multicentricity as high as 75%, though the findings in the latter paper are open to different interpretations. Lagios, using very strict criteria for defining 'multicentric foci of carcinoma', found an incidence of 21%.

Lagios (1977) defined multicentric *in situ* carcinoma as a focus of non-invasive carcinoma located 5 cm or more beyond the border of residual tumour or the excision biopsy cavity margin. The 5 cm distance was an arbitrary definition used to make certain that the second lesion was in another quadrant or in the central retroareolar area. He defined multicentric invasive carcinoma as two foci of invasive carcinoma of different histological pattern or with their own *in situ* component. He also required that the tumours contain a central area of hyalinization and that one is located 5 cm or more from the border of a reference tumour mass or the border of an excision biopsy cavity.

Cheatle and Cutler (1931) pointed out that as long as there are normal ducts between two separate tumour sites, the two tumours must have developed independently, if metastases are excluded. Egan (1982) used the same criteria in a reivew of 161 clinical, radiographic, and histopathological whole breast studies. Our view is that careful step-sectioning of the tumours and the intervening breast parenchyma can reveal or exclude direct spread and that the 5 cm distance proposed by Lagios (1977) is perhaps too strict.

In cases of invasive carcinomas of similar histological type, each tumour should show areas of *in situ* carcinoma. If no *in situ* carcinoma is demonstrated, the two tumours could still be independent primaries, but this cannot be proven. With the knowledge that in a large majority of invasive ductal and lobular carcinomas, an *in situ* component can be identified, a search for this in order to prove the site of origin is clearly important. In medullary and, to a lesser extent, in mucoid carcinomas, an *in situ* component is much less frequently found. If the separate tumours have a distinctly different histological picture (lobular, ductal, medullary, mucoid, etc.) they can be accepted as independent primaries even in the absence of an *in situ* component.

Care must be taken in deciding the histological type since carcinomas can show extreme degrees of heterogeneity in different areas and, furthermore, mixtures of subtypes of invasive ductal carcinoma, as well as invasive carcinoma of indeterminate nature also exist (Azzopardi, 1979). Intraductal carcinoma and cancerization of lobules surrounded by or adjacent to invasive ductal carcinoma should be considered to be parts of a single tumour. Although this might seem fairly obvious, it is not always made clear in the literature.

There are several different methods of demonstrating multicentric breast carcinomas: (1) the quadrant biopsy technique in which random samples of the quadrants of the breast are examined histologically (Tellem *et al.*, 1962); (2) several millimetres thick serial sections of the whole breast are examined macroscopically and areas selected for histological examination (Cheatle and Cutler, 1931); (3) large blocks of breast embedded in paraffin and subserial sections are examined histologically (Gallager and Martin, 1969); (4) whole mounts of breast stained, mounted in plastic, and viewed under the dissecting microscope (Wellings *et al.*, 1975); (5) Egan (1982) used a correlated clinical, radiographic, and pathological approach to study whole breasts. After freezing the breast and slicing it in serial sections, areas were selected for histological study after specimen radiography.

In the study of multicentricity of breast carcinomas, only serial slicing, preferably with step-sectioning visualizes the entire breast parenchyma and shows the relationship between separate tumours. For this reason the work of Wellings *et al.* (1975), Egan (1982), and especially Lagios (1977) is particularly valuable.

Bilateral primary breast carcinomas

Having discussed the multicentric nature of unilateral breast carcinomas, one concludes that bilaterality is probably an expression of multicentricity. The criteria for the diagnosis of a contralateral carcinoma are essentially similar to those used in the diagnosis of unilateral multicentric ones, as discussed by Robbins and Berg (1964).

Because clinical data alone (including the time interval between the presentation of the tumours) cannot determine the primary or secondary nature of a contralateral carcinoma, pathological criteria are essential for the diagnosis. The main criterion is the presence of contiguous *in situ* ductal or lobular carcinoma. Medullary and mucoid carcinomas are exceptions because they contain *in situ* components relatively rarely. Metastatic carcinomas are not associated with *in situ* elements.

The location of the carcinoma in the second breast is also important; metastases from one breast to the other usually occur through lymphatics. Metastatic foci are generally located in the adipose tissue rather than in the breast parenchyma and are found close to the midline or in the tail of the breast, when there is retrograde spread from the lymph nodes of the second axilla. Metastases tend to be multiple and to grow in an expansile fashion as opposed to the common stellate pattern of the primary lesion, but there are exceptions: medullary carcinoma, mucoid carcinoma, and some types of ductal carcinoma NOS also have a rounded outline.

Robbins and Berg (1964) pointed out that contiguous *in situ* change is a more important criterion than the difference of histological type, because the latter is open to errors in both directions. Qualheim and Gall (1957) reported structural heterogeneity in close to 30% of breast tumours. On the other hand, similarity of the tumours does not necessarily indicate that one is a metastasis: the association with an *in situ* component can prove its primary nature. A breast carcinoma also has to be distinguished from a metastasis from a different organ. The tumours which most commonly metastasize to the breast in Britain are bronchial carcinoma, especially oat cell carcinoma, and malignant melanoma of the skin. Apart from obvious histological differences, elastosis, which is so characteristic a feature of primary breast carcinomas, is not present in metastatic tumours (Azzopardi, 1979).

Leukaemic or lymphomatous deposits should be distinguished from an undifferentiated carcinoma. Mucin stains or immunohistochemical stains for epithelial membrane antigens and prekeratin can reveal the epithelial deriva- tion of the tumour, while stains for the common leucocyte antigen or immunoglobulins can indicate the lymphomatous nature. Such stains, as well as electronmicroscopy, are invaluable at times in distinguishing convincingly between invasive lobular carcinoma and a malignant lymphoma.

SECOND CANCER IN FEMALE GENITAL TRACT

Multiple cancers of the cervix, vagina, and vulva

The portio vaginalis of the cervix, vagina, vulva, and anus are covered by a continuous layer of stratified squamous epithelium. The reported multicentric carcinomas occurring in this area are usually explained on the basis of exposure to a common carcinogen and a common susceptibility to malignant change. The vast majority, over 90%, of carcinomas in these regions are of squamous type which explains why most of the reported multiple cancers of the lower genital tract also belong to this histological type.

To prove the independent origin of multiple squamous carcinomas requires colposcopic and histopathological study, without which the general criteria for the diagnosis of a second cancer established by Warren and Gates (1932) cannot be applied. The combined colposcopic and histological study has to show that each lesion is separated from another by tumour-free tissue; this includes a demonstration that they are not linked by a continuous field of squamous carcinoma *in situ*. Furthermore, in order to exclude a metastatic origin, the tumours should show adjacent dysplasia or carcinoma *in situ* of the surface epithelium. If a tumour shows only microinvasion, metastasis is unlikely. This applies to verrucous carcinoma, a specific type of squamous carcinoma which is locally infiltrative but practically never associated with metastasis (Kraus and Perez-Mesa, 1966).

Rare types of primary malignant tumours, like adenocarcinomas and malignant melanomas, can present as a 'second' cancer and must then be distinguished from metastatic lesions. The most common sources of metasta- sis in the lower genital tract are the cervix, endometrium, ovary, rectum, urethra, bladder, and kidney (Way, 1980). Malignant melanomas of the anus, vulva and vagina, should show 'junctional activity' for acceptance of their local origin.

The fact that similar histological types of adenocarcinoma can occur in different parts of the female genital tract warrants careful clinical and pathological study to exclude metastatic origin. Adenocarcinoma of the endocervix, for example, exhibits a variety of histological patterns and it is difficult sometimes, on histological grounds alone, to distinguish it from one originating in the endometrium. However, features such as an abundance of intracellular mucin, a fibrous appearance of the stroma, and the presence of endocervical adenocarcinoma *in situ* favour the endocervix as a primary site; while the absence of intracellular mucin, the presence of endometrial stroma around the malignant glands, and the coexistence of atypical endometrial hyperplasia favour an endometrial origin (Clement and Scully, 1982). A highly differentiated, rare type of endocervical adenocarcinoma is the 'adenoma malignum' which shows an association with the Peutz–Jegher's syndrome. In this syndrome, adenocarcinoma of the duodenum can develop (McGowan *et al.*, 1980).

Histologically similar, so-called clear cell carcinomas can occur in the vagina, cervix, endometrium, and ovary. In the first two sites it occurs in a younger age group and most commonly in females exposed prenatally to diethylstilboestrol (Herbst *et al.*, 1974).

Bilateral ovarian cancers and cancers involving the ovary and the uterine corpus

As in other organs, if multiple cancers are of different histological type, it is relatively easy to fulfil Warren and Gates's third criterion. However, if the tumours belong to the same histological type, the exclusion of metastasis is very difficult. In most cases, the macroscopic picture and histological step-sectioning can exclude direct spread but not metastasis. Obviously, the possibility of metastasis is much less in minimal cancer than in advanced cancer. In cases of advanced cancers, only precancerous lesions adjacent to each tumour can provide satisfactory evidence of their local, independent origin. The problem is that precancerous lesions are not well defined for the three major categories of ovarian cancer: malignant germ cell tumours, granulosa cell tumours, and common epithelial carcinomas.

Precancerous lesions of *germ cell type* include the following two examples. (1) The dysgenetic gonad of a phenotypic female with a karyotype containing a Y chromosome (Scully, 1981). There is a 25% chance of developing a malignant germ tumour by the age of 30 years. Most often this tumour is a gonadoblastoma which is an *in situ* form of malignancy. However, in about 50% of the cases with gonadoblastoma there is, in addition, dysgerminoma and less often other types of malignant germ cell tumour (immature teratoma, embryonal carcinoma, endodermal sinus tumour, choriocarcinoma). (2) The dermoid cyst (benign cystic teratoma): 1-2% of dermoid cysts are associated with cancer, most commonly a squamous cell carcinoma.

The precursor of *granulosa cell tumours* is not known but proliferating granulosa cells within atretic follicles have been suggested. This, however, does not explain granulosa cell tumours developing in postmenopausal women, because atretic follicles containing granulosa cells have not been reported beyond the menopause. The known precursor lesions of the common carcinomas of the ovary are endometriosis, benign Brenner tumours, mucinous cystadenomas, and serous cystadenomas. Mostoufizadeh and Scully (1980) described atypical hyperplasia and carcinoma *in situ* in cases of ovarian endometriosis. However, it is thought that only a small percentage of endometrioid carcinomas arise in endometriosis. The association of a benign Brenner tumour with a malignant one, according to Scully (1982), also suggests that it was the site of origin of the malignant component.

The malignant change occasionally found in *mucinous cystadenomas* and *serous cystadenomas* is suggestive of their precancerous potential. Ovarian cancer is bilateral in 30–50% of cases, but only 20–25% of these are Stage I cancers without extra-ovarian spread. Since lymphatic pathways between the ovaries are probably of minor importance in the spread of the disease, it must be assumed that the bilaterality of most Stage I cases is a manifestation of multicentric origin (Scully, 1979). In more advanced stages, unless there is an adjacent precancerous lesion, the primary or metastatic origin cannot be determined.

Ovarian carcinomas have to be distinguished from metastatic carcinomas. Adenocarcinomas of the gut, breast, and endometrium sometimes metastasize to the ovaries. Apart from metastatic signet ring cell carcinoma of both ovaries (Krukenberg tumour), a rare primary Krukenberg tumour also exists (Joshi, 1968). The exclusion of metastasis from an intestinal adenocarcinoma in cases of mucinous or endometrioid adenocarcinoma of the ovary can be very difficult. The presence of accompanying mucinous cystadenoma is in favour of an ovarian origin for the malignant tumour. The presence of foci of squamous differentiation practically excludes a metastasis from the intestine. Clear cell carcinoma has to be distinguished from metastatic renal carcinoma. The presence of mucin and hobnail cells in the former is helpful.

The precancerous lesion of carcinoma of the endometrium is atypical hyperplasia (Koss *et al.*, 1981). The coexistence of atypical hyperplasia with endometrial carcinoma is helpful in cases where the primary or secondary nature of an adenocarcinoma in the uterus is in doubt.

Simultaneous involvement of the endometrium and the ovary by carcinoma is a relatively uncommon event (Eifel *et al.*, 1982). It is known that the ovaries, the fallopian tubes, the uterine corpus, and the cervix can give rise to the same histological types of metaplastic changes and of epithelial neoplasms (Hendrickson and Kempson, 1980). To explain this phenomenon, Lauchlan (1968) has introduced the term 'extended mullerian system'. The theory of the extended mullerian system helps to understand the simultaneous development of histologically similar tumours in more than one anatomic site.

Eifel *et al.* (1982) emphasized that the simultaneous presence of morphologically identical ovarian and uterine epithelial neoplasms need not be interpreted as *prima facie* evidence that one neoplasm is metastatic from the other. They produced evidence that simultaneously occurring low grade endometrioid neoplasms of the ovary and endometrium are separate primary tumours. They emphasized that step-sectioning of the myometrium, adnexa, and ovarian hilar regions is necessary to exclude myometrial and lymphatic permeation and to prove that non-invasive Grade II or III uterine endometrioid carcinomas associated with identical ovarian tumours are likely to represent simultaneous primaries. In cases of papillary, clear-cell, and mucinous carcinomas occurring both in the ovaries and in the endometrium, metastasis was more likely since there was already deep myometrial and lymphatic invasion at the time of presentation.

PRIMARY BILATERAL TESTICULAR CANCER

Men with a testicular tumour have a greater risk of developing another tumour in the remaining testis. The risk is only 0.7% in cases of scrotal testis, but it is as high as 15% in the presence of inguinal and 30% in the cases of abdominal cryptorchidism (Gilbert and Hamilton, 1940). The reported incidence of bilateral testicular cancer varies between 1% and 3.1% (Abeshouse *et al.*, 1955; Mostofi and Price, 1973; Pugh, 1976; Aristizabal *et al.*, 1978). This variation in incidence is due to the inclusion or exclusion of lymphomas and the different number of cryptorchid cases in different series.

Although non-Hodgkin's lymphomas are the tumours which most commonly involve both testes, they generally represent secondary rather than primary tumours (Aristizabal *et al.*, 1978). Only an estimated 10% of testicular lymphomas truly represent localized primary disease (Woolley *et al.*, 1976). Primary testicular origin of lymphomas can be accepted only if thorough staging shows that the tumour is localized to the testis.

The other major group of testicular tumours which can involve both testes are the germ cell tumours. Aristizabal *et al.* (1978) found that all combinations of tumour types may occur simultaneously or sequentially. Seminoma is the most common germ cell tumour to be bilateral. Spermatocytic seminoma may be multicentric as well as occasionally bilateral.

The diagnosis of primary bilateral testicular cancer requires the exclusion of the possibility that the tumour in the second testis is the result of metastasis. Most workers view bilateral testicular cancers as independent primaries (Abeshouse *et al.*, 1955; Moertel, 1966; Mostofi and Price, 1973; Pugh, 1976). The absence of demonstrable vascular and lymphatic communications between the two testes, the occurrence of bilateral tumours of different histological types, the rarity of metastases from extragenital sites except for prostatic carcinomas and lymphomas, the presence of the tunica albuginea as a barrier against direct spread, all strongly support this concept, although concrete proof refuting the possibility of metastasis is difficult to obtain.

Even the different histological appearance of bilateral tumours cannot be used as absolute evidence of a double primary tumour. In cases of testicular germ cell tumours, the microscopic appearance of the metastasis is sometimes very different from that of the primary neoplasm. The exception is the pure seminoma, which usually metastasizes as seminoma. When seminoma is combined with a teratomatous tumour, it is usually, though not always, the latter which metastasizes. There are several instances of mature teratoma in the metastases of immature teratomatous tumours (Bär and Hedinger, 1976). The presence of mature teratoma in the metastases in cases without mature teratoma in the primary tumour can be explained by the possibility of maturation of the malignant teratomatous tissue (Mostofi, 1980). The reverse phenomenon is, of course, even commoner. Mixed germ cell tumours containing choriocarcinoma almost always metastasize as pure choriocarcinoma (Bär and Hedinger, 1976).

Azzopardi *et al.* (1961), studying burned out testicular tumours, noted the presence of intratubular malignant germ cells. Skakkebaek (1978) who used the term 'carcinoma *in situ*' for these lesions, noted their presence adjacent to seminoma, embryonal carcinoma, and teratocarcinoma. Mostofi (1980) described an intratubular stage of yolk sac tumour and choriocarcinoma. The finding of *in situ* malignant germ cell proliferation adjacent to infiltrative germ cell neoplasm provides the most conclusive evidence of a primary, rather than metastatic, origin for bilateral testicular germ cell tumours.

Tumour markers such as alpha-foetoprotein (AFP) and human chorionic gonadotrophins (HCG), measured by radioimmunoassay or localized by immunocytochemical techniques, are useful in the staging, detection of recurrence, prognosis, and management of testicular cancer (Javadpour, 1979). Mostofi (1980), showed that β-HCG was demonstrable in choriocarcinoma, any germ cell tumour with foci of choriocarcinoma or containing syncytiotrophoblast. AFP was present in yolk sac tumours and in tumours with yolk sac or embryonal carcinoma components. Mostofi pointed out that syncytiotrophoblast or yolk sac elements may be present in only small amounts, easily missed in HE sections, but highlighted by immunoperoxidase techniques. This can explain the elevated serum levels of HCG in cases of pure seminoma and of HCG or AFP in teratomatous tumours without overt chorionic or yolk sac elements.

DISCUSSION OF CRITERIA

Most statistical studies on multiple cancer are based on data from tumour registries and consequently rely on the variable criteria of the reporting physician. Greenberg (1959) addressed himself to this problem, using the data of the Connecticut Tumor Registry. His criteria were stringent: (1) The cancer must have been identified as a second primary cancer by the reporting hospital. (2) The second cancer must have been in a different anatomical site from the first cancer. (3) An interval of at least five years must have elapsed between the diagnosis of the first primary cancer and the subsequent diagnosis of the second primary cancer.

Schoenberg (1977), in an excellent monograph, summarized the data of the Connecticut Tumor Registry. The criterion he used for defining a second primary cancer was that the tumour be so designated by the reporting physician. We agree with Moertel (1966) that the following objections can be raised to the validity of the data used by Greenberg and Schoenberg: (1) In some cases the diagnosis of cancer was based on purely clinical grounds without surgical, necropsy, or histological confirmation. (2) A patient was accepted as having a second primary cancer when it was so stated by the attending physician, regardless of the criteria used to reach this conclusion. (3) When pathological material was obtained from each neoplasm, this was not reviewed to confirm that the second lesion was indeed a primary cancer rather than a metastasis.

These statistical studies were, therefore, in some respects not stringent enough in their criteria, while on the other hand, Greenberg's five-year rule did not recognize the existence of synchronously presenting double primary malignancies, let alone those presenting less than five years later, some of which at least are genuinely primary.

The problem of the diagnosis of a second primary malignancy can be approached in two ways. If one is strict in the criteria adopted, one can be certain that one is correctly diagnosing a second primary malignancy, but there is bound to be a major element of underdiagnosis of dual cancers. If the criteria adopted are less stringent, the net will include many more instances of presumptive dual cancers but the reliability of the diagnosis is correspondingly diminished. An attempt to compromise is obviously necessary in order to include the majority of the dual cancers, while excluding cases in which an apparent second primary tumour may merely represent a metastasis.

General criteria for diagnosis of independent primaries can be adopted, which have more or less general applicability to different organs and tumours. In this chapter, while adopting Warren and Gates's (1932) general criteria, much more emphasis is placed on the *special* criteria which have been largely ignored in past discussion of this complex topic. It requires a detailed knowledge of the differing appearances, evolutions, and biological behaviour of hundreds of tumour entities and of the innumerable pitfalls with which histopathology is beset.

The *first* criterion of Warren and Gates, that each tumour must have definite features of malignancy, is acceptable as it stands, but it is suggested that there is a good case for identifying any geographically separate *in situ* tumours as distinct 'second' cancers, while recognizing that invasive cancers should still have pride of place. Study of microinvasive and *in situ* carcinomas will in future yield even more valuable information about multiple cancers than is available from the study of advanced cancers.

The *second* criterion, that each tumour must be anatomically distinct, is acceptable as long as it is understood that multiple blocks and serial reconstruction are sometimes needed to exclude three-dimensional continuity with certainty. If two invasive cancers are linked through an *in situ* component, they should *not* be regarded as independent tumours.

The *third* criterion, that the probability of one tumour being a metastasis from the other must be excluded as far as possible, is the most difficult to apply. Since most carcinomas have an *in situ* phase, demonstration of this in a given tumuour is crucial to prove the independent site of origin. The ultimate test of an independent cancer will be proof that it is composed of a different clone of cells. Some of the features of apparent multiple cancers which must be assessed are as follows:

1. Anatomical location in relation to each other.
2. General configuration of the lesion.
3. Evidence of *in situ* tumour, dysplasia, and other known preinvasive lesions.
4. Evidence of discontinuity in three dimensions, even by an *in situ* component.
5. Distinct histological types as indicated by morphology, structural and cytological differentiation, cytochemistry and ultrastructure.
6. Distinctive antigenic, enzymatic and other determinants (e.g. keratin, vimentin, thyroglobulin, calcitonin, immunoglobulins, acid phosphatase).
7. Special features applicable to individual tumours (e.g. elastosis in breast carcinomas, junctional activity in melanomas, dense-core granules in endocrine tumours, osmiophilic lamellar bodies in alveolar cell carcinoma).

On a more general theme, the question needs asking: is a clinical cancer the result of proliferation of a single transformed cell or is it the result of a coalescence of multiple microscopic cancers? The answer depends on whether one believes that an *in situ* or invasive carcinoma results from the proliferation of a single clone of cells or from a coalescence of multiple clones. If the latter were true, then single clinical cancers would in a sense be 'multiple' biologically. Most recent work points to the monoclonal origin of the majority of cancers. The so-called field theory of origin of cancers is not true in the sense of 'recruitment' of new cells into cancer cells, but only in the sense that tumour derived from a single cell can spread laterally and replace normal cells.

The term 'multicentric origin' is regrettably used by some to indicate multiple points of invasion from an *in situ* lesion. On the polyclonal theory of carcinogenesis, these have often been interpreted as multiple cancers. This view is no longer tenable, if one accepts, as one must, the monoclonal origin of tumours. The term multicentric origin in this sense is best discontinued. Multicentric origin is best reserved to describe two or more tumours, spatially distinct, not joined by *in situ* tumour and derived from different clones of cells. It is for this reason that we have stressed the importance of *in situ* carcinoma in establishing the primary, as opposed to the metastatic, origin of a given tumour.

The fact that most of the second cancers occur in the same organ or system affected initially is not difficult to understand in the light of knowledge that a whole organ is exposed to the same carcinogenic influences. Extensive areas of, say, the bladder epithelium may thus be altered: multiple areas of dysplasia and *in situ* carcinoma may be found and the intervening, morphologically normal, epithelium may also have been 'initiated' in the neoplastic process. When 'progression' occurs, as it probably does in several steps, more areas become morphologically abnormal and eventually multiple invasive cancers may result.

Most clinical cancers are, therefore, monoclonal unicentric cancers, even though they may show multiple points of invasion. Conversely, multiple cancers of one organ are relatively common and become increasingly common if a patient both survives his first cancer and lives into the indefinite future. Fortunately this last event is unlikely!

REFERENCES

Abeshouse, B. S., Tiongson, A., and Goldfarb, M. (1955). Bilateral tumours of testicles: review of the literature and report of a case of bilateral simultaneous lymphosarcoma. *Journal of Urology*, **74**, 522.

Agrez, M. V., Ready, R., Ilstrup, D., and Beart, R. W. (1982). Metachronous colorectal malignancies. *Diseases of Colon and Rectum*, **25**, 569.

Allen, A. C., and Spitz, S. (1953). Malignant melanoma: a clinicopathological analysis of the criteria for diagnosis and prognosis. *Cancer*, **6**, 1.

Appleman, H. D., and Helwig, E. B. (1976). Gastric epithelioid leiomyoma and leiomyosarcoma (leiomyoblastoma). *Cancer*, **38**, 708.

Aristizabal, S., Davis, J. R., Miller, R. C. *et al.* (1978). Bilateral primary germ cell testicular tumours. Report of four cases and review of the literature. *Cancer*, **42**, 591.

Auerbach, O., Gere, J. B., Forman, J. B. *et al.* (1957). Changes in the bronchial epithelium in realtion to smoking and cancer of the lung. *New England Journal of Medicine*, **256**, 97.

Auerbach, O., Stout, A. P., Hammond, E. C., and Garfinkel, L. (1967). Multiple primary bronchial carcinomas. *Cancer*, **20**, 699.

Azzopardi, J. G. (1979). Problems in breast pathology. In *Major problems in pathology*, Vol. 11. London: W. B. Saunders.

Azzopardi, J. G., Mostofi, F. K., and Theiss, E. A. (1961). Lesions of testis observed in certain patients with widespread choriocarcinoma and related tumours. *American Journal of Pathology*, **38**, 207.

Balch, C. M., Murad, T. M., Soong, S. J. *et al.* (1978). Prognostic histopathological features comparing Clark's and Breslow's staging methods. *Annals of Surgery*, **188**, 732.

Barclay, T. H. C., and Schapira, D. V. (1983). Malignant tumours of the small intestine. *Cancer*, **51**, 878.

Bär, W., and Hedinger, Chr. (1976). Comparison of histologic types of primary testicular germ cell tumours with their metastases. *Virchows Archiv A. Pathological Anatomy and Histology*, **370**, 41.

Blackshaw, A. J. (1980). Non-Hodgkin's lymphomas of the gut. In *Recent advances in gastrointestinal pathology*. London: W. B. Saunders, p. 214.

Bonikos, D. S., Hendrickson, M., and Bensch, K. G. (1977). Pulmonary alveolar cell carcinoma. Fine structure and *in vitro* study of a case and critical review of this entity. *American Journal of Surgical Pathology*, **1**, 93.

Boyd, D. P., Meissner, W. A., Verlkoff, C. L., and Gladding, T. C. (1954). Primary melanocarinoma of the oesophagus. Report of a case. *Cancer*, **7**, 266.

Breslow, A. (1975). Tumour thickness, level of invasion and node dissection in stage I cutaneous melanoma. *Annals of Surgery*, **182**, 572.

Bridge, M. F., and Perzin, K. H. (1975). Primary adenocarcinoma of the jejunum and ileum. A clinicopathological study. *Cancer*, **36**, 1876.

Bussey, H. J. R., Wallace, M. H., and Morson, B. C. (1967). Metachronous carcinoma of the large intestine and intestinal polyps. *Proceedings of the Royal Society of Medicine*, **60**, 208.

Cahan, W. G. (1977). Multiple primary cancers of the lung, oesphagus and other sites. *Cancer*, **40**, 1954.

Carney, J. A. (1979). The triad of gastric epithelioid leiomyosarcoma, functioning extra-adrenal paraganglioma and pulmonary chondroma. *Cancer*, **43**, 374.

Chaudhry, A. P., Hampel, A., and Gorlin, R. J. (1958). Primary malignant melanoma of the oral cavity: a review of 105 cases. *Cancer*, **11**, 923.

Cheatle, G. L., and Cutler, M. (1931). *Tumours of the breast: their pathology, symptoms, diagnosis and treatment*. Philadelphia: J. B. Lippincott.

Clark, W. H. Jr., From, L., Bernardino, E. A., and Mihm, M. C. (1969). The histogenesis and biologic behaviour of primary human malignant melanomas of the skin. *Cancer Research*, **29**, 705.

Clement, P. B., and Scully, R. E. (1982). Carcinoma of the cervix; histologic types. *Seminars in Oncology*, **9**, 251.

Coffman, B., Crum, E., and Forman, W. B. (1983). Two primary carcinomas of the lung: adenocarcinoma and a metachronous squamous cell carcinoma. *Cancer*, **51**, 124.

Coleman, W. P., Loria, P. R., Reed, R. J., and Krementz, E. T. (1980). Acral lentiginous melanoma. *Archives of Dermatology*, **116**, 773.

Collins, W. T., and Gall, E. A. (1952). Gastric carcinoma: a multicentric lesion. *Cancer*, **5**, 62.

Cook, M. G., Eusebi, V., and Betts, C. M. (1976). Oat cell carcinoma of the oesophagus: a recently recognised entity. *Journal of Clinical Pathology*, **29**, 1068.

Cooney, T., Benediktsson, H., and Mukai, K. (1980). Immunohistochemical evaluation of a complex endocrinopathy. *American Journal of Surgical Pathology*, **4**, 491.

Cormier, W. J., Gaffey, T. A., Welch, J. M. *et al.* (1980). Linitis plastica caused by metastatic lobular carcinoma of the breast. *Mayo Clinic Proceedings*, **55**, 747.

Dawson, I. M. P., Cornes, J. S., and Morson, B. C. (1961). Primary malignant lymphoid tumours of the gastrointestinal tract. *British Journal of Surgery*, **49**, 80.

Dodge, O. G. (1961). Gastro-oesophageal carcinoma of mixed histological type. *Journal of Pathology and Bacteriology*, **81**, 459.

Dutz, W. (1978). The non-lymphomatous mucosa in primary gastrointestinal lymphoma: an aetiological clue? (abstract) Twelfth Congress of the International Academy of Pathology and Third World Congress of Academic and Environmental Pathology, Jerusalem.

Egan, R. L. (1982). Multicentric breast carcinomas: Clinical-radiographic-pathologic whole organ studies and 10 year survival. *Cancer*, **49**, 1123.

Eggleston, J. C., Tockman, M. S., Baker, R. R. *et al.* (1982). *In situ* and microinvasive squamous cell carcinoma of the lung. *Clinics in oncology*, Vol. 1. London: W. B. Saunders, p. 499.

Eifel, P., Hendrickson, M., Ross, J. *et al.* (1982). Simultaneous presentation of carcinoma involving the ovary and the uterine corpus. *Cancer*, **50**, 163.

Fidler, I. J., Gersten, D. M., and Hart, I. R. (1978). The biology of cancer invasion and metastasis. *Advances in Cancer Research*, **28**, 149.

Fisher, E. R., Gregorio, R. M., and Fisher, B. (1975). The pathology of invasive breast cancer. A syllabus derived from the findings of the National Surgical Adjuvant Breast Project (Protocol No. 4). *Cancer*, **36**, 1.

Foulds, L. (1969). *Neoplastic development*, Vol. 1. London: Academic Press.

Foulds, L. (1975). *Neoplastic development*, Vol. 2. London: Academic Press.

Freeman, C., Berg, J. N., and Cotlow, S. J. (1972). Occurrence and prognosis of extra nodal lymphomas. *Cancer*, **29**, 252.

Friedell, G. H., Parija, G. C., Nagy, G. K., and Soto, E. A. (1980). The pathology of human bladder cancer. *Cancer*, **45**, 1823.

Gallager, H. S., and Martin, J. E. (1969). Early phases in the development of breast cancer. *Cancer*, **24**, 1170.

Gilbert, J. B., and Hamilton, J. B. (1940). Studies in malignant testis tumours III. Incidence and nature of tumours in ectopic testes. *Surgery, Gynecology and Obstetrics*, **71**, 731.

Godwin, I. D. II. (1975). Carcinoid tumours. An analysis of 2837 cases. *Cancer*, **36**, 560.

Golby, M., and Codling, B. W. (1969). Coincidental carcinoma of oesophagus and stomach. *British Journal of Surgery*, **56**, 601.

Greenberg, R. A. (1959). The occurrence of primary multiple cancers. Thesis, Yale University, New Haven.

Gromet, M. A., Epstein, W. L. and Blois, M. S. (1978). The regressing thin malignant melanoma. A distinctive lesion with metastatic potential. *Cancer*, **42**, 2282.

Heald, R. J., and Bussey, H. J. R. (1975). Clinical experiences at St Mark's Hospital with multiple synchronous cancers of the colon and rectum. *Diseasees of the Colon and Rectum*, **18**, 6.

Hendrickson, M. R., and Kempson, R. L. (1980). Surgical pathology of the uterine corpus. In *Major Problems in Pathology*, Vol. 12. Philadelphia: W. B. Saunders.

Herbst, A. L., Robboy, S. I., Scully, R. E., and Poskanzer, D. C. (1974). Clear cell adenocarcinoma of the vagina and cervix in girls: analysis of 170 registry cases. *American Journal of Obstetrics and Gynecology*, **119**, 713.

Holmes, E. C., Clark, W., Morton, D. L. *et al.* (1976). Regional lymph node metastases and the level of invasion of primary melanoma. *Cancer*, **37**, 199.

Iida, F., Murata, F., and Nagata, T. (1978). Histochemical studies of mucosubstances in metaplastic epithelium of the stomach with special reference to the development of intestinal metaplasia. *Histochemistry*, **56**, 229.

Isaacson, P. (1979). Middle East lymphoma and α-chain disease. An immunohistochemical study. *American Journal of Surgical Pathology*, **3**, 431.

Jass, J. R. (1983). A classification of gastric dysplasia. *Histopathology*, **7**, 181.

Javadpour, N. (1979). Serum and cellular biologic tumour markers in patients with urologic cancer. *Human Pathology*, **10**, 557.

Joshi, V. V. (1968). Primary Krukenberg tumour of the ovary. Review of literature and a case report. *Cancer*, **22**, 1199.

Katzenstein, A-LA., Prioleau, P. G., and Askin, F. B. (1980). The histologic spectrum and significance of clear cell change in lung carcinoma. *Cancer*, **45**, 943.

Kerl, H., Hödl, S., Kresbach, H., and Stettner, H. (1982). Diagnosis and prognosis of the early stages of cutaneous malignant melanoma. *Clinics in Oncology*, **1**, 433.

Kleinsasser, O., and Glanz, H. (1982). Microcarcinoma and microinvasive carcinoma of the vocal cords. *Clinics in Oncology*, **1**, 479.

Kornberg, R., Harris, M., and Ackerman, B. (1978). Epidermotropically metastatic malignant melanoma. *Archives of Dermatology*, **114**, 67.

Koss, L. G. (1979). Mapping of the urinary bladder: its impact on the concepts of bladder cancer. *Human Pathology*, **10**, 533.

Koss, L. G., Schreiber, K., Oberlander, S. G. *et al.* (1981). Screening of asymptomatic women for endometrial cancer. *Obstetrics and Gynaecology*, **57**, 681.

Kraus, F. T., and Perez-Mesa, C. (1966). Verrucous carcinoma. Clinical and pathologic study of 105 cases involving oral cavity, larynx, and genitalia. *Cancer*, **19**, 26.

Kreyberg, L., Liebow, A. A., and Uehlinger, E. A. (1967). *International histological classification of tumours*. Number 1, *Histological typing of lung tumours*. Geneva: WHO.

Kuiper, D. H., Gracie, W. A. Jr., and Pollard, H. M. (1970). Twenty years of gastrointestinal carcinoids. *Cancer*, **25**, 1424.

Lagios, M. D. (1977). Multicentricity of breast carcinoma demonstrated by routine correlated serial subgross and radiographic examination. *Cancer*, **40**, 1726.

Lauchlan, S. C. (1968). Conceptual unity of the müllerian tumour group. A histologic study. *Cancer*, **22**, 601.

Lauren, P. (1965). The two histological main types of gastric carcinoma: diffuse and so-called intestinal type carcinoma. An attempt at a histoclinical classification. *Acta Pathologica et Microbiologica Scandinavica*, **64**, 31.

LeGal, Y., and Bauer, W. G. (1961). Second primary bronchogenic carcinoma. *Journal of Thoracic and Cardiovascular Surgery*, **41**, 114.

Lewin, K. J., Ranchod, M., and Dorfman, R. F. (1978). Lymphomas of the gastrointestinal tract. A study of 117 cases presenting with gastrointestinal disease. *Cancer*, **42**, 693.

Liebow, A. A., and Castleman, B. (1971). Benign clear cell ('sugar') tumors of the lung. *Yale Journal of Biology and Medicine*, **43**, 213.

Lund, H. Z. (1965). How often does squamous cell carcinoma metastasize? *Archives of Dermatology*, **92**, 635.

McDonald, D. F., and Thorson, T. (1956). Clinical implications of transplantability of induced bladder tumours to intact transitional epithelium of dogs. *Journal of Urology (Baltimore)*, **75**, 690.

McGowan, L., Young, R. H., and Scully, R. E. (1980). Peutz–Jeghers syndrome with 'adenoma malignum' of the cervix. *Gynecologic Oncology*, **10**, 125.

McGrath, E. J., Gall, E. A., and Kessler, D. P. (1952). Bronchogenic carcinoma, a product of multiple sites of origin. *Journal of Thoracic Surgery*, **24**, 271.

McGuirt, W. F., Matthews, B., and Kaufman, J. A. (1982). Multiple simultaneous tumours in patients with head and neck cancer. A prospective sequential panendoscopic study. *Cancer*, **50**, 1195.

Melicow, M. M. (1952). Histological study of vesical urothelium intervening between gross neoplasms in total cystectomy. *Journal of Urology*, **68**, 261.

Ming, S. C., Goldman, H., and Freiman, D. G. (1967). Intestinal metaplasia and histogenesis of carcinoma of the human stomach. *Cancer*, **28**, 1418.

Mobley, D. F., and Martinez, A. J. (1968). Two histologically different primary carcinomas of the lung. A review of the literature and presentation of a case. *Cancer*, **22**, 287.

Moertel, C. G. (1966). Multiple primary malignant neoplasms. Their incidence and significance. *Recent Results in Cancer Research*, **7.**

Moertel, C. G., Dockerty, M. B., and Baggenstoss, A. H. (1961). Multiple primary malignant neoplasms. I. Introduction and presentation of data. *Cancer*, **14**, 221.

Monnier, P., Savary, M., Pasche, R., and Anani, P. (1982). Endoscopic morphology of microinvasive squamous cell carcinoma of the oesophagus. *Clinics in Oncology*, **1**, 559.

Morgan, A. D., and Mackenzie, D. H. (1964). Clear-cell carcinoma of the lung. *Journal of Pathology and Bacteriology*, **87**, 25.

Morson, B. C., and Konishi, F. (1980). Dysplasia in the colorectum. In *Recent Advances in Gastrointestinal Pathology*. London: W. B. Saunders, p. 331.

Morson, B. C., Sobin, L. H., Grundmann, E. *et al.* (1980). Precancerous conditions and epithelial dysplasia in the stomach. *Journal of Clinical Pathology*, **33**, 711.

Moseley, H. S., Giuliano, A. E., Storm, F. K. *et al.* (1979). Multiple primary melanoma. *Cancer*, **43**, 939.

Mostofi, F. K. (1980). Pathology of germ cell tumors of testis. A progress report. *Cancer*, **45**, 1735.

Mostofi, F. K., and Price, E. B. Jr. (1973). *Tumors of the male genital system.* (Fascicle 8) *Atlas of tumour pathology*, Second Series. Washington, DC: Armed Forces Institute of Pathology.

Mostoufizadeh, M., and Scully, R. E. (1980). Malignant tumors arising in endometriosis. *Clinical Obstetrics and Gynecology*, **23**, 951.

Nakamura, K., Sugano, H., and Takagi, K. (1968). Carcinoma of the stomach in incipient phase; its histogenesis and histological appearances. *Gann*, **59**, 251.

Pangalis, G. A., and Rappaport, H. (1977). Common clonal origin of lymphoplasmacytic proliferation and immunoblastic lymphoma and intestinal alpha-chain disease. *Lancet*, **2**, 880.

Pearse, A. G. E. (1974). The APUD cell concept and its implications in pathology. *Pathology Annual*, **9**, 27.

Piccone, V. A., Klopstock, R., LeVeen, H. H., and Sika, J. (1970). Primary malignant melanoma of the oesophagus associated with melanosis of the entire oesophagus. First case report. *Journal of Thoracic and Cardiovascular Surgery*, **59**, 865.

Platz, H., Fries, R., Hudec, M. *et al.* (1982). Prognostic relevance of minimal invasion in carcinomas of the oral cavity: a retrospective DOSAK study. *Clinics in Oncology*, **1**, 467.

Pugh, R. C. B. (1976). Bilateral tumours. In *Pathology of the Testis* (ed. R. C. B. Pugh). Oxford: Blackwell, p. 150.

Qualheim, R. E., and Gall, E. A. (1957). Breast carcinoma with multiple sites of origin. *Cancer*, **10**, 460.

Ranchod, M., and Kempson, R. L. (1977). Smooth muscle tumours of the gastrointestinal tract and retroperitoneum. A pathologic analysis of 100 cases. *Cancer*, **39**, 255.

Rappaport, H., Ramot, B., Hulu, N., and Park, J. K. (1972). The pathology of so-called Mediterranean abdominal lymphoma with malabsorption. *Cancer*, **29**, 1502.

Robbins, G. F., and Berg, J. W. (1964). Bilateral primary breast cancers. *Cancer*, **17**, 1501.

Rohwedder, J. J., and Wheatherbee, L. (1974). Multiple primary bronchogenic carcinoma with a review of the literature. *American Review of Respiratory Diseases*, **109**, 435.

Rosai, J. (1981). *Ackerman's surgical pathology*, Vol. 1. St Louis: C. V. Mosby, p. 672.

Rossmann, P., and Vortel, V. (1961). Pulmonary metastases imitating alveolar-cell carcinoma. *Journal of Pathology and Bacteriology*, **81**, 313.

Schmoeckel, C., Bockelbrink, A., Bockelbrink, H., and Braun-Falco, O. (1982). Prognostic criteria in malignant melanoma. *Clinics in Oncology*, **1**, 455.

Schoenberg, B. S. (1977). *Multiple primary malignant neoplasms. The Connecticut experience, 1935–1964.* Berlin: Springer-Verlag.

Schwartz, M. (1961). A biomathematical approach to clinical tumour growth. *Cancer*, **14**, 1272.

Scully, R. E. (1979). *Tumors of the ovary and maldeveloped gonads.* (Fascicle 16) *Atlas of tumour pathology.* Washington, DC: Armed Forces Institute of Pathology, p. 413.

Scully, R. E. (1981). Neoplasia associated with anomalous sexual development and abnormal sex chromosomes. *Paediatric and Adolescent Endocrinology*, **8**, 203.

Scully, R. E. (1982). Minimal cancer of the ovary. *Clinics in Oncology*, **1**, 379.

Skakkebaek, N. E. (1978). Carcinoma *in situ* of the testis: frequency and relationship to invasive germ cell tumours in infertile men. *Histopathology*, **2**, 157.

Slaughter, D. P., Southwick, H. W., and Smejkal, W. (1953). Field cancerization in oral stratified squamous epithelium. Clinical implications of multicentric origin. *Cancer*, **6**, 963.

Smith, R. A. (1966). Development and treatment of fresh lung carcinoma after successful lobectomy. *Thorax*, **21**, 1.

Soga, J., and Tazawa, K. (1971). Pathologic analysis of carcinoids: histologic re-evaluation of 62 cases. *Cancer*, **28**, 990.

Suckow, E. E., Yokoo, H., and Brock, D. R. (1962). Intraepithelial carcinoma concomitant with oesophageal carcinoma. *Cancer*, **15**, 733.

Tellem, M., Prive, L., and Meranze, D. R. (1962). Four quadrant study of breast removed for carcinoma. *Cancer*, **15**, 10.

Tisell, L. E., Angervall, L., Dahl, I. *et al.* (1978). Recurrent and metastasizing gastric leiomyoblastoma (epithelioid leiomyosarcoma) associated with multiple pulmonary chondro-hamartomas: long survival of a patient treated with repeated operations. *Cancer*, **41**, 259.

Unger, S. W., Wanebo, H. J., and Cooper, P. H. (1981). Multiple cutaneous malignant melanomas with features of primary melanoma. *Annals of Surgery*, **193**, 245.

Ushigome, S., Spjut, H. J., and Noon, G. P. (1967). Extensive dysplasia and carcinoma *in situ* of esophageal epithelium. *Cancer*, **20**, 1023.

Van den Heule, B., Van Kerkem, C., and Heimann, R. (1979). Benign and malignant lymphoid lesions of the stomach. A histological reappraisal in the light of the Kiel classification for non-Hodgkin's lymphomas. *Histopathology*, **3**, 309.

Warren, S., and Gates, O. (1932). Multiple primary malignant tumours. A survey of the literature and a statistical study. *American Journal of Cancer*, **16**, 1358.

Way, S. (1960). Carcinoma of the vulva. *American Journal of Obstetrics and Gynecology*, **79**, 692.

Way, S. (1980). Carcinoma metastatic in the cervix. *Gynecological Oncology*, **9**, 298.

Wayte, D. M., and Helwig, E. B. (1968). Melanotic freckle of Hutchinson. *Cancer*, **21**, 893.

Wellings, S. R., Jensen, H. M., and Marcum, R. G. (1975). An atlas of subgross pathology of the human breast with special reference to possible precancerous lesions. *Journal of National Cancer Institute*, **55**, 231.

Williams, E. D., and Celestin, L. R. (1962). The association of bronchial carcinoid and pluriglandular adenomatosis. *Thorax*, **17**, 120.

Woolley, P. V., Osborne, C. K., Levi, J. A. *et al.* (1976). Extranodal presentation of non-Hodgkin's lymphomas in the testis. *Cancer*, **38**, 1026.

Yesner, R., Gerstl, B., and Auerbach, O. (1965). Application of the World Health Organization classification of lung carcinoma to biopsy material. *Annals of Thoracic Surgery*, **1**, 33.

Chapter

12

JAMES A RECABAREN, MICHAEL P. OSBORNE, and
JEROME J. DeCOSSE

Individuals at High Risk –
Preventive Measures

The purpose of identifying those individuals at risk for multiple cancers is that of prevention. Prevention may involve removal of a carcinogenic influence, but elimination of a risk factor is not always possible, as in the case of genetic susceptibility, endogenous hormonal influence or established dietary patterns. Risk factors for tumors in which multiple cancers may occur are listed in Table 1. The precise contribution of each different risk factor to multiple cancer is unknown, but their role is discussed in detail in other chapters.

BIOMARKERS OF ENHANCED RISK FOR MULTIPLE CANCERS

The most reliable markers for those at high risk for multiple primary carcinoma are in those tumors associated with specific etiologic factors. Thus, individuals with genetic or immunodeficiency syndromes are at high risk for multiple primary cancers (see Chapter 9) and the patient treated for a previous malignancy has an historical marker of high risk.

Age is not a risk factor for multiple cancers unless part of a genetic syndrome. The average age of individuals with simultaneous carcinomas is 62 for men and 58 for women; these ages are similar to those of similar sporadic cancers in the general population. The ages for the first metachronous cancer in men and women are 58 and 52 years respectively (Moertel, 1966).

The influence of socio-economic status on the risk of multiple primary cancers is similar to that for cancer in general. The association between lower socio-economic group and a higher incidence of some cancers is well established (Levin *et al.*, 1974). This association is most often seen in carcinoma of the cervix, stomach, and esophagus but there is little correlation

Table 1 Contribution of cancer-associated risk factors in malignancy

Factor	Sites considered in estimate	Range of total cancer burden associated with factor	
Genetic	All – primarily reproductive/digestive	5% (5–30%)	(Anderson, 1974)
Environmental			
Diet	Digestive tract	80–90%	(Higginson and Muir, 1976)
Tobacco	Upper aerodigestive tract, lungs, bladder, kidney, pancreas	30–50%	(Doll and Peto, 1981)
		20–30%	(Doll and Peto, 1981)
Alcohol	Upper digestive tract, larynx, liver	3–5%	(Doll and Peto, 1981)
Medical – Drugs and therapeutic radiation	Breast, endometrium, ovary, thyroid, bone, lung, blood (leukemia)	1– 4%	(Penn and Starzl, 1972; Arseneau *et al.*, 1972)
Previous cancer	Any organ, but primarily reproductive/ digestive	Less than 5%	(Schoenberg, 1975)

with cancers of the breast or colon, two organ systems commonly associated with multiple cancers. Differences in cancer risk with socio-economic status are generally attributed to environmental differences.

Marital status does not affect the risk of multiple cancers, although married persons generally experience a lower mortality from cancer when compared to single persons. (Self-selection may contribute to this finding since those in poor health, a previous cancer or with high risk factors are less likely to marry.) The differences in risk for breast cancer and cervical cancer in married females is related to reproductive history. Multiple head and neck cancers also have a higher incidence in single males, probably related to individual lifestyle.

There are differences in incidence of multiple cancers between ethnic groups. Spanish Americans in the United States have the highest risk of multiple primary breast cancers: whites have an intermediate risk and blacks the lowest risk. American Indian populations do not have an increased risk of multiple primary malignancies, but the number of individuals studied is small (Newell, 1980).

Identification of those at high risk for multiple primary cancers is difficult except in individuals with a history of a previous malignancy or a genetic predisposition to cancer. In the individual without a contributing history, it is difficult to isolate any specific risk categories.

(a) In some cases, precursor lesions of multiple cancer may be identified. Adenomatous polyps of the colon, mucosal dysplasia in ulcerative colitis, dysplasia of the cervix, and atypical lesions of the breast are common examples and may be markers of exposure to carcinogenic agents.

(b) Chromosomal abnormalities may be identified in cells at risk for cancer. These changes are deemed the result of carcinogenic exposure and can be detected by studies of chromosomal morphology, cell kinetics, and DNA synthesis. Abnormal DNA synthesis has been demonstrated by increased tritiated thymidine incorporation into colonic mucosal cells of patients with an increased risk of cancer (Lipkin *et al.*, 1980).

(c) A biomarker such as intraluminal CEA can be produced by altered protein synthesis in those at risk for large bowel cancer (Lipkin *et al.*, 1980). Aneuploidy may be demonstrated by precursor cells. Glutamate–pyruvate transaminase allele linkage has been suggested to be associated with a genetic susceptibility to breast cancer (Lynch, 1981).

(d) Screening procedures are available for those at risk for multiple cancers. These may range from breast self-examination to mammography, colonoscopy or fecal occult blood studies. Biomarkers such as calcitonin in MEN syndromes are markers for high risk of medullary carcinoma of the thyroid and other associated cancers (Ewing *et al.*, 1982).

(e) A fecal mutagen is said to be detectable in increased amounts in individuals at high risk for colon cancer (Bruce *et al.*, 1977) which increases in concentration with anaerobic incubation of feces but loses its mutagenic effect when oxidized. This substance can be quantitated in fecal samples and may have potential as a monitor of risk for colon carcinoma (Wilkens *et al.*, 1980).

CANCER PREVENTION

The prevention of cancer may be based on primary epidemiologic measures, removal of a causative carcinogen, or secondary administration of preventive agents. The detection of individuals at high risk for multiple cancers is the basis of any cancer prevention program; and, as noted above, is based on the presence of premalignant lesions, carcinogenic exposure or increased genetic susceptibility.

Environmental carcinogens require both monitoring and regulation and, if possible, elimination from exposure to the population. Increased susceptibility states must be recognized; these include genetic syndromes and cancer families. Individuals and family members are at high risk and require strict surveillance for early detection of cancer (Albano *et al.*, 1982).

The control of cancer using substances that can inhibit, delay or reverse carcinogenesis is known as chemoprevention. The agents are varied and both natural and synthetic substances have been used (Table 2). There are several mechanisms by action by these agents; some are truly preventive, whereas others modify an existing precancerous lesion. The mechanism of action of the chemopreventive agents can be divided into major categories: induction of gene suppression, detoxification of carcinogens, blocking oxidative damage to DNA, stimulation of the immune response, and antagonism of putative hormonal promoters (Griffen, 1980; DeCosse, 1982).

Table 2   Potential chemopreventive agents (after DeCosse, 1982)

Natural	Vitamins A, C, E
	Vitamin precursors (β-carotene)
	Coumarin
	Indoles
	Flavones
	Plant sterols
	Selenium salts
Synthetic	Phenolic antioxidants (butylated hydroxyanisole, BHA)
	Prostaglandin synthesis inhibitors (indomethacin)
	Retinoids
	Antihormones

Substances used as preventive agents are in two main groups: natural agents which include vitamins, flavones, indoles, and sterols; synthetic agents which include vitamin analogues, antioxidants, phenols, and prostaglandin inhibitors. Of particular interest are the retinoid group of synthetic vitamin A analogues which are necessary for proper growth and differentiation of all epithelial cells in the body. They may function in a similar manner to steroid hormones, with epithelial organs as target tissues. In the absence of retinoids, squamous metaplasia results and tissues develop with a predominance of keratinized squamous cells.

Epithelial systems with retinoid dependence include the tracheobronchial tree, mammary gland, gastrointestinal system, urinary tract, pancreatic ducts, and the reproductive system (Sporn and Newton, 1981). Dysplastic lesions at these sites are considered to be premalignant, but represent a histologic state that is reversible with the administration of retinoid substances. The ability of retinoids to suppress malignant transformation can occur even after exposure to a carcinogen and initial molecular damage. This can be deemed an 'anti-promoting' effect and retinoids apparently do not have any effect on the initiating phase.

Human deficiency states have also been associated with high risk of malignancy (Wald *et al.*, 1980). Vitamin A-deficient animals show an enhanced risk of lung, bladder, and large bowel malignancy (Muller-Salamin *et al.*, 1979). Epidemiologic studies suggest that a similar mechanism may be present in the human lung cancer model (Shekelle *et al.*, 1981). Low dietary intake of β-carotene has been associated with increased susceptibility to lung, bladder, and stomach cancer (Peto *et al.*, 1981).

In cell culture studies, the retinoids appear to modulate the effects of the regulation of cell division. These effects may be enhancing (Wilson and Reich, 1978) or suppressing transforming growth factors (Todaro and De Larco, 1978). The development of malignancy has been associated with cellular transforming polypeptides. The ability of retinoids to act even after experimental carcinogen exposure, and to reverse premalignant or even early malignant transformation, makes these substances promising agents in the developing field of chemoprevention. New synthetic retinoids, with less toxic effects, are now available for further study.

Phenolic antioxidants inhibit carcinogen formation by modification of mixed function microsomal oxidase activity. They increase detoxification of various carcinogens by their antioxidant properties. The phenols also can block oxidative damage to the DNA molecule. Nucleophilic antioxidant agents such as butylated hydroxyanisole can competitively bind with electrophilic carcinogens, and are effective in experimental models. They prevent the activation of hydrocarbons to their carcinogenic–electrophilic intermediates.

Various trials of inhibitors of promoter substance have been reported, and promising agents include indomethacin (Narisawa, 1981). Ascorbic acid has the ability to inhibit the formation of colonic carcinogenic agents. The vitamin blocks the synthesis of nitroso compounds from the nitrate precursors in the stomach, and decreases the concentration of fecal mutagens in the colonic contents (Mirvish *et al.*, 1972).

EXPERIMENTAL CHEMOPREVENTION IN SELECTED ORGAN SYSTEMS

Colorectal cancer

Colorectal cancer was until recently the most frequent cancer in the Western world. Environmental factors are thought to be important in this high incidence, and epidemiologic studies of migrating populations have supported this observation. The diets of economically developed countries have been blamed as the cause of increased large bowel cancer rates and increased consumption of meats, proteins, fats, and refined foods low in fiber is suspected as promoting carcinogenesis. These foods also modify the intestinal microflora and possibly contribute to fecal mutagens (see Chapter 6).

A number of dietary compounds have been shown to promote or inhibit colon carcinogenesis in the animal model. Increased consumption of vegetable or animal fats promotes, while diets high in fiber or cellulose inhibit, tumor formation (Eyers and DeCosse, 1981). Fat increases bile excretion and changes the microflora of the colonic contents. The intestinal microflora are presumed to be capable of synthesis of mutagens from products of bile acids, sterols, and nitroso compounds. Dietary fiber conversely has the capacity to bind bile acids, fats and minerals (Zn, Fe, Ca, Cu, Mg) and decrease colonic transit time (Levine, 1981).

Chemoprevention of large bowel cancer has been studied in both laboratory and clinical situations. In the animal model, experimental carcinogenesis has been inhibited with BHT, disulphiram, sodium selenite, retinoid derivatives, ascorbic acid, and α-tocopherol (DeCosse, 1982). With the exception of retinoids, the majority of these products are antioxidants. Ascorbic acid and α-tocopherol also block the formation of nitroso compounds and decrease fecal mutagen levels (Bruce and Dion, 1980).

Clinically, ascorbic acid was tested in a randomized double blind trial in patients with hereditary polyposis of the colon (Bussey *et al.*, 1982). Reduction in number and area of rectal polyps was observed, and labeling studies of removed polyps suggested a suppression of DNA synthesis. The mechanism of action by ascorbic acid in this study was suggested to be both systemic and local.

Breast cancer

Several potential chemopreventive agents have been investigated in experimental breast cancer models. Selenium has been demonstrated to be moderately effective (Harr *et al.*, 1972). Sporn and his co-authors have demonstrated the effects of vitamin A and its derivatives (retinoids) in reducing experimental mammary carcinoma induced by 7,12-dimethylbenzanthracene (DMBA) and 1-methyl-1-nitrosurea (MNU) (Sporn *et al.*, 1976a,b; Moon *et al.*, 1976, 1977, 1979). These effects do not appear to be influenced by the hormonal status of the animal (Thompson *et al.*, 1982). Simultaneously, Jordan (1976) showed the chemopreventive effect of the antiestrogen, tamoxifen (Nolvadex) in the DMBA model.

(a) *Selenium*

Various factors appear to influence the ability of selenium to prevent experimental mammary cancer. These include dietary concentration of selenium (Harr *et al.*, 1973), dietary fat intake (Ip, 1981), and hormonal influences (Welsch *et al.*, 1981a). Selenium has been shown to be an effective inhibitor of both the initiating and promoting phases of DMBA (Welsch *et al.*, 1981a) and NMU carcinogenesis (Thompson and Becci, 1980).

(b) *Vitamin A and retinoids*

Currently studies are attempting to improve efficacy of such agents while reducing toxicity. Increased selective pharmacological targeting has become possible by chemical synthetic manipulation of the polar-end terminus of the retinoid molecule (Grubbs *et al.*, 1977a; Moon *et al.*, 1979). Studies have reported that the timing and duration of exposure are important (Thompson *et al.*, 1979; McCormick *et al.*, 1980), and it has been shown that retinoids can inhibit DNA synthesis *after* exposure to the carcinogen (Mehta and Moon, 1980).

Some experiments suggest that retinoids may have an adverse effect and promote mammary carcinogenesis (Welsch and De Moog, 1983). *In vitro* studies have also supported this view (Wilson and Reich, 1978; Levine and Ohucki, 1978) but the influence of dose on this phenomenon is unclear (Schroder and Black, 1980).

(c) *Antiestrogens, ovariectomy or prolactin inhibition*

Antiestrogens (Jordan *et al.*, 1980; Turcot-Lemay and Kelley, 1980; Welsch *et al.*, 1982), ovariectomy (McCormick *et al.*, 1982), and prolactin suppression

(Welsch *et al.*, 1980, 1981b, 1982) are all able to reduce the rate of mammary cancer in selected experimental models.

(d) *Combined chemopreventive agents*

Recent research has examined the potential for combined regimens. Studies include the additive effects of selenium and vitamin A (Ip and Ip, 1981; Thompson *et al.*, 1981) or the synergistic effects of retinoid treatment with either prolactin suppression (Welsch *et al.*, 1980), ovariectomy (McCormick *et al.*, 1983) or hormone inhibition by antiestrogens with immune stimulation (Welsch and De Moog, 1983).

Future directions of research in chemoprevention will require the development of more potent analogues with fewer side-effects, the study of the effects of those agents on human tissues *in vitro* and *in vivo* and recognition of factors which influence those effects.

Gastric cancer

In Western society, gastric cancer has steadily decreased in frequency. The etiologic factors are unknown, but diets high in nitroso compounds are suspect. Gastric carcinogenesis experiments in laboratory animals have shown that nitroso-containing diets are converted to mutagenic substances. The carcinogen is a nitrosourea derivative and its mutagenic activity can be blocked by administered ascorbic acid (Weisburger *et al.*, 1980).

Changes in dietary practices may account for the changing incidence of gastric cancer. The increased availability of fresh fruits and vegetables has increased vitamin C dietary levels in the United States. In areas of endemic gastric cancer, dietary modification and supplemental vitamin C could be evaluated as a chemopreventive agent (Weisburger *et al.*, 1980).

Urological cancer

Carcinogenic agents have induced multiple epithelial tumors in the urinary bladders of laboratory animals, and initiation can be blocked by subsequent exposure to 13-*cis*-retinoic acid with reduction in the number of tumors formed (Grubbs *et al.*, 1977b). Clinical investigations with oral 13-*cis*-retinoic acid in patients with resected multiple superficial bladder cancers have been inconclusive.

Skin cancer

Human keratoacanthomas, multiple basal cell carcinomas, and solar keratosis have been treated successfully by retinoids (Haydey *et al.*, 1980). Hydrocarbon initiation of skin tumors in laboratory animals has been reversed with antioxidant (BHA) administration (Slaga & Bracken, 1977). The mode of action of the antioxidants is to decrease covalent bonding of the electrophiles to the DNA molecule. Orally administered 13-*cis*-retinoic acid is being used in the treatment of therapy-resistant acne but cutaneous and mucosal toxicity are common (Peck *et al.*, 1979). This toxicity may limit widespread use for cancer chemoprevention.

Lung cancer

Tracheobronchial epithelia have been shown to undergo metaplastic changes in retinoid-deficient animals (Muller-Salamin *et al.*, 1979). In the United Kingdom, vitamin A levels of patients with lung cancer show a statistically significant deficiency when compared to age-matched controls (Shekelle and Lepper, 1981). However, vitamin A deficiency cannot be interpreted as an etiologic factor, since individuals with a vitamin A deficiency in the United Kingdom are rare, and lung cancer is endemic. The deficiency could be a contributing factor to the carcinogenesis, but not a major etiologic factor. Restoration of vitamin A levels might be considered as a potential means of chemoprevention.

Oropharyngeal cancers

Leukoplakia and erythroplasia are thought to be precursor lesions to carcinoma, with the non-keratinizing red lesions at higher risk. Investigation in the animal model shows inhibition of leukoplakia and epidermoid carcinoma after retinoid administration (Shklar *et al.*, 1980). A phase I–II study of 13-*cis*-retinoic acid formulated in a lozenge has shown modest benefit in inhibition of oral leukoplakia (Shah *et al.*, 1983).

CONCLUSION

Genetic susceptibility, environmental carcinogen exposure, the presence of premalignant lesions or a history of previous malignancy are true markers of high risk of multiple cancer. The purpose of identifying these markers is the early detection and ultimately the prevention of multiple malignancy.

At present, the greatest potential for chemoprophylaxis lies with malignancies of epithelial origin, such as breast, colon and lung cancers and prevention research is active in these areas. Until chemopreventive agents are developed, we must persist with epidemiologic measures and removal of causative carcinogens.

REFERENCES

Albano, W. A., Recabaren, J. A., Lynch, H. T., and Organ, C. H. (1982). Natural history of hereditary cancer of the breast and colon. *Cancer,* **50,** 360.

Anderson, D. E. (1974). The role of genetics in human cancer. *Ca–A Cancer Journal for Clinicians,* **24,** 130.

Arseneau, J. C., Sponzo, R. W., Levin, D. L. *et al.* (1972). Nonlymphomatous malignant tumors complicating Hodgkin's disease. *New England Journal of Medicine,* **287,** 1119.

Bruce, W. R., and Dion, P. W. (1980). Studies relating to a fecal mutagen. *American Journal of Clinical Nutrition,* **33,** 2511.

Bruce, W. R., Varghese, A. J., Funer, R. *et al.* (1977). A mutagen in the feces of normal humans. *Origins of Human Cancer,* Cold Springs Harbor Laboratory, p. 1641.

Bussey, H., DeCosse, J. J., Deschner, E. *et al.* (1982). A randomized trial of ascorbic acid in polyposis coli. *Cancer,* **50,** 1434.

DeCosse, J. J. (1982). Potential for chemoprevention. *Cancer,* **50,** 2550.

Doll, R., and Peto, R. (1981). The causes of cancer: quantitative estimates of avoidable risks of cancer in the United States today. *Journal of the National Cancer Institute,* **66,** 1191.

Ewing, H. P., Newsome, E. D., and Hardy, J. D. (1982). Tumor markers. *Current Problems in Surgery,* **19,** 79.

Eyers, A. A., and DeCosse, J. J. (1981). *Nutrition in gastrointestinal disease.* New York: Churchill Livingstone, p. 59.

Griffen, A. C. (1980). Cancer chemoprevention. *Journal of Cancer Research and Clinical Oncology,* **98,** 1.

Grubbs, C. J., Moon, R. C., Sporn, M. B., and Newton, D. L. (1977a). Inhibition of mammary cancer by retinyl methyl ether. *Cancer Research,* **37,** 599.

Grubbs, C. J., Moon, R. C., Squire, R. A. *et al.* (1977b). 13-cis-retinoic acid: inhibition of bladder carcinogenesis induced in rats by N-butyl-N-(4-hydroxy-butyl) nitrosamine. *Science,* **198,** 743.

Harr, J. R., Exon, J. H., Weswig, P. M., and Whanger, P. D. (1973). Relationship of dietary selenium concentration; chemical cancer induction and tissue concentration of selenium in rats. *Clinical Toxicology,* **6,** 487.

Harr, J. R., Exon, J. H., Whanger, P. D., and Weswig, P. M. (1972). Effect of dietary selenium on N-2 fluorenyl-acetamide (FAA)-induced cancer in vitamin-E supplemented, selenium depleted rats. *Clinical Toxicology,* **5,** 187.

Haydey, R. P., Reed, M. L., Dzubow, L. M., and Shupack, (1980). Treatment of keratoacanthomas with oral 13-cis-retinoic acid. *New England Journal of Medicine,* **303,** 560.

Higginson, J., and Muir, C. S. (1976). The role of epidemiology in elucidating the importance of environmental factors in human cancer. *Cancer Detection and Prevention,* **1,** 79.

Ip, C. (1981). Factors influencing the anticarcinogenic efficacy of selenium in dimethylbenzanthracene-induced mammary tumorigenesis in rats. *Cancer Research,* **41,** 2683.

Ip, C., and Ip, M. M. (1981). Chemoprevention of mammary tumorigenesis of a combined regimen of selenium and vitamin A. *Carcinogenesis,* **2,** 915.

Jordan, V. C. (1976). Effect of tamoxifen (ICI 46474) on inhibition and growth of DMBA-induced rat mammary carcinomata. *European Journal of Cancer,* **12,** 419.

Jordan, V. C., Allen, K. E., and Dix, C. J. (1980). Pharmacology of tamoxifen in laboratory animals. *Cancer Treatment Reports,* **64,** 745.

Levin, D. L., Devesa, S. S., Godwin, J. D. *et al.* (1974). *Cancer rates and risks.* Washington, DC: National Cancer Institute, p. 58.

Levine, L., and Ohucki, K. (1978). Retinoids as well as tumor promoters enhance decyclation of cellular lipids and prostaglandin production in MDCK cells. *Nature,* **276,** 275

Levine, R. (1981). *Nutrition in gastrointestinal disease.* New York: Churchill Livingstone, p. 1.

Lipkin, M., Sherock, P., and DeCosse, J. (1980). Risk factors and preventive measures in control of cancer of the large intestine. *Current Problems in Cancer,* **4,** 1.

Lynch, H. T. (1981). *Genetics and breast cancer.* New York: Van Nostrand Reinhold, p. 9.

McCormick, D. L., Burns, F. J., and Albert, R. E. (1980). Inhibition of rat mammary carcinogenesis by short dietary exposure to retinyl acetate. *Cancer Research,* **40,** 1140.

McCormick, D. L., Mehta, R. G., Thompson, C. A. *et al.* (1982). Enhanced inhibition of mammary carcinogenesis by combined treatment with *N*-(4-hydroxyphenyl), retinamide and ovariectomy. *Cancer Research,* **42,** 508.

McCormick, D. L., Sowell, Z. L., Thompson, C. A., and Moon, R. C. (1983). Inhibition by retinoid and ovariectomy of additional primary malignancies in rats following surgical removal of the first mammary cancer. *Cancer,* **54,** 594.

Mehta, R. G., and Moon, R. C. (1980). Inhibition of DNA synthesis by retinyl acetate during chemically induced mammary carcinogenesis. *Cancer Research,* **40,** 1109.

Mirvish, S. S., Wallcate, L., Eagen, M., and Shubik, R. (1972). Ascorbate–nitrite reaction: possible means of blocking the formation of carcinogenic *N*-nitroso compounds. *Science,* **177,** 65.

Moertel, G. G. (1966). *Multiple primary malignant neoplasms.* Berlin: Springer-Verlag.

Moon, R. C., Grubbs, C. J., and Sporn, M. B. (1976). Inhibition of 7,12-dimethylbenz(a)anthracene-induced mammary carcinogenesis by retinyl acetate. *Cancer Research,* **36,** 2626.

Moon, R. C., Grubbs, C. J., Sporn, M. B., and Goodman, D. G. (1977). Retinyl acetate inhibits mammary carcinogens induced by *N*-methyl-*N*-nitrosurea. *Nature,* **267,** 620.

Moon, R. C., Thompson, H. J., Becci, P. J. *et al.* (1979). *N*-(4-hydroxyphenyl) retinamide, a new retinoid for prevention of breast cancer in the rat. *Cancer Research,* **39,** 1339.

Muller-Salamin, Matter, A., and Lasnitzki, I. (1979). Interaction of retinoic acid and 3-methylcholanthrene on the fine structure of mouse prostate epithelium *in vitro.* *Journal of the National Cancer Institute,* **63,** 485.

Narisawa, T. (1981). Inhibition of the development of methyl nitrosourea-induced rat colon tumors by indomethacin treatment. *Cancer Research,* **41,** 1954.

Newell, G. R. (1980). Multiple primary cancers: suggested etiologic implications. *Cancer Bulletin,* **32,** 160.

Peck, G. L., Olsen, T. G., Yoder, F. W. *et al.* (1979). Prolonged remissions of cystic and conglobate acne with 13-*cis*-retinoic acid. *New England Journal of Medicine,* **300,** 329.

Penn, I., and Starzl, T. E. (1972). A summary of the status of the de novo cancer in transplant recipients. *Transplantation Proceedings,* **4,** 719.

Peto, R., Doll, R., Buckley, J. D., and Sporn, M. B. (1981). Can dietary beta-carotene materially reduce human cancer rates? *Nature,* **290,** 201.

Schoenberg, B. S. (1975). *Multiple primary malignancies: the Connecticut experience.* New York: Springer-Verlag.

Schroder, E. W., and Black, P. M. (1980). Retinoids: tumor preventers or tumor enhancers. *Journal of the National Cancer Institute,* **65,** 671.

Shah, J. P., Strong, E. W., DeCosse, J. J. *et al.* (1983). Effect of retinoids on oral leukoplakia. *American Journal of Surgery* (in press).

Shekelle, R. B., and Lepper, M. (1981). Dietary vitamin A and risk of cancer in the Western Electric study. *Lancet,* **2,** 1185.

Shklar, G., Flynn, E., Szabo, G. *et al.* (1980). Retinoid inhibition of experimental lingual carcinogenesis: ultrastructure observations. *Journal of the National Cancer Institute,* **65,** 1307.

Slaga, J. J., and Bracken, W. M. (1977). The effects of antioxidants on skin tumor initiation and aryl hydrocarbon hydroxyphyl. *Cancer Research,* **37,** 1631.

Sporn, M. B., and Newton, D. L. (1981). *Inhibition of tumor induction and development.* New York: Plenum Press, p. 71.

Sporn, M. B., Dunlop, N. M., Newton, D. L., and Henderson, N. (1976a). Relationships between structure and activity of retinoids. *Nature* **263,** 110.

Sporn, M. B., Dunlop, N. M., Newton, D. L., and Smith, J. M. (1976b). Prevention of chemical carcinogenesis by vitamin A and its synthetic analogs (retinoids). *Federation Preceedings,* **35,** 1332.

Thompson, H. J., and Becci, P. J. (1980). Selenium inhibition of N-methyl-N-nitrosurea-induced mammary carcinogenesis in the rat. *Journal of the National Cancer Institute,* **65,** 1299.

Thompson, H. J., Becci, P. J., Brown, C. C., and Moon, R. C. (1979). Effect of the duration of retinyl acetate feeding on inhibition of 1-methyl-1-nitrosurea-induced mammary carcinogenesis in the rat. *Cancer Research,* **39,** 3977.

Thompson, H. J., Meeker, L. D., and Becci, P. J. (1981). Effect of combined selenium and retinyl acetate treatment on mammary carcinogenesis. *Cancer Research,* **41,** 1413.

Thompson, H. J., Meeker, C. D., Tagliagerro, A. R., and Becci, P. J. (1982). Effect of retinyl acetate on the occurrence of ovarian hormone-responsive and non-responsive mammary cancers in rats. *Cancer Research,* **42,** 903.

Todaro, G. J., and De Larco, J. E. (1978). Growth factors produced by sarcoma virus transformed cells. *Cancer Research,* **38,** 4147.

Turcot-Lemay, L., and Kelley, P. A. (1980). Characterization of estradiol, progesterone, and prolactin receptors in nitrosomethylurea-induced mammary tumors and effects of antiestrogen treatment on the development and growth of these tumors. *Cancer Research,* **40,** 3232.

Wald, N., Idle, M., and Boreham, J. (1980). Low serum-vitamin A and subsequent risk of cancer. *Lancet,* **1,** 813.

Weisburger, J. H., Marguardt, H., Mower, H. F. *et al.* (1980). Inhibition of carcinogenesis. Vitamin C and the prevention of gastric cancer. *Preventive Medicine,* **9,** 353.

Welsch, C. W., and DeMoog, J. V. (1983). Retinoid feeding, hormone inhibition, and/or immune stimulation and genesis of carcinogen-induced rat mammary carcinomas. *Cancer Research,* **43,** 585.

Welsch, C. W., Brown, C. K. Goodrich-Smith, M. *et al.* (1980). Synergistic effect of chronic prolactin suppression and retinoid treatment in the prophylaxis of N-methyl-N-nitrosourea induced mammary tumorigenesis in female Sprague–Dawley rats. *Cancer Research,* **40,** 3095.

Welsch, C.W., Goodrich-Smith, M., Brown, C.K. *et al.* (1982). 2-Bromo-a-ergocryptine (CB-254) and tamoxifen (ICI 45,474) induced suppression of genesis of mammary carcinomas in female rats treated with 7,12-dimethylbenzanthracene (DMBA): a comparison. *Oncology*, **39**, 88.

Welsch, C. W., Goodrich-Smith, M., Brown, C. K. *et al.* (1981a). Selenium and the genesis of murine mammary tumors. *Carcinogenesis*, **2**, 519.

Welsch, C. W., Goodrich-Smith, M., Brown, C. K., and Roth, L. (1981b). The prophylaxis of rat and mouse mammary gland tumorigenesis by suppression of prolactin secretion: a reappraisal. *Breast Cancer Research and Treatment*, **1**, 225.

Wilkins, T. D., Lederman, M., Van Tassell *et al.* (1980). Characterization of a mutagenic bacterial product in human feces. *American Journal of Clinical Nutrition*, **33**, 2513.

Wilson, E. L., and Reich, E. (1978). Plasminogen activator in chick fibroblasts: induction of synthesis by retinoic acid; synergism with viral transformation and phorbol ester. *Cell*, **15**,

Part 3

Patterns of multiple primary cancer

Risk Factors and Multiple Cancer
Edited by B.A. Stoll
© 1984 John Wiley and Sons Ltd.

Chapter

13 A. R. HARWOOD

Multiple Cancers of the Respiratory Tract

This chapter discusses the clinical evidence for multiple cancers of the respiratory tract based both on the literature and on the Princess Margaret Hospital experience. In addition, respiratory tract carcinogenesis will be examined at the cellular level, and the selective vulnerability of different respiratory tract epithelia will be discussed. The final section will review the possibilities for reducing the mortality rate from second respiratory tract cancers.

CRITERIA FOR DIAGNOSIS AND METHODS OF ANALYSING DATA

The increased risk of a second primary malignancy in a patient with cancer is classed according to whether it is previous, synchronous, or metachronous. *Previous* is the diagnosis of malignant disease prior to the current diagnosis. *Synchronous* is applied to neoplasms diagnosed at the same time as, or within six months of, identifying the primary lesion. (The six month interval has been used traditionally on the basis that any neoplasm identified within a six month interval was probably present at the time of the initial cancer.) *Metachronous* is applied to second cancers that develop six months or more after the diagnosis of the primary cancer.

Criteria for diagnosis of second cancers are discussed in Chapter 11 but the gross and histologic criteria utilized at our institute for diagnosis of second primary respiratory tract squamous cell carcinomas are as follows:

1. The neoplasm must be clearly malignant histopathologically.
2. Each neoplasm must be geographically separate and distinct and the lesions should be separated by normal-appearing mucosa. If a second

neoplasm is contiguous to the initial primary tumor or is separated by mucosa with intra-epithelial neoplastic change, the two should be considered as confluent growths rather than multicentric carcinomas.

3. The possibility that the second neoplasm represents a metastasis should be excluded.

We have found most difficulty in distinguishing a new primary carcinoma of the lung from a solitary metastasis. Solid cancers of the head and neck (particularly at an early stage) rarely metastasize to the lungs, and when metastases occur they are frequently multiple and peripheral. In contrast, a primary bronchogenic carcinoma will tend to be a single central lesion. Bronchoscopy and mediastinoscopy will frequently be positive in a primary bronchogenic carcinoma but negative in a metastatic lesion. Metastatic lesions rarely spread to the mediastinum whereas primary bronchogenic carcinomas frequently do so. Finally, it is extremely common for a primary bronchogenic carcinoma to spread through the blood stream to the brain, a metastatic site extremely uncommon for a primary head and neck cancer.

A difficult problem is that of a single pulmonary lesion arising in a patient with previous head and neck cancer which is controlled, and where bronchoscopy and mediastinoscopy are found to be negative. Under these circumstances we advise excision of the lesion, and histopathological assessment will usually determine whether the lesion is a carcinoma which has arisen primarily from the bronchial epithelium and abuts the bronchial lumen (frequently in association with adjacent carcinoma *in situ*), or is a blood-borne metastasis in the pulmonary substance with none of the above features.

When a new lesion develops in the *same* location as the original primary tumor, we classify this as recurrence of the original tumor rather than a new primary lesion. This is irrespective of the time after treatment that this new lesion develops.

In our data, the frequency of second respiratory tract primaries remains constant with time for up to 10 years following the diagnosis of the initial primary cancer of the upper respiratory tract. If one were frequently confusing metastatic lesions with second primaries, one would expect more second primaries to be seen in the first few years after diagnosis of the initial primary. This is not the case, and indicates that an inability to distinguish between second primaries and metastatic lesions has not been a major problem in our series.

The majority of publications in the literature calculate the *crude* risk of developing a second respiratory tract malignancy. This entails dividing the number of second primaries by the total number of first primary cases and determining a crude percentage risk. This represents an underestimate of the risk for the patient who survives, because this calculation takes no account of patients dying of their initial primary cancer or intercurrent disease, and who are, therefore, not at risk to a secondary respiratory tract tumor (Wagenfeld *et al.*, 1980).

This underestimation of the risk of second primaries will become progressively more severe with worsening of the prognosis of the initial primary malignancy. For example, in T1 glottic cancer the majority of patients are cured of their disease, and the crude risk of second respiratory tract malignancy (6.5%) is very similar to the actuarial figure, which takes into account causes of death other than second respiratory tract cancer (6.5% in 5 years and 12.2% at 10 years) (Wagenfeld *et al.*, 1980). In contrast, in supraglottic cancer where the cure rate of the primary disease is much lower, the crude incidence of second primaries was 12.3% but the actuarial incidence was 19% at 5 years (Wagenfeld *et al.*, 1980). We have, therefore, used an actuarial method to give an accurate estimate of the risk of a survivor of the original primary cancer developing a second respiratory tract malignancy.

The actuarial approach is analogous to the calculation of actuarial survival rates (Cutler and Ederer, 1958). This approach enables one to use all information for every patient, irrespective of the follow-up time. The period of analysis is divided into a number of equal intervals (half yearly) and the probability of not developing a second primary in each of the intervals calculated. In the calculation, patients dying without a second respiratory tract malignancy are considered as being withdrawn from observation (censored) at the middle of the interval during which they died. The probability of avoiding a second respiratory tract malignancy up to a particular time was obtained by taking a cumulative product of the individual interval probabilities up to that time.

This method of calculation, therefore, concentrates on the *rate* of development of a second respiratory tract neoplasm for the patients who survived their first primary cancer, and is an essential requirement to determine high risk groups for intervention programs. By comparing such data with observed numbers of cases in a matched population of the same sex and age, one can estimate the increased incidence of second respiratory tract malignancies in patients with primary cancer.

Other investigators have analysed data on population-based tumor registries. Schoenberg (1977) examined the Connecticut Tumor Registry, a large well-defined group of people suffering from primary cancer, and looked for the proportion developing a subsequent second malignancy. It was possible from the registry to obtain simultaneous controls from the same population who had not developed a second malignancy. He analysed the data in terms of observed tumors/expected tumors, using the person–years approach. This adjusts for age and sex distribution as well as for the survival experience of patients with a first primary cancer. A population-based tumor registry analysis gives a general overview of the second malignancy risk in an overall population, as compared to a hospital-based registry which might be biased due to referral patterns.

Comparison of our data with those of Schoenberg shows very similar correlations between the initial primary cancer (e.g. larynx) and the subsequent second malignancies which develop (e.g. carcinoma of the lung). From the point of view of the clinician dealing with the head and neck cancer patient, the specific information about risk and incidence rates from hospital-based analysis is of more practical and direct use than broader based tumor registry experience, which is of more use to government agencies planning a general population-based intervention program.

SECOND RESPIRATORY TRACT CANCER – BY SITE

This section will discuss the site of the initial primary cancer in relation to the subsequent risk of developing a second respiratory tract cancer.

Laryngeal cancer

Laryngeal carcinoma can primarily arise at one of three sites – the glottic larynx (the primary tumor originates on the vocal cord), the supraglottic larynx (originating above the vocal cord), and the subglottic larynx (originating below the vocal cord). Primary subglottic carcinomas are extremely rare and will not be considered further. In view of the major differences in risk of second respiratory tract primaries between a tumor arising from the glottic larynx and a tumor arising from the supraglottic larynx, they will be considered separately.

Glottic carcinoma

Between 1965 and 1979 we saw 1319 patients with glottic carcinoma, and the number and type of previous malignancies in this group is shown in Table 1. The commonest previous malignancy is cancer of the skin or lip, possibly because skin cancer is extremely common in the population at large. Of interest is the relatively high frequency of antecedent bladder cancer and Schoenberg (1977) noted a similar relationship between previous carcinoma of the bladder and subsequent carcinoma of the lung. Carcinoma of the bladder is a smoking-related disease and as the cure rate is relatively high following treatment, this may explain the association noted.

The incidence of previous lung or oropharyngeal malignancy prior to glottic carcinoma is extremely low at 0.5% (in comparison with its high rate of metachronous incidence following the diagnosis of glottic carcinoma). The reason for this difference is unclear but may be related to the selective

Table 1 Previous and synchronous second malignancies in 1319 patients with glottic cancer

Previous	Patients	Synchronous	Patients
Skin or lip	29		
Bladder	13	Nasopharynx	1
Colon and rectum	7	Oropharynx	1
Oral cavity	2	Oral cavity	3
Lung	5	Lung	4
Prostate	5		
Total	61	*Total*	9

vulnerability of respiratory tract epithelium to inhaled carcinogens as discussed later. An alternative reason for the low incidence of previous cancer of the lung is likely to be the poor survival of lung cancer patients. Table 1 shows the coincident second respiratory tract malignancies in patients presenting with glottic carcinoma; again, approximately 0.5% of glottic cancer cases have a synchronous lung or oropharyngeal tumor.

Table 2 shows the metachronous second respiratory tract primaries in 1319 cases of glottic carcinoma, with a crude incidence of 7.8%. No difference in

Table 2 Metachronous second respiratory tract malignancies in 1319 patients with glottic carcinoma

	Patient number	Patients dead of second cancer
Lung	72	55 (76% of total lung cancer cases)
Oropharynx	13	3
Hypopharynx	3	1
Supraglottic larynx	3	1
Oral cavity	10	3
Sinuses and nasopharynx	2	2
Total	103/1319 (7.8% of total patient number)	65

second respiratory tract malignancies is found by stage of the primary cancer (Wagenfeld *et al.*, 1980). By far the most common tumor is in the lung, representing 70% of the total incidence of second respiratory tract primaries, other common sites of second primaries being the oral cavity and oropharynx. In contrast to other reports (Lawson and Som, 1975), second tumors in the larynx are extremely uncommon in our series as are tumors in the nasopharynx, nasal cavity, and sinuses. Bronchogenic carcinoma is the commonest cause of death among the second respiratory tract malignancies and, in our experience, *more patients with T1 glottic cancer die of bronchogenic carcinoma than of their original primary cancer in the larynx.*

Using the actuarial method of calculation, the incidence of second respiratory tract primaries in a patient treated for glottic carcinoma is 1.3% per year and is constant with time up to 10 years (Wagenfeld *et al.*, 1980). Expressing this another way, if one presents with glottic carcinoma to our institution and is cured of the original primary and the patient does not die of intercurrent disease (unrelated to the second respiratory tract tumor), then the risk of developing a second respiratory tract tumor is 6.5% within 5 years and 12.2% within 10 years (Wagenfeld *et al.*, 1980).

Within 5 years of diagnosis 5% of the survivors will have died, and within 10 years 12% of the survivors will have died, solely as a result of the second respiratory tract tumor. Table 2 shows that 76% of the bronchogenic carcinoma patients died from their disease. (This is less than the 95% death rate from second respiratory tract neoplasms in the lung noted in our earlier report (Wagenfeld *et al.*, 1980), presumably due to shorter follow-up time in our more recently diagnosed cancers of the lung.)

Comparing the observed number of second respiratory tract malignancies in the glottic cancer patients with the expected number in a sample of the same age and sex distribution taken from the general Ontario population, glottic carcinoma patients have 3.6 times the expected incidence of second respiratory tract neoplasms over the control group (Wagenfeld *et al.*, 1980). In the review of the Connecticut Tumor Registry (Schoenberg, 1977), of 1731 patients with laryngeal cancer accumulating 6745 person years of observation, statistically significant excesses of second respiratory tract tumors were observed; in particular, cancer of the tongue (7 cases observed versus 1 expected) and cancer of the lung (27 cases observed versus 10 expected).

The report of Berg *et al.* (1970), accumulating 4287 person-years of risk of glottic cancer patients seen at Memorial Hospital, New York, found a three-fold increase in observed-to-expected incidence of metachronous cancer of the lung. No other site showed an increase in observed-to-expected cancer incidence in this group of patients. Thus, overall data from three major series show a consistent three- to fourfold observed-to-expected incidence of metachronous cancer of the lung for patients treated for glottic carcinoma.

Table 3 Previous and synchronous second malignancies in 515 patients with supraglottic carcinoma

Previous	Patients	Synchronous	Patients
Lung	2	Lung	4
Oral cavity	4	Oral cavity	1
Oropharynx	2	Oropharynx	3
Glottic Larynx	1		
Skin and lip	5		
Bladder	1		
Total	15	*Total*	8

Supraglottic carcinoma

Between 1965 and 1979 we saw 515 patients with supraglottic carcinoma. The number and type of previous malignances is shown in Table 3. Of supraglottic carcinoma patients 2% had had a previous second respiratory tract tumor, the commonest being an oral cavity tumor. This incidence is higher than that seen with glottic carcinomas but lower than that for hypopharyngeal cancer.

Table 3 shows the synchronous second respiratory tract malignancies and Table 4 the metachronous second respiratory tract malignancies for primary supraglottic carcinoma. Table 4 clearly shows that the most common metachronous second primary is in the lung, followed by oral cavity and oropharyngeal malignancies, the overall crude risk being 10%. Using the actuarial method of calculation the incidence of second respiratory tract

Table 4 Metachronous second respiratory tract malignancies in 515 patients with supraglottic cancer

	Patient number	Patients dead of second cancer
Lung	35	26 (72% of total lung cancer cases)
Oral cavity	5	2
Oropharynx	8	1
Hypopharynx	3	2
Total	51/515 (10% of total patient number)	

primaries in a patient treated for supraglottic carcinoma is actually 4% per year which is constant with time (Wagenfeld *et al.*, 1981). This a threefold greater risk than the glottic carcinoma patients and 14 times the expected rate seen in the normal population of the same age and sex in Ontario (Wagenfeld *et al.*, 1981).

Expressing the results in another way, if one presents to our institute with supraglottic carcinoma and is cured of the primary tumor and does not die of intercurrent disease, then the risk of developing a second respiratory tract tumor is 19% at five years. To further illustrate the problem, Figure 1 shows the survival data for supraglottic carcinoma (Wagenfeld *et al.*, 1981). Approximately one-third of patients are alive and well at five years, one-third die of intercurrent disease. The intercurrent disease death rate is twice the expected

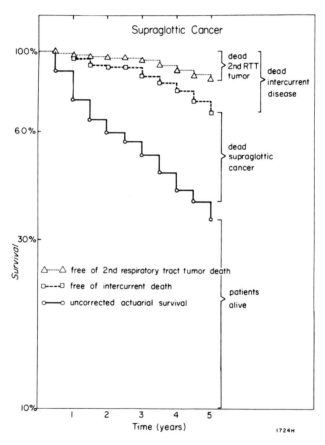

Figure 1   Survival data supraglottic cancer. (Reproduced with permission of the Editor, *Archives of Otolaryngology*).

rate (when compared to a matched population of the same age and sex in Ontario). This increase in intercurrent disease death rate is almost entirely due to the 14-fold increase of second respiratory tract neoplasms (Wagenfeld *et al.*, 1981).

Schoenberg (1977) in his analysis did not subdivide his laryngeal cancer patients into glottic and supraglottic types. Berg *et al.* (1970) who did so showed findings very similar to our own; they found second cancers to be three times as frequent in the supraglottic as compared to the glottic larynx cancer patients. In a prospective study, Schottenfeld *et al.* (1974) also found the risk of second respiratory tract primaries in patients with primary supraglottic cancer to be 5.4 times that of glottic cancer patients. Since the Princess Margaret Hospital series used primary irradiation (with surgery in reserve) for the primary cancer while the Memorial series used primary surgery, the observation of a similar risk of second primaries in the two series suggests both that irradiation is having little effect in inducing second primaries, and also that laryngectomy is not protecting the patient from developing a second respiratory tract primary.

It is not clear why there should be such a major difference in the incidence of second respiratory tract tumors between two regions of the larynx which are within 0.5 cm of one another. One possible explanation is that the supraglottic patient not only smokes heavily but also is frequently a heavy alcohol consumer compared to the glottic cancer patient, and the combination of the two carcinogenic agents may be responsible in part for this observation.

Cancer of the hypopharynx

The experience with previous, synchronous and metachronous respiratory tract cancers in 164 patients with cancer of the hypopharynx is shown in Table 5 (T. Keane, personal communication, 1982). Previous malignancies in the oral cavity, oropharynx and larynx are more common (6.7% incidence) than in glottic carcinoma and the reason for this is unclear, especially as no previous cancers of the lung are noted. The crude incidence of synchronous and metachronous second respiratory tract primaries is 8.5%, only slightly higher than in laryngeal cancer, and again cancers of the lung predominate.

The actuarial risk of the hypopharyngeal cancer patient cured of the primary tumor subsequently developing a second respiratory tract tumor is approximately 3% per year. Unfortunately Schoenberg (1977), Berg *et al.* (1970), and Schottenfeld *et al.* (1974) did not separate hypopharyngeal cancer from cancer of the pharynx which also includes oropharyngeal carcinoma. There are, therefore, no other data to support our findings with respect to second respiratory tract cancers associated with primary cancer of the hypopharynx.

Table 5   Previous, synchronous, and metachronous second respiratory carcinomas in 164 patients with cancer of the hypopharyx

	Patients
Previous	
Larynx	4
Oral cavity	6
Oropharynx	1
Total	11/164 (6.7%)
Synchronous and metachronous	
Lung	10
Oropharynx	3
Oral cavity	1
Total	14/164 (8.5%)

Cancer of the oropharynx is reviewed here for purposes of comparison. Between 1970 and 1979, 372 patients with cancer of the tonsil received radical irradiation at the Princess Margaret Hospital (P. Garrett, personal communication, 1982). The incidence of previous, synchronous and metachronous second respiratory tract malignancies in cancer of the tonsil is shown in Table 6. The incidence of previous malignancies is similar to that seen in cancer of the supraglottic larynx, while the incidence of synchronous and metachronous second respiratory tract malignancies (6.1%) includes a higher proportion of oral cancers.

Using the actuarial method of calculation the risk of second primaries is 13% at 5 years and 27% at 10 years for a rate of approximately 3% per year (P. Garrett, personal communication, 1982). The rate is constant with time and shows no evidence of levelling off. This rate is similar to the rate observed in cancer of the supraglottic larynx and hypopharynx. Others (Berg *et al.*, 1970; Schoenberg, 1977) have observed a similarly increased incidence of second respiratory tract tumors in patients with primary carcinoma of the pharynx.

Cancer of the nose, sinuses, and nasopharynx

Between 1974 and 1979, 313 patients with cancer of the nose, paranasal sinuses, and nasopharynx have been seen at the Princess Margaret Hospital (F. Beale, D. Payne, personal communication, 1982). Only one previous second respiratory tract malignancy has been seen and only three synchronous and metachronous second respiratory tract malignancies have been

Table 6   Previous, synchronous, and metachronous second respiratory tract carcinomas in 372 patients with cancer of the oropharynx

	Patients
Previous	
Lung	1
Oral cavity	2
Hypopharynx	1
Larynx	4
Total	8/372 (2.1%)
Synchronous and metachronous	
Lung	10
Oral cavity	7
Hypopharynx	1
Larynx	5
Total	23/372 (6.1%)

observed to date for a crude incidence of 1% (Table 7). There would, therefore, appear to be no increased incidence of second respiratory tract malignancies in this group of patients, an observation noted also by others (Schoenberg, 1977; Schottenfeld *et al.*, 1974).

The reason why cancer at these sites, which are part of the upper respiratory tract, is not associated with an increased incidence of second malignancies is unclear. It is interesting too that no second malignancy in the nose, sinuses and nasopharynx is observed in our other patient groups and presumably different etiologic factors are responsible for tumors at this site. One factor is that cancers at the other sites are clearly related to smoking and

Table 7   Previous, synchronous, and metachronous second respiratory tract carcinomas in 313 patients with cancers of the nasal cavity, sinuses, and nasopharynx

	Patients
Previous	
Lung	1
Synchronous and metachronous	
Lung	2
Larynx	1
Total	4/313 (1%)

alcohol consumption whereas cancers of the nose, sinuses and nasopharynx are not clearly related to these carcinogens. Also, since these latter areas are exposed to cigarette smoke but not to the local effects of alcohol, the influence of cocarcinogens may be an important factor.

A marked increase in second respiratory tract primaries occurs also in patients with a primary cancer of the oral cavity (Chapter 14). The actuarial rate of 3.2% per year is constant with time up to 10 years following diagnosis of the primary cancer of the floor of the mouth. This is similar to the findings noted by us in patients with cancers of the supraglottic larynx, hypopharynx and oropharynx.

Lung cancer

The commonest second primary carcinoma in a patient with a bronchogenic carcinoma is a second cancer within the lung. These may be considered to be synchronous or metachronous using the definitions previously discussed. Specific criteria for the diagnosis of a synchronous second bronchogenic carcinoma have been described in detail by Martini and Melamed (1975) and are discussed in Chapter 11.

The incidence of synchronous second lung tumors varies in the literature from 0.19% to 0.43% (Rohwedder and Weatherbee, 1974; Paulson, 1975). One of the major problems in obtaining an accurate estimate of the risk of second respiratory tract tumors in a patient with bronchogenic carcinoma, is the extremely poor cure rate of the initial primary lung cancer. Only 5% of patients survive and are thus at risk of developing a second primary. To obtain an accurate estimate of the risk to those who survive a first bronchogenic carcinoma (still a significant number of patients because of the high incidence of the disease) it is essential to use the actuarial method of calculating the risk described above.

Unfortunately the majority of publications have confined themselves to describing the crude risks of second primaries in such patients without taking into account the survival of the patients or the length of follow-up. For example, the crude risk of a second respiratory tract primary in a patient previously treated for a bronchogenic carcinoma has been described as being of the order of 0.2–3.9% (Martini and Melamed, 1975, Paulson, 1975, Rohwedder and Weatherbee, 1974, Smith *et al.*, 1976). Clearly, for reasons already discussed, such crude estimates are grossly underestimating the risk of second primaries in survivors with cancer of the lung because the majority of patients are not at risk long enough to develop the second primary.

Berg *et al.* (1970) found a 1.8 observed to expected incidence ($p=0.05$) of second primaries in patients initially treated for cancer of the lung (1058 patients accumulating 1172 years at risk). Unfortunately insufficient years at risk were accumulated by these patients to quantify precisely the risk of the second primary.

The problem was investigated by Shields and Robinette (1973) who studied 2836 male patients treated for cancer of the lung of whom 535 survived 5 years and 156 for 10 years or more. Forty-one patients developed a second lung tumor, roughly 8% of the 5-year survivors and 26% of the 10-year survivors developing a second primary bronchogenic carcinoma. This would give an approximate actuarial risk of between 1.5 and 2.6% second respiratory tract primary tumors per year following treatment. The majority of patients who developed second primary tumours after initial bronchogenic carcinoma have been found to be heavy smokers (Smith *et al.*, 1976). It is relevant that Auerbach *et al.* (1967) found a 3.5 to 14.5% incidence of multiple primary cancers of the lung in an autopsy series.

It is apparent, therefore, that despite relatively poor documentation of the problem in the literature, survivors following treatment of a primary bronchogenic carcinoma carry a risk of a second lung tumor of the same order of magnitude as of a second primary in the laryngopharynx or oral cavity.

It is interesting to note that in primary oral cavity cancer, the commonest second primary is in the oral cavity, while it is cancer of the lung for the other upper respiratory sites considered. Others (Schoenberg, 1977) have noted similar patterns. The reasons for this must in some way be related to the patient's lifestyle.

In summary, our own data and those in the literature show an extremely strong correlation between first primary cancers of the head and neck and subsequent development of second respiratory tract malignancies, except for cancers of the nose, paranasal sinuses, and nasopharynx. The risk of second respiratory tract primaries and the type vary with the site of the original primary cancer and the reasons for this are still unclear.

What is quite clear for the clinician dealing with head and neck cancer patients is that following its cure, we face almost an epidemic of second respiratory tract cancers. Over the long term this may be as important in terms of survival as the initial primary cancer. It is quite apparent that urgent steps must be taken to try to deal with this problem.

RESPIRATORY CARCINOGENESIS

The respiratory tract consists of the conducting airway (nose, nasopharynx, oral cavity, oropharynx, larynx, and tracheobronchial tree) and the respiratory epithelium which consists of 60–90 m^2 of alveolar surface. This entire system is exposed continually to environmentally inhaled carcinogens (urban, domestic or occupational). Some of these, such as cigarette smoke and asbestos fibres, are clearly oncogenic as reviewed elsewhere (Chretien, 1982).

These substances may act as elementary components, or they may cause complex reactions by interaction with other carcinogens, producing additive or synergistic carcinogenic effects. For example, tobacco smoke contains numerous carcinogens with synergistic effects (Chretien, 1982). Because of the physical conditions in the alveoli, penetration by tobacco smoke deep into the lung followed by a long retention occurs especially with deep inhalation and retention of the breath in the lung for a few seconds. This slow clearance of the compartment leads to a long contact time between the carcinogenic components of tobacco smoke and the respiratory structures.

Effects at the cellular level

Among the more than 30 types of cells that constitute the airway and alveolar structures, bronchial cells are the most vulnerable to inhaled carcinogens. The reason for this is unclear although extensive autopsy studies on the tracheobronchial tree (Auerbach *et al.*, 1980) and short-term organ culture studies of human bronchial mucosa (Morais *et al.*, 1982) have been carried out to determine the cellular effects of cigarette smoking and other inhaled carcinogens. A model for the pathogenesis of bronchogenic carcinoma has been set up (Nasiel *et al.*, 1982). This model includes epithelial injury, squamous metaplasia, various degrees of atypical metaplasia or dysplasia, carcinoma *in situ* and invasive carcinoma. This is illustrated in Figure 2.

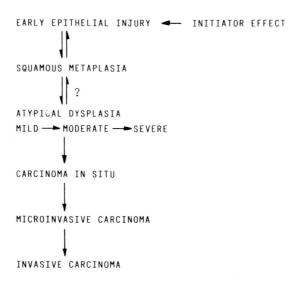

Figure 2   Model of pathogenesis of bronchogenic carcinoma.

The initiation phase is characterized by epithelial injury with basal cell hyperplasia and loss of degenerated columnar cells resulting in an unpro tected non-ciliated low epithelium. Because of loss of cilia, the inhalation carcinogens are not properly removed, resulting in increased exposure of the target cells to the carcinogens. Squamous metaplasia then develops. The next important step is the development of cellular and epithelial atypia which is of a mild, moderate or severe variety. This then progresses to carcinoma *in situ* and ultimately to invasive carcinoma.

This step-wise progression of squamous cell carcinoma of the lung probably takes 10–20 years or more, and the sequential changes can be identified cytologically (Nasiel *et al.*, 1982). It is probable that different elements of cigarette smoke produce different effects (initiator and promotion) at different phases in the step-wise progression. Chemopreventive agents would exert their effect prior to the development of severe atypia and carcinoma *in situ*, as it is probable that once these stages are reached the process is irreversible.

Unfortunately there is far less knowledge available on the cellular processes involved in the induction of non-squamous cell carcinoma of the lung.

Selective vulnerability of respiratory tract epithelium

Cancers of the lung are more commonly found in the main bronchi than in the lower respiratory tract and alveoli, while primary tracheal cancers are very rare. We have noted above that in a patient presenting with cancer of the larynx, the commonest second primary is in the lung, whereas in a patient presenting with primary cancer in the oral cavity, the commonest second primary site is in the oral cavity. On the other hand, patients presenting with cancers of the nose or nasopharynx have a low incidence of second respiratory tract malignancies.

Several hypotheses have been presented to explain this selective localization of cancer induced by inhaled substances (Chretien, 1982):

1. The surface area for deposition of particles in bronchi is much less than in the alveolar surface, and thus the concentration of potential carcinogens is much higher. Higher concentrations of inhaled carcinogens could occur due to differences in local clearance of the carcinogen or to differences in regional ventilation depositing greater concentrations of carcinogen in a particular area.
2. The lung parenchyma could be quickly cleared of its particles by alveolar macrophages, whereas macrophages remain for a long time in the bronchial tree where the particles may be released.
3. Enzymes responsible for transformation of chemically inhaled carcinogen into active carcinogens reside in bronchial cells rather than in the alveoli.

However, so far there is no satisfactory explanation for the selective vulnerability of certain cells compared to others in the respiratory tract. A great deal of further research into respiratory tract anatomy, physiology, biochemistry, and immunology is required.

POSSIBILITIES FOR REDUCING MORTALITY

We have shown that second respiratory tract malignancy is an increasing and major problem in patients who are cured of malignant diseases of the upper respiratory tract. In some areas such as supraglottic laryngeal carcinoma, cancer of the oropharynx and oral cavity, this is a major source of morbidity and mortality, and in early glottic carcinoma more patients are now dying of their second respiratory tract malignancy than of their initial cancer.

Since second respiratory tract malignancies now represent an important cause of death in these patients, it is vitally important either to detect them earlier (and improve the cure rate) or to try and prevent them developing. Since patients presenting with a cancer of the upper respiratory tract represent such an extremely high risk group of patients for subsequent development of second respiratory tract malignancies, there is great potential for education, screening, and chemoprevention programs in these patients.

Alterations in lifestyle and chemoprevention

There is overwhelming evidence to implicate cigarette smoking as the major etiologic factor in the development of second respiratory tract malignancies in patients with cancer of the upper respiratory tract (Berg *et al.*, 1970). Alcohol is also an important risk factor which, if combined with smoking in a sustained joint exposure, enhances the risk in a synergistic fashion (Schottenfeld *et al.*, 1974). Measures to reduce smoking and intake of alcohol are discussed in Chapter 5.

Stopping smoking and the use of intensive screening programs are at best only a partial solution to the problem of second respiratory tract tumors. Chemopreventive agents are natural or synthetic substances administered to prevent, inhibit or reverse one or more of the stages of carcinogenesis (DeCosse, 1982). Chemoprevention focuses on inhibition or reversal of tumor promotion and is discussed fully in Chapter 12 of this book.

Screening

When the patient with cancer of the upper respiratory tract presents to the physician, irreversible changes have occurred in the respiratory tract epithelium which will lead to a second respiratory tract cancer within the next 5–10 years in a significant fraction of the patients even if the patient immediately stopped smoking. It is currently not known whether such changes can be reversed by chemoprevention agents but it is likely that a significant fraction cannot. Therefore, since the majority of patients on routine follow-up who develop a second respiratory tract tumor will die of it (as noted earlier) this raises the question of screening and diagnosis of the second tumor at an earlier phase in its development, in the hope that the mortality rate of the second tumor is reduced.

A number of screening programs for cancer of the lung in high risk groups (although not to date, of patients with a primary tumor of the upper respiratory tract) are under way and will be briefly reviewed. The only available reliable tests for identifying presymptomatic lung cancer are chest X-ray and sputum cytology.

Mayo Lung Project (Sanderson and Fontana, 1982)

This project seeks to evaluate the effect of four-monthly chest X-ray and sputum cytology testing compared to a non-screened control group in a high risk population of patients (males, 45 years or more, 1 pack a day smokers). The initial screening test in 10,938 patients revealed 92 cases of lung cancer, 59 being detected by chest X-ray, 16 by cytology, and 17 by both. One-half underwent 'curative' resections and half were found to be Stage I.

Of the remaining group, 4,624 patients were randomized to the 'screening' arm and 4598 to the control arm. At the time of last reporting, 110 cases of cancer of the lung had been detected in the screened arm as compared to 78 in the control arm. More than three times as many Stage I cases were found in the screened arm as compared to the control arm and they were principally of the squamous cell carcinoma subtype. To date, there have been 39% fewer deaths in the screened group from squamous cell carcinoma and adenocarcinoma compared to the control group (17 versus 28). However, no reduction in deaths has been seen from undifferentiated carcinoma. Overall compliance in this screening program is 80%.

These data have to be interpreted very cautiously as one may merely be picking up the tumor earlier in the screened group, but not improving overall survival. Another puzzling aspect of this study is the greater number of lung cancer cases seen in the screened group as compared to the control group. Nevertheless, screening does seem to diagnose squamous cell carcinoma of the lung at an earlier stage possibly permitting its more effective treatment. Small cell undifferentiated lung cancer does not seem to be detected early enough by screening to benefit the patient. To date in this project, mortality from lung cancer is not significantly different between the control group and the surveillance group.

Memorial Sloan Kettering Lung Project (Martini, 1982)

This project is slightly different from the Mayo Lung Project in that high risk patients were screened either by an annual chest X-ray or by an annual chest X-ray plus sputum cytology at four-monthly intervals. Begun in 1974, 10,140 patients were entered into the study and 55 cancers of the lung were found on initial evaluation and 114 on subsequent follow-up for an incidence of 3 per 1000 per year. Of these patients, 38% had clinical Stage I disease, and 54 of the 65 Stage I patients are alive and well. The routine chest X-ray was useful in picking up early peripheral lesions, while sputum cytology was useful for finding early major bronchial lesions.

In a small series of 27 patients seen at the Memorial Hospital with early or 'occult' lung cancer, none has had recurrence of his original tumor following excision. Unfortunately, in this group 45% developed a second cancer of which 32% were second lung cancers. To date there is no difference in survival rate between the control and the screened arms.

Johns Hopkins Lung Project (Levin *et al.*, 1982)

This project was undertaken in conjunction with the two previously discussed projects. High risk groups (male, over age 45 years, 1 package of cigarettes per day) were randomized to annual chest X-ray (control group) or annual chest X-ray plus annual sputum cytology (screened group). A total of 10,387 men were entered into this study and at the first screening 70% of lung cancers were resectable in the screened group compared to 42.5% in the control group. To date, however, with more than 20,000 person-years of observation in each group (average four years follow-up), no difference is seen in lung cancer mortality between the control and screened groups. Possible reasons for this lack of demonstrable decrease in mortality (even though early cases have been detected) include insufficient passage of time, ineffective therapy or the multifocal nature of cancer of the lung.

In summary, three major screening programs have failed to show any significant benefit to date from the routine use of screening in high risk groups of patients.

It is well known that some bronchial carcinomas shed malignant cells into the sputum for many months before a lesion becomes detectable by conventional bronchoscopy or chest X-ray (Pearson *et al.*, 1967). This situation not infrequently arises in screening programs of high risk patients, and when it occurs the upper respiratory tract must be carefully assessed and, if found to be negative, fiberoptic bronchoscopy is carried out (Marsh *et al.*, 1982). If the visual search is negative, differential bronchial brushing is carried out to ascertain the positive lobe and appropriate treatment is undertaken.

In a small proportion of patients no localized malignancy can be detected and these patients require careful follow-up. A new way of localizing occult tumors of this type employs a haematoporphyrin derivative (HPD) which localizes in tumors and can be visualized by its property of fluorescence under ultraviolet light. In a series of 10 patients with early tumors of the airways (including lesions of 1 to 1.5 mm) definite tumor fluorescence could be demonstrated in all (King *et al.*, 1982; Balchum, 1982). This approach may, therefore, be of benefit in this specific patient group and there is also a possibility that this technique may be of therapeutic benefit.

New techniques of this type are essential because as a result of screening programs in high risk patients, many more occult primaries which are difficult to detect by conventional means will become apparent. Locating such small tumors, and their treatment at this stage, will result in a higher cure rate. However, it must be emphasized that this method of assessment and treatment is at an extremely early stage of development at present and requires extensive further experience before it becomes a routine method of assessment. Such techniques of early diagnosis, even if they do not improve survival rates, would at least reduce the morbidity of treatment by detecting the disease at a stage that may not require major pulmonary resections.

CONCLUSION

The clinician treating cancer of the head and neck is facing an epidemic of second respiratory tract malignancies of such a magnitude that it is progressively replacing the initial primary cancer as the major cause of death in these patients. Until very recently, this has been a neglected area in the management of the head and neck cancer patient and a major effort is required to combat this problem.

It is apparent from this review that no single strategy will deal with this problem. What is required is a coordinated attack encompassing the following strategies:

1. An effective method is needed to recognize patients who are at greatest risk of developing a second respiratory tract malignancy.
2. The patient must be encouraged to stop smoking, or, at least, smoke a safer cigarette.
3. Intensive screening programs are required in these patients, in an attempt to diagnose the second malignancy earlier and thus treat it more effectively, rather than waiting for symptoms to arise.
4. Chemoprevention programs need to be initiated in these patients as soon as the primary treatment is completed and successful.

REFERENCES

Auerbach, O., Hammond, E. C., and Garfinkel, L. (1980). Changes in bronchial epithelium: then and now. In *A safe cigarette. Banbury Report*, No. 3. (eds G. B. Gori and F. G. Bock). Cold Spring Harbor Laboratory, p. 141.

Auerbach, O., Stout, A. P., and Hammond, E. C. (1967). Multiple primary bronchial carcinomas. *Cancer*, **20**, 699.

Balchum, O. J., Dowan, O. R., Profio, A. E., and Huth, G. C. (1982). Fluorescence bronchoscopy for localizing early bronchial cancer and carcinoma *in situ*. *Recent Results in Cancer Research*, **82**, 97.

Berg, J. W., Schottenfeld, D., and Ritter, F. (1970). Incidence of multiple primary cancers. III. Cancers of the respiratory and upper digestive system as multiple primary cancers. *Journal of the National Cancer Institute*, **44**, 263.

Chretien, J. (1982). Inhalation carcinogenesis: an overview. *Recent Results in Cancer Research*, **82**, 1.

Cutler, S. J., and Ederer, F. (1958). Maximum utilization of the life table method in analyzing survival. *Journal of Chronic Diseases*, **8**, 699.

DeCosse, J. J. (1982). Potential for chemoprevention. *Cancer*, **50**, 2550.

King, E. G., Dovan, A., Man, G. *et al.* (1982). Hematoporphyrin derivative as a tumor marker in the detection and localization of pulmonary malignancy. *Recent Results in Cancer Research*, **82**, 90.

Lawson, L., and Som, M. (1975). Second primary cancer after irradiation of laryngeal cancer. *Annals of Otology and Rhinolaryngology*, **84**, 771.

Levin, M. L., Tockman, M. S., Frost, J. K., and Ball, W. C. (1982). Lung cancer mortality in males screened by chest X-ray and cytologic sputum examination. A preliminary report. *Recent Results in Cancer Research*, **82**, 138.

Marsh, B., Frost, J., and Erozan, Y. (1982). Bronchoscopic localization of radiologically occult cancer. *Recent Results in Cancer Research*, **82**, 87.

Martini, N. (1982). Results of Memorial Sloan Kettering lung project. In *Recent Results in Cancer Research*, **82**, 174.

Martini, N., and Melamed, M. R. (1975). Multiple primary lung cancer. *Journal of Thoracic and Cardiovascular Surgery*, **70**, 606.

Morais, R., Watters, C., Binda, A. *et al.* (1982). Epithelial lesions induced by alpha particules and cigarette smoke condensates in organotypic culture of human bronchus. *Recent Results in Cancer Research*, **82**, 21.

Nasiel, M., Carlens, E., Auer, G. *et al.* (1982). Pathogenesis of bronchial carcinoma with special reference to morphogenesis and the influence on the bronchial mucosa of 20 methylcholanthrene and cigarette smoking. *Recent Results in Cancer Research*, **82**, 53.

Paulson, D. L. (1975). *Journal of Thoracic and Cardiovascular Surgery*, **70**, 611.

Pearson, F. G., Thompson, D. W., and Delarue, N. C. (1967). Experience with the cytologic detection, localization, and treatment of radiographically undemonstrable bronchial carcinoma. *Journal of Thoracic and Cardiovascular Surgery*, **54**, 371.

Peto, R. (1981). Trends in US cancer onset rates. In *Quantification of occupational cancer*. Banbury Report, No. 9. (eds R. Peto, and M. Schneiderman). Cold Spring Harbor Laboratory, p. 269.

Rohwedder, J. J., and Weatherbee, (1974). Multiple primary bronchogenic carcinoma with a review of the literature. *Annual Review of Respiratory Diseases*, **109**, 435.

Sanderson, D., and Fontana, R. (1982). Results of the Mayo lung project: an interim report. *Recent Results in Cancer Research*, **82**, 179.

Schoenberg, B. S. (1975). A program for the conquest of cancer 1802. *Historical Medicine*, **30**, 3.

Schoenberg, B. S (1977). Multiple primary malignant neoplasms. *Recent Results in Cancer Research*, **58.**

Schottenfeld, D., Gantt, R. C., and Wynder, E. L. (1974). The role of alcohol and tobacco in multiple primary cancers of the upper digestive system, larynx and lung: a prospective study. *Preventive Medicine*, **3**, 277.

Shields, T. W., and Robinette, C. D. (1973). Long term survivors after resection of bronchial carcinoma. *Surgery, Gynecology and Obstetrics*, **136**, 759.

Smith, R. A., Nigam, B. K., and Thompson, J. M. (1976). Second primary lung carcinoma. *Thorax*, **31**, 503.

Wagenfeld, D. J. H., Harwood, A. R., Bryce, D. P. *et al.* (1980). Second primary respiratory tract malignancies in glottic carcinoma. *Cancer*, **46**, 1883.

Wagenfeld, D. J. H., Harwood, A. R., Bryce, D. P. *et al.* (1981). Second primary respiratory tract malignant neoplasms in supraglottic carcinoma. *Archives of Otolaryngology*, **107**, 135.

Risk Factors and Multiple Cancer
Edited by B.A. Stoll
© 1984 John Wiley and Sons Ltd.

Chapter

14 PETER J. FITZPATRICK, BARRY S. TEPPERMAN, and GERRIT DeBOER

Multiple Cancers of Mouth, Pharynx, and Oesophagus

Goodner and Watson (1956) reported that half of 126 patients with oesophageal carcinoma had a primary growth also in the oral cavity or pharynx. On the other hand, Shibuya *et al.* (1982) reported from Japan that only 28 of 339 (8.3%) patients with oesophageal carcinoma had more than one primary neoplasm. Of 32 tumours 11 were in the mouth or pharynx and 12 in the stomach. Institutional figures may be biased by selection, and Schoenberg's (1977) analysis of 25 years' data in the Connecticut Tumor Registry confirms the association of multiple primary neoplasms throughout the upper resiratory and alimentary tracts. He cites a 49.3% risk for second malignancies in these regions among patients with an index tumour in the oral cavity.

There is an increased risk of similar tumors arising in anatomically related organs due to the effect of the same carcinogens. There may also be other subtle (but as yet unrecognized) relationships between cancers in different organs. In order to assess the magnitude of the problem we have investigated the prevalence of additional cancers developing in patients with one primary squamous cell carcinoma in the mouth, pharynx, or oesophagus.

MATERIAL AND METHODS

Retrospective analysis was carried out on 6203 cases of squamous cell carcinoma arising from the anterior floor of the mouth to the lower oesophagus, and seen at Princess Margaret Hospital between January 1958 and May 1982. The primary tumour arising in the upper alimentary tract, for which the patient was first referred to our hospital, was called the index lesion (Table 1), and the other malignancies (with the exception of skin tumors that

Table 1   Multiple primary cancers in patients with index squamous carcinomas in the upper alimentary tract. (Princess Margaret Hospital, 1958–82)

Index tumour			Additional tumours			
	Patients		Prior + synchronous	Metachronous		Total
	Total	Index		Aliment. or resp.	Other	
Mouth	2891	349	136	211	77	288
Pharynx	1843	226	104	107	45	152
Oesophagus	1469	73	59	14	8	22
Total	6203	648	299	332	130	462

were omitted from the survey) were related to it according to their time of appearance. They were classified as prior, synchronous or metachronous depending on whether they developed before, concurrently or subsequent to the index tumour, and the majority involved the upper alimentary or respiratory tract. All were identified by the criteria described by Warren and Gates (1932), which require that all tumours be confirmed histologically, that each be geographically distinct, and that no tumour may be a metastasis of another.

Follow-up information has been recorded within the last year for approximately 80% of the patients reviewed. Because of the possibility that incomplete follow-up could bias the results (i.e. the frequency of second primaries might not be the same in patients lost to follow-up as in those followed up to date), the overall expected numbers of subsequent cancers were calculated in two different ways. For deceased patients, the period at risk for developing second cancers ran up to the date of death. For patients last known to be alive, the first approach used the actual last date each patient was seen. The second method assumed that all living patients were at risk up to 31 May, 1982 which was the most recent follow-up date for any patient.

Actuarial and relative survival rates were calculated from the time of diagnosis of the index cancer by the Berkson–Gage method and compared by the Wilcoxon–Gehan statistic. Slopes were fitted by the method of least squares. Patient groups were compared by Student's t test and contingency table analysis by the use of Yates's corrected chi-square statistic. The expected number of primary neoplasms by site was calculated by applying age- and sex-specific population incidence rates to the years at risk experienced by the patient population. Incidence rates for the Province of Ontario averaged over the three years 1969 to 1971 were used (Statistics Canada, 1978). Risk ratio confidence limits were calculated and tested as Poisson variates by the approximation of Bailar. In the case of cancers in the floor of mouth data were obtained from a detailed retrospective chart review (Fitzpatrick and Tepperman, 1982).

Table 2   The five-year crude survival rates (CSR) for 3428 patients with upper alimentary tract squamous cancers (1958–72)

	Patients	Median age	Sex ratio	5 yr CSR %
Mouth	1678	64.9	2.1 : 1	34.8
Oropharynx	631	61.5	2.7 : 1	23.1
Hypopharynx	381	64.6	2.4 : 1	20.1
Oesophagus	738	65.9	2.1 : 1	4.4

RESULTS

Table 2 shows the overall five-year crude survival rates for 3428 patients with upper alimentary tract squamous carcinomas seen between 1958 and 1972. They range from 4.4% for oesophagus to 34.8% for oral cavity. Since the development of a second independent cancer requires that the patient has survived the first tumour, the short survival in most patients with oesophageal cancer accounts for the small number of subsequent primaries observed.

Among 6203 patients with a primary squamous carcinoma of the upper alimentary tract, 648 patients (10.4%) developed two or more independent tumours (Table 3). Altogether, 761 additional malignancies were observed, with up to five cancers being seen in individual patients. There were 279 patients with a prior or synchronous cancer, 76 and 83 of which respectively were in the upper alimentary or respiratory tracts (Table 4). Among the 409 patients who developed 462 metachronous tumours, there were 208 in the

Table 3   Analysis of 648 patients with a squamous cell carcinoma in the upper alimentary tract with two or more independent tumours. Each tumour constitutes a separate case, yielding a total of 761 additional malignancies

	Additional cancers					
	1	2	3	4	5	Patients
Oral	286	55	5	2	1	349
Pharynx	203	17	5	1	0	226
Oesophagus	65	8	0	0	0	73
Total						648
						Cases
Prior and synchronous	191	78	21	4	5	299
Metachronous	363	82	9	8	0	462
Total	554	160	30	12	5	761

Table 4 Analysis of 279 patients with other malignancies prior or synchronous to the index tumour

Index tumour		Additional tumour prior or synchronous											Cases
Site	Patients	Mouth	Pharynx	Oesophagus	Larynx	Lung	GI	Breast	Gyn	GU	Lymphoma	Other	Total
Mouth	125	37	5	6	21	17	4	10	9	12	11	4	136
Pharynx oro + hypo	96	13	7	3	22	12	16	7	9	8	4	3	104
Oesophagus	58	5	0	0	7	4	11	10	4	6	6	6	59
Total	279	55	12	9	50	33	31	27	22	26	21	13	299

Table 5 Analysis of 409 patients who developed metachronous malignancies following the index tumour

Index tumour		Additional tumour metachronous											Cases
Site	Patients	Mouth	Pharynx	Oesophagus	Larynx	Lung	GI	Breast	Gyn	GU	Lymphoma	Other	Total
Mouth	251	87	34	24	10	56	26	7	4	20	9	11	288
Pharynx oro + hypo	138	27	11	18	4	47	20	4	4	6	6	5	152
Oesophagus	20	2	4	1	5	2	1	0	0	3	2	2	22
Total	409	116	49	43	19	105	47	11	8	29	17	18	462

same anatomic region of the mouth, pharynx or oesophagus, and 124 in the larynx or lung (Table 5).

There is a substantially higher risk of developing a second primary cancer subsequent to the diagnosis and treatment of the index tumour in the upper alimentary tract. Overall the observed-to-expected ratio was 2.48, specifically 2.32 for males and 2.89 for females (Table 6). The greatly elevated risk was for upper alimentary or respiratory tumours but not for cancers at other sites. The risk was greatest for patients with index tumours in the pharynx, somewhat less for those in the mouth and only slight for those in the oesophagus.

For both males (Table 7) and females (Table 8) the excess number of additional cancers is approximately twice that expected in the normal population, and the observation that the excess incidence of second primaries is greater in women than in men may be accounted for by the higher proportion of smokers (and thus a higher expected incidence of these cancers) in the normal male population during the period under discussion.

A more detailed statistical assessment of risk for multiple primary malignancies is not possible for those patients with *prior* or *synchronous* cancers. This is because of the impossibility of extrapolating back in time for an accurate estimate of the size or characteristics of the baseline population at risk for comparison.

CARCINOMA OF THE FLOOR OF THE MOUTH

There have already been reports on second cancers in the subgroup of 377 patients with squamous cell carcinoma of the floor of the mouth seen between

Table 6   Risk of subsequent malignancy after primary squamous carcinoma in upper alimentary tract. (Because of incomplete records the observed to expected ratios for other cancers developing subsequent to the index tumour were calculated from two dates. The patient years at risk for the actual follow-up date and using 31 May 1982 for all patients known to be alive were 14,792.62 and 19,624.72 years).

		Female	Male	*Total*
	Observed	144	318	462
Follow-up	Actual date Expected	49.84	136.82	186.66
	O/E	2.89	2.32	2.48
	31 May 1982 Expected	71.19	187.67	258.86
	O/E	2.02	1.69	1.78

Table 7 The greatly increased risk for developing other upper alimentary or respiratory tract tumours in males. For other malignancies the risk is the same as in the normal population

Subsequent site		Index site (males)			
		Mouth	Pharynx	Oesophagus	*Total*
Upper digestive	O	145	83	9	237
or respiratory	E	24.952	10.726	3.232	38.910
	O/E	5.81	7.74	2.78	6.09
95% Confidence limits		4.90–6.84	6.16–9.59	1.27–5.29	5.34–6.92
Other[a]	O	47	28	6	81
	E	64.181	25.432	8.300	97.913
	O/E	0.732	1.10	0.723	0.827
95% Confidence limits		0.538–0.974	0.73–1.59	0.265–1.57	0.657–1.028
Total[a]	O	192	111	15	318
	E	89.133	36.158	11.532	136.82
	O/E	2.15	3.07	1.30	2.32
95% Confidence limits		1.86–2.48	2.53–3.70	0.73–2.15	2.08–2.59

[a]Minus skin tumours.

1958 and 1975 at the Princess Margaret Hospital (Fitzpatrick and Tepperman, 1982; Tepperman and Fitzpatrick, 1981). There were 300 men and 77 women for a 3.9 : 1 ratio. The median age was 60 (30–92) years; 59% were in the sixth and seventh decades.

Use of alcohol and tobacco, both aetiological agents, was common in this population. Among 312 patients whose habits were recorded, 241 (77.2%) smoked tobacco, 192 (61%) abused alcohol, and 163 (52%) indulged both habits. Other possible predisposing factors included poor oral hygiene (11%), poorly fitting dentures (8%), and leucoplakia (8%). Patients were staged retrospectively according to the UICC TNM classification (UICC, 1978). Two-thirds of the patients (235) had tumours less than 4 cm in size (T_1–T_2), and in two-thirds (242) lymph nodes were not palpable (N_0). Radiation was the first planned treatment alone for 330 patients (87.5%) and combined with surgery in 20 (5%).

The overall actuarial 5-year and 10-year survival rates were 39.9% and 23.3%, respectively (Figure 1). The median disease-free period was 9 months, and the median survival time 36 months, for patients dying from this cancer. Neither patient nor treatment factors correlated with outcome and only the clinical stage of the cancer was found to be correlated with survival.

Table 8 The greatly increased risk for developing other upper alimentary or respiratory tract tumours in females. For other malignancies the risk is the same as in the normal population

		Mouth	Pharynx	Oesophagus	*Total*
			Index site (females)		
Subsequent site		Mouth	Pharynx	Oesophagus	*Total*
Upper digestive	O	66	24	5	95
or respiratory	E	2.350	0.961	0.385	3.696
	O/E	28.09	24.97	12.99	25.70
95% Confidence limits		21.72–35.73	16.00–37.16	4.22–30.31	20.79–31.42
Other[a]	O	30	17	2	49
	E	29.593	11.636	4.916	46.145
	O/E	1.01	1.46	0.407	1.06
95% Confidence limits		0.68– 1.45	0.85– 2.34	0.049–1.470	0.79– 1.40
Total[a]	O	96	41	7	144
	E	31.943	12.597	5.301	49.841
	O/E	3.01	3.25	1.32	2.89
95% Confidence limits		2.43– 3.67	2.43– 4.42	0.53 –2.72	2.44– 3.40

[a]Minus skin tumours.

The most important prognostic parameter was the presence of cervical node metastases at the time of diagnosis and, if present, the extent of the primary tumour or the regional nodes did not significantly influence length of survival. Among patients whose cervical metastases were successfully treated, the 5-year survival rate was 32.8%, and the median survival time 30 months. This compares to 17.5%, with one-half of the patients dying within 15 months, if the metastases were not controlled ($p = 0.001$).

Second cancers may develop in patients who survive their first malignancy long enough to develop them. A total of 123 new cancers developed in 101 of the 377 patients (27%) after treatment. Eighty-two of these (66.7%) were second cancers in the respiratory or upper alimentary tracts, arising in 63 men and 19 women. Their mean age (60 ± 11.5 years) was similar to that (59.3 ± 12.4) of patients in whom no other cancer developed. The sex ratio was also similar in the two groups (3.3 : 1 and 4.1 : 1), but the sex ratio for second oral cavity tumours (1.4 : 1) differed sharply from that of second cancers in other sites (6.6 : 1; $p = 0.009$). Tobacco and alcohol use were comparable in both groups.

It should be noted that patients with second cancers had smaller floor of mouth tumours (75% staged as T_1 or T_2 versus 57%; $p = 0.011$), and fewer

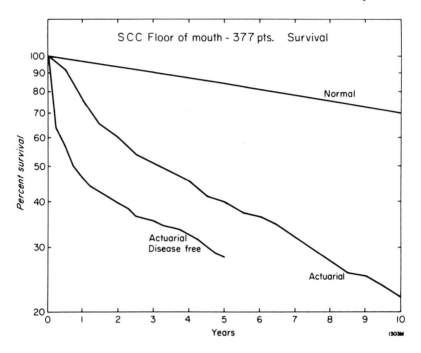

Figure 1   Survival in squamous carcinoma of the floor of the mouth. The five-year survival rate is 40%, but patients continue to die at a greater rate than the normal population. Only one-half the patients are disease-free at nine months. (Courtesy of the Editor, Journal Canadian Association of Radiologists.)

regional node metastases (79% versus 59% N_0; $p = 0.0004$). These differences are reflected in the longer survival of those with second cancers, 48.7% compared with 36.6%.

The distribution of new tumours is shown in Table 9. The major individual sites were the tonsil in 12, the hypopharynx in 7, and the larynx in 6. Comparison with the expected incidence of five cases in all sites demonstrates a significant excess of new cancers in all upper aerodigestive sites for men, and in all sites except the oesophagus for women.

New cancers are still being diagnosed up to 210 months after treatment of the index cancer of the floor of the mouth. The actuarial rates of onset of second malignancies were calculated from the time of diagnosis of the index cancer in order to delineate the period of maximum risk (Figure 2). For at least the first 10 years of follow-up, in any of the subsites analysed, a constant proportion of survivors develop new tumours. Although estimates are less reliable beyond this point, the risk for new primaries appears constant at

3.6% per year in all sites. Thus, more cases of subsequent primaries are anticipated.

In the full series of 377 patients with carcinoma of the floor of the mouth, 19 had previously been treated for respiratory and upper digestive tract cancers, 16 of them within the preceding three years. These included four lung and three oropharyngeal cancers. In six patients (7.3%), second tumours developed within irradiated tissues but distant from the index cancer, four within two years of treatment.

Half of those patients not developing second cancers died within three years (Figure 2). Beyond the fifth year after treatment for cancer of the floor of the mouth, patients without a second cancer die at the same rate as a sex- and age-matched normal population, approximately 3% per year. This is presumptive evidence of cure.

Table 9   Second upper alimentary or respiratory tract malignancy after primary squamous carcinoma of the floor of the mouth. (Published with permission of the Editor, *Lancet*)

| | Cases | | | Relative risk | |
| | Observed | Expected | | | 95% Confidence |
Sites	(O)	(E)	O/E		limits
Full series (n=377; 1665.12 person years at risk)					
All sites	82	4.92	16.67		13.26– 20.70
Oral cavity	29	0.38	76.32		50.84–109.05
Upper respiratory	19	0.65	29.23		17.46– 45.32
Lung	24	3.55	6.75		4.33– 10.05
Oesophagus	10	0.33	30.58		14.64– 56.24
Males (N=300; 1276.51 person years at risk)					
All sites	63	4.69	13.43		10.32– 17.19
Oral cavity	17	0.35	48.57		28.29– 77.79
Upper respiratory	15	0.62	24.19		13.55– 39.96
Lung	21	3.42	6.14		3.80– 9.39
Oesophagus	10	0.30	33.14		15.87– 60.95
Females (N=77; 388.61 person years at risk)					
All sites	19	0.23	82.61		50.43–130.87
Oral cavity	12	0.03	342.95		193.45–654.78
Upper respiratory	4	0.04	112.50		30.27–238.03
Lung[a]	3	0.13	22.41		4.50– 65.46
Oesophagus[b]	0	0.03	0		0 –145.14

[a]p=0.02. [b]NS=not statistically significant. Probability for all other values less than 10^{-5}.

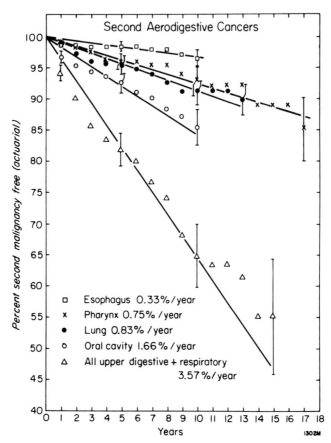

Figure 2 The rate of onset for a second malignancy in patients with squamous carcinoma of the floor of the mouth. It remains constant from the time of successful treatment of the first cancer. (Published with permission of the Editor, *Lancet.*)

Despite a better initial prognosis because of the earlier stage of their index tumours, patients who later developed second cancers had an excess mortality in the same perod (5.2% per year), attributable entirely to the second tumour. To date, 30 of the 82 patients (37%) with second respiratory or upper alimentary tract neoplasms have died from this second cancer, whereas only two succumbed to floor of mouth cancer. New tumours distal to the oral cavity have a worse outcome, with a 52% crude survival rate, compared to 85% for second tumours within the mouth ($p = 0.028$). Among the 19 patients who had had a prior respiratory or upper alimentary tract cancer, five (26%) died from their first cancer and two from their second (the index tumour of this study).

DISCUSSION

Most of our patients were treated by irradiation. Although the oncogenic effect of ionizing radiation is well known, we were not able to identify with certainty any cases of radiation-induced tumours. Radiation carcinogenesis has been reported with doses as low as 6 cGy (BEIR III, 1980), but the risk of radiation-induced malignancy decreases at therapeutic doses because of death rather than transformation in susceptible cells (Kogelnik *et al.*, 1975). For epithelial malignancies there is a delay of several years before radiation oncogenesis becomes clinically evident.

Comparing the results of radical irradiation and surgery in patients rendered free of squamous carcinomas in the head and neck for at least five years, Kogelnik indicated that radiation reduced the prevalence of second malignancies in the treated field, presumably by sterilizing dysplasia and subclinical neoplasia. In a review of 272 patients under 30 years of age with head and neck tumors, of whom 58 were followed for 10 years or more, no second primaries were observed (Clark *et al.*, 1982). Alcohol or tobacco use was not prevalent among these patients and radiation carcinogenesis cannot be postulated.

Neither the oesophagus nor lung is irradiated in treating oral or pharyngeal tumours and thus it is impossible for radiation to have played any role in the development of second malignancies at those sites (Tables 4 and 5). Subsequent cancers developing after radiotherapy may result from an inadequate dose or treatment volume, or the failure to sterilize a field of multicentric subclinical mucosal neoplasia, rather than from radiation oncogenesis. The multicentric origin is associated with interacting aetiologic associations, including prolonged exposure to tobacco and alcohol.

Our results clearly underestimate the magnitude of the problem because patients still alive or lost to follow-up continue to be at risk and patients dying of their primary tumour or of unrelated causes would have been at risk had they survived longer. Patients with a pharyngeal first tumour have a greater risk than those with oral or oesophageal tumours for developing other primary carcinomas in the upper alimentary or respiratory tracts. The risk is greater for both sexes but more dramatic for women when compared to the general population. This effect probably stems from the fact that males have a higher incidence of these cancers because more of them smoked in the past. In terms of patient years at risk, female patients have a somewhat lower risk than the males ($95/5208.8 = 0.0182$ cases per patient year at risk compared to $237/9583.5 = 0.0247$).

These observations suggest that all patients with carcinomas of the head and neck should be investigated further for the possibility of an associated tumour in the lung or upper aerodigestive tract. Examination under anaesthetic, with multiple blind biopsies and sampling from suspicious leucoplakic oerythroplakic mucosa may be necessary for the early diagnosis of unsuspected tumours.

When there are synchronous malignancies the treatment priority is for the most potentially lethal tumour. In this review, 279 patients had a prior or synchronous cancer with 76 and 83 in the upper alimentary and respiratory tracts respectively (Table 4). In general, the further along the aerodigestive tract the worse the prognosis. For metachronous malignancies the second tumour is treated as though it existed alone, if the first is controlled. Among the 409 patients who developed 462 metachronous tumours there were 208 and 124 in the upper alimentary and respiratory tracts respectively (Table 5). Clearly the epithelial cancers in the upper alimentary and respiratory tracts are multicentric and must reflect the influence of common carcinogens.

There is good epidemiological evidence to implicate tobacco and its by-products from combustion as being carcinogenic to the upper respiratory and alimentary tract mucosa, and alcohol as a promoter for carcinogenesis in the upper alimentary tract (see Chapter 5). Factors which were considered to be of aetiological importance in the past (such as the use of snuff, syphilis, or the presence of achlorhydric anaemia in the Plummer–Vinson syndrome) must be rare. In many patients the diagnosis was suggested by their physique and in particular their plethoric facial appearance. Perhaps surprisingly, our clinical notes, although recording chronic oral and pharyngeal inflammation, seldom described frank corrugated leucoplakia or granular erythroplasia.

CONCLUSION

Survival rates alone do not adequately reflect the outcome of the first cancer in the upper alimentary tract, and the development of multiple squamous cell carcinomas is common following successful treatment. The risk for new primary cancers among patients who survive a first squamous cancer in the upper alimentary tract is constant, and excessive (13–21 times normal) and regardless of time. Only control of the first cancer identifies patients at risk to develop a second. With earlier diagnosis, and the better treatment of the first cancer, second cancers become the major threat to survival; so long as this remains true, overall survival rates cannot improve regardless of therapeutic expertise. In order to detect second cancers at an early and potentially curable stage, we advocate meticulous and lifelong clinical surveillance.

Acknowledgements

This chapter represents the combined efforts of many people, since the patients were treated by various staff members of the Princess Margaret

Hospital and referred by many surgeons. Miss Evelyn Eisenreich provided the secretarial skills. To all these, we offer our grateful thanks.

Acknowledgement is also made to the Lancet and the Journal of the Canadian Association of Radiologists where some of the material in this chapter was originally published.

REFERENCES

BEIR III (1980). National Research Council Advisory Committee on the Biological Effects of Ionizing Radiation: *The effect on populations of low levels of ionizing radiation.* Washington, DC: National Academy of Science.

Clark, R. M., Rosen, I. B., and Laperriere, N. L. (1982). Malignant tumors of the head and neck in a young population. *American Journal of Surgery*, **144**, 461.

Fitzpatrick, P. J., and Tepperman, B. S. (1982). Carcinoma of the floor of the mouth. *Journal of the Canadian Association of Radiologists*, **33**, 148.

Goodner, J. T., and Watson, W. L. (1956). Cancer of the esophagus. Its association with other primary cancers. *Cancer*, **9**, 1248.

Kogelnik, H. D., Fletcher, G. H., and Jesse, R. H. (1975). Clinical course of patients with squamous cell carcinoma of the upper respiratory and digestive tracts with no evidence of disease five years after initial treatment. *Radiology*, **115**, 423.

Moertel, C. G. (1977). Multiple primary malignant neoplasms. *Cancer*, **40**, 1786.

Schoenberg, B. S. (1977). *Multiple primary malignant neoplasms: the Connecticut Tumor Registry*, 1939–61. Berlin: Springer-Verlag.

Shibuya, H., Takagi, M., Horuichi, J. *et al.* (1982). Carcinomas of the oesophagus with synchronous or metachronous primary carcinoma in other organs. *Acta Radiologica (Oncology)*, **21**, 39.

Statistics Canada, Health Division (1978). *New primary sites of malignant neoplasms in Canada – 1975.* Ottawa: Ministry of Industry, Trade and Commerce.

Tepperman, B. S., and Fitzpatrick, P. J. (1981). Second respiratory and upper digestive tract cancers after oral cancer. *Lancet*, **2**, 547.

UICC (1978). *TNM Classification of malignant tumors*, 3rd edn. Geneva.

Warren, S., and Gates, O. (1932). Multiple primary malignant tumors: A survey of the literature and statistical study. *American Journal of Cancer*, **51**, 1358.

Chapter

15 HUGH R. K. BARBER

Cancers of Breast, Uterus, and Ovary

INTRODUCTION

A higher than expected association of multiple primary cancers involving the breast, ovary, endometrium, or colon has been reported by various investigators. There is about a twofold increase in risk of a second primary in the ovaries following breast cancer, while estimates of the relative risk of subsequent breast cancer in ovarian cancer patients have ranged from 1.4 to 4.

Women with endometrial cancer have a relative risk of 1.2–2.0 for a second primary cancer in the breast, and this appears most frequently in women over 60 within 10 years of the endometrial cancer. Women with breast cancer probably have a slightly elevated risk for endometrial cancer but the magnitude of this association (as well as that between breast cancer and subsequent ovarian cancer) is hard to evaluate since removal of the uterus and ovaries may be undertaken in the course of treatment for breast cancer.

There are reports of an increased risk for cancer of the colon and rectum among breast cancer patients, and also an elevated risk for breast cancer among patients with cancer of the colon and rectum. It seems established that multiple primary cancers involving the breast, endometrium, and ovary occur more frequently than would be expected by chance, but the association between breast and colon and rectal cancer is somewhat less certain.

In addition, cancers of the breast, ovary, endometrium, and colon tend to occur in the same geographic areas more frequently than would be expected by chance. Mortality rates for breast, colon, and ovarian cancers are correlated in various countries around the world. In the United States, high mortality rates for breast cancer, colon cancer, and ovarian cancer, and (to a

315

certain extent) endometrial cancer tend to be found in the same regions of the country.

Various explanations have been offered for the association of these cancers both in individuals and geographic areas. For instance, in an individual or in a geographic area there may be etiologic agents for more than one cancer, e.g. a high fat diet, abnormal hormone levels, or reduced fertility. In an individual, the presence of one tumor may predispose to another, and for instance, the presence of an ovarian cancer may increase the risk of breast cancer because of the higher levels of hormones secreted from the ovary. It might be useful to investigate whether a specific histologic type of ovarian cancer is associated with an increased risk of breast cancer.

DIET AND MULTIPLE CANCERS

It has been reported that migrants to the United States develop more bowel cancer, and eventually more breast, endometrial, or ovarian cancer, when they come from regions where these cancers are uncommon (see Chapter 8). It is believed that there is a correlation between risk for these cancers and the average consumption of dietary protein and fat in the Western world. No major cancer is common everywhere in the world, and we know that high rates are rarely genetic, because migrants from one culture to another tend to show a shift in cancer patterns once they have settled in the new country.

It is likely that diet has an indirect role, modifying carcinogenesis, and several mechanisms are advanced to explain this effect (see Chapter 6). For example, it is theorized that excess dietary fat may promote carcinogenesis by its influence on bile acid production and/or gut microflora development in colon cancer; and on the secretion of endocrine glands in breast and endometrial cancers and possibly also in ovarian cancer.

For some years it has been suspected that dietary differences may explain much of the international variation in breast and endometrial cancer rates. Both have been shown to be highly correlated with total fat consumption in populations. This association for breast cancer has also been shown to hold true in Japan where combinations of fat and pork consumption could explain more than 80% of the variance in the breast cancer rates.

Fat consumption is, of course, highly correlated with dietary variables such as meat and total calorie consumption and with economic development. These variables are themselves correlated highly with breast and endometrial cancer rates. There are, however, other observations which link dietary fat, meat and/or total calories to breast and endometrial cancer. The associations between height and/or weight and breast and endometrial cancer, indirectly implicate dietary excess in their etiology. Diet has been reported to have an influence on the age of first menses and significant differences in age of first menses do exist among different populations. Age of menarche has been shown to relate closely to body fatness; menses occur when a critical level of body fat is reached. Animal data suggest that dietary fat may be more important than other sources of calories in determining estrus.

There is evidence also that vegetarian women have an earlier menopause than non-vegetarian women. This could be due to the lower body weight of vegetarian women or to some other factor associated with a vegetarian diet. It appears, therefore, that total dietary energy and perhaps other dietary factors influence duration of menstrual life and may, thereby, affect breast and endometrial cancer rates. Vegetarian Seventh Day Adventist women have lower than average rates of both breast and endometrial cancer. These observations could be explained totally in terms of lower than average body weight of vegetarians, although, in addition to eating less meat, vegetarians generally eat less total fat and have a higher ratio of polyunsaturated to saturated fat in their diet, and so perhaps other factors could be implicated.

Observations made of positive associations between breast and endometrial cancer and dietary fat, meat and total calories may relate to their effect on estrogen production. A consistent positive association has been demonstrated between plasma and urinary estrogen levels and body weight in postmenopausal women. The main sources of estrogen postmenopausally are adrenal and ovarian androgens (mainly androstenedione) which are converted to estrogen (mainly estrone) in peripheral tissues, particularly adipose tissue. The amount of androgen converted to estrogen is, therefore, a function of adipose tissue mass and indirectly of dietary energy intake (see Chapter 10).

Recent studies of endocrine status suggest that the diet may be an important determinant also of endogenous prolactin production. Postmenopausal vegetarian women have lower plasma prolactin levels than non-vegetarian women in addition to lower excretion of estrogen in their urine. These observations suggest that it may be possible to explain the geographic variations in the incidence of breast and endometrial cancer through the influence of dietary factors and endocrine status. If true, this observation has important preventive implications.

The association between cancers of the breast and endometrium and fat intake is still a source of controversy. It may be that the low socio-economic groups in Western countries are obese because of their high carbohydrate intake whereas patients from suburbia have an increased obesity because of the amount of fat in the diet. This emphasizes the limitations of epidemiology especially in dealing with nutritional factors that could have had their influence years ago. It is more pertinent to obtain information from a country such as Japan, where a trend in Westernization of diet can be satisfactorily recorded and where it has been shown that women with cancer of the endometrium eat a more Westernized diet than their respective controls.

Metabolic and animal studies are needed to define the relationship between nutrition and cancers of the breast and endometrium in various populations.

The role of nutrition as it may affect production and storage of hormones, and the interaction of hormones with cellular receptors, are difficult to unravel, particularly because these factors may operate differently in various age groups.

In searching for an explanation for the increased incidence of ovarian cancer as well as that of breast and endometrial cancer in the Japanese, it is suggested that change in the diet following the Second World War may offer an explanation. Prior to the Second World War the Japanese had a diet that was very low in cholesterol. However, after the war, particularly as they became more affluent, the Japanese nation took on a more Westernized diet and shifted from a low cholesterol diet to one that was high in fat. Obviously, there are other changes in lifestyle, but this and the decrease in the size of their families stand out as areas that need further investigation.

It has also been noted that there is an increasing incidence of endometrial cancer in the age group 30 to 39, in the United States, Great Britain, and Israel. In populations with a relatively high level of nutrition, perhaps some increase in cholesterol and saturated fats (or some other factors that physicians are completely unaware of) may be causing more endometrial cancer at an earlier age.

CANCER OF THE BREAST

Epidemiology

One out of every 11 women will develop breast cancer during her life but breast cancer is not a chance event that occurs randomly through the population. Black females in the United States have a lower incidence than white females. Breast cancer occurs more frequently among Jews than among non-Jews, and less often than expected among American Indians and Mexican Americans. Members of the upper social classes are affected more frequently than those in the lower classes, the risk being about twice as great. Males represent 1% of cases.

Within the United States, mortality rates are higher in urban areas than in rural localities, and are higher in the north than in the south. This excess in the north is restricted to postmenopausal women and is only partly explained by the socio-economic differences between the north and the south. Premenopausal breast cancer appears to be distributed relatively uniformly throughout the United States.

Breast cancer has a low incidence in Japan and other Asian and African countries compared to the white population in the United States. Low rates are found in most African and Asian countries, intermediate rates in southern Europe and South American countries, and high rates in North America and northern European countries.

There is also a remarkable difference in the way incidence rates change with age in these areas. In North America and northern European countries where the risks for breast cancer are relatively high, the incidence rates increase with age over the entire age span. There is only slight levelling off of this increase around 45–54 years of age, and a somewhat slower rate of increase after age 55 years than before age 45 years.

In countries with intermediate risk such as Greece, the incidence rate tends to *plateau* after about age 50 years, whereas in low risk countries, such as Japan, the incidence rate *declines* after age 50 years. It has been reported that among migrants to Israel, the shape of the age-specific incidence curves for European born Jews is similar to the North American–northern European curves; whereas among Asian and African born immigrants there is a plateau after age 50 years.

Risk factors

Risk factors for breast cancer in females include: old age, living in North America or northern Europe, upper socio-economic class, urban-living, white, nulliparity or age at first live delivery over 30, obese body build, early menarche, late menopause, history of cancer in one breast, history of fibrocystic disease, first degree relative with breast cancer, history of primary cancer of the ovary or endometrium; history of excessive radiation to the chest.

(1) Women over age 40 have more than 80% of the breast cancers that are clinically detected. The highest incidence of breast cancer occurs after the age of 35, with 83% of the cases occurring after the age of 50, and only 1.5% under the age of 30.

(2) Approximately 25% of all patients with breast cancer manifest a familial history defined as two or more first degree relatives with verified breast cancer. Approximately one-third of such familial occurrence (about 7% of all breast cancer patients) demonstrate evidence of a hereditary etiology when subjected to meticulous medical–genetic study. Hereditary forms of breast cancer differ from their sporadic counterparts in the following clinical features: significant early age of onset; excess of bilaterality; vertical transmission.

Emphasis is on mothers and sisters and on premenopausal and bilateral cancers, when considering familial risk factors. Thus, the premenopausal patient with a family history of breast cancer has a 3.5 times increased risk if her mother has had cancer of the breast, while it is 5 times if the mother and grandmother have had it, and 9 times if two close relatives with premenopausal bilateral breast cancer have been identified.

(3) The risk is increased 1.5 times in women who have had their menarche before age 12, and 2 times when the menopause has occurred after age 55.

(4) Nulliparous women and those with their first live birth after the age of 34 are most liable to develop breast cancer. Women who are over 30 when they gave birth to their first child have a 1.5 times increased risk over the normal population.

(5) Women who already have had carcinoma of one breast are probably at the highest risk for development of a new primary breast carcinoma. This risk has been estimated at 4 to 15 times the risk of breast cancer in someone not similarly affected.

(6) Patients with a hyperplastic type of fibrocystic disease are at increased risk of breast cancer. This is no longer controversial, and one of the reasons for previous differences in opinion regarding this association is probably the ubiquitous use of the term fibrocystic disease to describe a variety of breast lesions.

(7) The risk is increased by excessive exposure of the breast to ionizing radiation, e.g. multiple fluoroscopies or radiation treatment for skin conditions over the breast. A result is that mammography tends to be underutilized by the medical community in general. But, using assumptions that are made in constructing a worst possible hypothesis, most conservative analyses estimate that between 3.5 and 7.5 cancers may be induced in a population of 1 million women per year exposed to 1 rad, after a latent period of 10 to 15 years. This theoretical number of potentially induced breast cancers is trivially low when compared to the natural incidence of breast cancer in women.

(8) The relationship of emotional stress to cancer is currently being studied and three related questions are being investigated. First, what effect may an event such as the loss of a loved one or a huge financial setback have on a person's susceptibility to cancer? Second, is there such a thing as a cancer-prone personality? Finally, how may the biologic changes that occur under stress affect the ability of the body's defense system to protect us from cancer-causing agents?

Recent research on stress and cancer suggests that there is a link between breast cancer and the release of emotions, particularly extreme suppression of anger and bottling up of feelings. Stress may bring about hormonal changes that interfere with the patient's immunologic defense system against cancer, and patients with lower immunologic competence may be at risk to a variety of cancers including breast cancer. Patients over age 60 are known to have a decrease in their immunologic competency, as do patients with thymic atrophy or decreased thymus-dependent T lymphocytes.

(9) In 1974, three case-control studies were published suggesting a causal association between the use of the antihypertensive drug reserpine and the development of breast cancer. Estimates of relative risk ranged from about 2 to 4. A plausible biologic mechanism for the association was the prolactin-stimulating property of reserpine. The associations which were originally reported are almost certainly overestimates.

(10) Recently there has been interest in whether exposure to hair dyes increases the risk of cancer including breast cancer. This interest stems from reports that permanent and semi-permanent hair dyes are mutagenic in bacteria test systems. Both retrospective cohort studies of hairdressers and women who dye their own hair, and case-control studies, have been undertaken, but results to date have been conflicting.

CANCER OF THE ENDOMETRIUM

Epidemiology

Carcinoma of the endometrium is now the most common gynecologic cancer in the United States and accounts for 8% of all female cancers. It has been calculated that about one woman in 32 will develop carcinoma of the endometrium. It is not clear whether the recent increase in prevalence of endometrial carcinoma is due to an increase in the aging population, better nutrition (more fat in the diet), or specific dysfunctional reproductive factors.

Cancer of the endometrium is predominantly a disease of the perimeno-pausal and postmenopausal age groups. However, 5% of the cases occur in women of less than 40 years of age and it has been found as early as age 16. Over 75% of cases occur after age 50 years.

The death ratios by age for cancer of the endometrium show that while the median survival of all age groups up to 64 is more than 10 years, between ages 65 and 74 the median survival time drops to 5.6 years, and for 75 and over it is 2.1 years. In the older age groups there are more adenosquamous cancers and these are associated with less differentiated glandular elements and more vascular involvement than are adenocarcinomas of the endometrium. Women over age 60 also have a thinner myometrium, and therefore, slight penetration into the myometrium brings the disease into close contact with the lymphatics that are near the serosa.

The mean age of patients with grade 1 tumors is 56 years, whereas for grade 3 it is 64 years and Reagan (1974) found that both grade and extent of lesion increase with age. Thus, increased extent of the lesion, increased anaplasia, increased depth of invasion, and more rapid growth may all contribute to the poor prognosis in the elderly.

Reproductive risk factors

The possibility of endocrinopathy in the background of patients with carcinoma of the endometrium is based on observations of obesity, nulliparity, and infertility in many of these patients; of the frequency of prior failure of ovulation and dysfunctional bleeding; and of the normal proliferative effect of estrogen upon the endometrium in all age groups.

Certain characteristics have been noted in patients under the age of 40 including very high incidence of infertility, disturbance of the menstrual cycle with menorrhagia, long periods of amenorrhea or abnormal menarche with marked irregularity of the periods, and a high incidence of polycystic ovaries or the Stein–Leventhal syndrome. Patients with the Stein–Leventhal syndrome have a chronically depressed FSH titer and a chronically elevated luteinizing hormone (LH) titer. There is often hyperthecosis of the ovaries and increased androstenedione and testosterone production.

Gurpide *et al.* (1977) have shown that androstenedione is converted to estrone in the peripheral fat by extraovarian aromatization and since these patients are often obese, the endometrium is subjected to an unopposed estrogen stimulation. Possibly related is the increasing incidence of endometrial cancer among young girls with a long history of anovulation. Many of these girls are markedly obese and may have a genetic or chromosomal abnormality.

Women with carcinoma of the endometrium tend to be overweight, although Mack *et al.* (1976) have reported that patients who received estrogen and developed endometrial cancer did not have this characteristic. In various studies the incidence of obesity varied from 21 to 64% according to the criteria used. Wynder *et al.* (1966) found that 21 to 50 pounds overweight increased the risk of endometrial cancer by about 3 times, and 50 pounds overweight increased it by about 10 times. This is discussed at the end of the chapter.

Single or nulliparous married women have a higher risk of endometrial cancer than those who are married or parous. Nulliparous women have cancer of the endometrium rates twice as high as those of women with one child and more than 3 times as high as those of women with 5 or more children. Patients with cancer of the endometrium tend to experience the menopause at a later age and one study showed that women whose menopause occurred at 52 or after, had 2.4 times the risk of patients whose menopause occurred prior to age 49.

Familial and racial risk factors

Patients with endometrial cancer more often report a history of cancer in first degree relatives than do other persons and the familial excess pertains both to endometrial cancer and to cancers at other sites. Breast cancer in particular seems to cluster with endometrial cancer, both in individuals and in families. It is not known whether the familial and/or individual coincidence derives from environmental risk factors that cluster in families or whether it is determined by cultural factors or inherited factors.

Lynch and Krish (1971) have collected evidence in some families of autosomal dominant inheritance of susceptibility to endometrial cancer. The famous cancer family G, studied since 1885, now comprises over 650 blood relatives. Eighteen members over 40 years of age have had endometrial adenocarcinoma, 53 have had colonic carcinomas; and the question is raised whether there is a cancer-susceptible genome interacting with an oncogenic virus. Recent work with the major histocompatibility complex would indicate that there may be an association. The counter argument to this is that families tend to have the same diet and are frequently exposed to the same carcinogens.

Cancer of the endometrium is rare among the Japanese who eat the traditional oriental low cholesterol diet but it is becoming more common among those on a Westernized diet. It is common among Jewish women in the West. In contrast to invasive cervical cancer, which is still more common in black than in white women (despite the drop in incidence in both groups), the incidence rate for endometrial cancer in white women is nearly double that for black women.

Incidence rates of endometrial cancer in other United States non-white groups are also lower than for whites but American born children of both Asian and Latin American migrants experience rates closer to those of their neighbors than to those of their cousins back home. However, the non-white rates have shown little of the dramatic rise in endometrial cancer rates shown by whites in recent years.

Other possible risk factors

Several studies have reported cases of corpus cancer after radiation but there has not been any increase among Japanese women who were exposed to the atomic bomb. Although there is no unequivocal study showing an increased risk from endometrial cancer in irradiated patients, there are reports of a twofold increase in risk in women either sterilized by radiation, or treated more than five years previously for cancer of the uterine cervix. In addition to adenocarcinoma of the endometrium, it appears that sarcomas of the corpus have also appeared in excess among radiated patients.

Many studies have reported a frequent association of diabetes mellitus and endometrial cancer and the reported rates of clinical diabetes in cancer of the endometrium patients range from 3 to 17%. Reports of glucose tolerance showing abnormal function range from 16.9 to 64% of cancer of the endometrium patients depending on the diagnostic standards used. The extent to which this relationship correlates also with obesity remains to be evaluated.

Hypertension has often been reported as a correlate of endometrial carcinoma and in various studies, from one-third to three-quarters of the patients with endometrial carcinoma were reported to be hypertensive to some degree. The relationship between hypertension and obesity remains to be clarified.

Associated pathology

Endometrial hyperplasia in the postmenopausal patient may be a precursor of cancer especially if it is related to a feminizing tumor. Gusberg (1947) has reported that in his experience, adenomatous hyperplasia is a clear cancer precursor. In an untreated group of about 100 patients followed between 5 and 10 years, approximately 12% developed endometrial cancer and he estimates that approximately 25% would develop cancer if left untreated for a 20-year period.

The association between endometrial polyps and carcinoma of the endometrium has often been observed. Way (1951) has suggested that a polyp in the postmenopausal patient is potentially dangerous and hysterectomy is indicated. This is particularly so in high risk patients with evidence of pituitary dysfunction and hyperestrogenism.

Leiomyomas, fibroids, and endometrial carcinoma are found together in about 30 to 35% of patients, but this is the incidence of fibroids normally occurring in this age group. Although adenocarcinoma which contains squamous elements might behave more aggressively than others, there is no reason for presuming it to be etiologically different.

Two conditions appear to predispose strongly to endometrial cancer, but each is sufficiently rare to make quantitation of the relationship difficult. First, a proportion of patients who experience a granulosa and/or thecal cell ovarian tumor can anticipate a subsequent endometrial malignancy, and the probability of a second cancer appears to be related to the prominence of the thecal cells (the most important source of estrogens). The second condition is the polycystic ovarian syndrome, an uncommon condition also characterized by unopposed production of estrogen precursors and non-ovulation. In a study of feminizing ovarian stromal tumors from the Ovarian Tumor Registry in which the endometrium was also available for review, adenocarcinoma of the endometrium was present in 23% of the cases and hyperplasia in an additional 65%, so that 88% of the endometria studied showed evidence of an estrogen effect. Similar observations have been made by Smith *et al.* (1942), Dockerty and Mussey (1951), and Mansell and Hertig (1955).

High risk patients

Knowledge gained from epidemiologic studies helps to identify the high risk group of women who are candidates for endometrial cancer. Garnet (1958) suggested that risk factors include obesity, nulliparity, reduced glucose tolerance, hypertension, hyperestrogenism, continuous uninterrupted estrogen stimulation, menses continuing beyond the age of 50, history of dysfunctional uterine bleeding, and a history of anovulation.

Garnet (1958) has suggested that a combination of at least five of the following factors is required to define hyperestrogenism – early menarche, delayed onset of ovulation, cessation of ovulation late in reproductive life, dysfunctional uterine bleeding, involuntary sterility, endometrial polyps and hyperplasia, habitual abortion, severe cystic disease of the breast, and any other findings associated with unopposed estrogen stimulation of the endometrium. These help to identify clinically the high risk patient.

A large number of reports have been published on the association between cancer of the endometrium and estrogen metabolism (see Chapter 10). Aleem *et al.* (1976) have reported that the total plasma estrogen level was significantly higher in patients with endometrial carcinoma and hyperplasia compared to a postmenopausal control group, and to a group of patients having uterine bleeding without histologic endometrial lesions. Furthermore, in obese endometrial carcinoma patients, the estrogen level was significantly higher than in the non-obese and control groups.

Three groups of women may be at risk to endometrial cancer from *exogenous* estrogen exposure – women who have taken sequential oral contraceptives, postmenopausal women who received estrogen replacement therapy, and girls with ovarian dysgenesis who received unopposed estrogen therapy at puberty. In addition, four groups of women seem to be at risk to endometrial cancer from *endogenous* estrogen sources – women with granulosa cell or thecal cell ovarian tumors, anovulatory women, obese postmenopausal women, and women with liver disease.

Smith *et al.* (1975) reported a 7.5 times increase relative risk of endometrial cancer associated with estrogen use, and similarly, Zeil and Finkle (1975) reported a 7.6 times increased relative risk. Horowitz and Feinstein (1978) on the other hand, have concluded that the relative risk is not increased.

Hammond *et al.* (1979) reported that the use of progesterone in adequate doses for a 10-day period each month protected against the development of carcinoma of the endometrium among estrogen users. It may be concluded that estrogen is a cancer promoter and that if it is withdrawn (or progesterone is given) the promoter effect is eliminated. In support of this is the finding in the progesterone studies that there was a fall in the incidence of carcinoma of the endometrium after estrogen was discontinued.

CANCER OF THE OVARY

Epidemiology

Carcinoma of the ovary accounts for about 4% of all female cancers and approximately 1 of every 70 newborn girls will develop carcinoma of the ovary. Part of the recent increase of ovarian cancer in the United States may be attributable to improved diagnostic facilities, but even when the increase in aged women in the population is taken into account, there is still an increase in incidence that has not been explained.

Ovarian cancer appears to be more often diagnosed in individuals to whom better medical care is available, and data from specific hospitals must, therefore, be cautiously evaluated in respect to socio-economic status. The low rate of ovarian cancer in Japan is real, because diagnostic facilities and vital statistics are equal to those of the Western world. It is also noteworthy that the incidence of ovarian cancer increases among Japanese women when they migrate to the United States, a finding which suggests that environmental rather than genetic factors are partially responsible for the low rate of this cancer among the Japanese.

Silverberg (1980) has shown that the death rates by age for cancer of the ovary demonstrate a steady increase as the population at risk gets older. For non-whites it is lower than for whites in each age group over 30 years. Trends by age and race since 1930 show that the death rates for all ages in white females rose slowly until late 1940s and have remained at the same level until recent years, when the rate have decreased.

Beral (1980) has reported that the downward trend in mortality at age 30–34 preceded that at age 35–39, which in turn preceded that at age 40–44. She raised the question whether this may not be due to the use of the contraceptive pill by these groups. This pattern is consistent with the so-called cohort effect, that is, with different generations of women having a different risk of ovarian cancer throughout their lives. In addition, Beral (1980) reported that in the United States and many other countries the figures suggest that women born in 1900–10 have an especially high risk of developing ovarian cancer.

The following demographic leads may provide some clues:

1. Ovarian cancer, particularly in postmenopausal women, is less common in Japan than in the Western world. Compared with Caucasian women, oriental women also have a low incidence of breast and ovarian cancer.
2. Among first-generation Japanese women in the United States, ovarian cancer occurs more commonly than in Japan.
3. Not only has there been an increase in the incidence of ovarian cancer in the Western world, there has also been some increase in Japan.
4. Cancer of the ovary tends to be somewhat more common in upper than in lower income groups in the West.
5. Ovarian cancer in New York City is more common among Jews than other religious groups, particularly in postmenopausal women.
6. There is a positive correlation between the incidence pattern of ovarian, mammary, and endometrial cancers.

7. In several studies ovarian cancer is more commonly reported among single and nulliparous women.
8. There is a greater incidence of ovarian cancer in the highly industrialized nations.
9. Much of the international variation cannot be accounted for by racial or genetic differences – migrants from one country to another rapidly acquire rates of ovarian cancer prevalent in the country of adoption. Thus, second generation Chinese living in the United States have similar ovarian cancer mortality rates to Whites in the United States, whereas first-generation Chinese have considerably lower rates.
10. It is suggested that some environmental or lifestyle factors account for the international variation in ovarian cancer incidence.
11. The difference in the average size family from one country to another may also offer an explanation for the difference in the incidence of ovarian cancer.
12. Ovarian cancer appears to be more common in women with obesity, gallbladder disease, cervical fibroids or Peutz–Jegher's syndrome.
13. The generation of women in the childbearing age during the Depression had fewer children but more ovarian cancer than the generation of women before and after the Depression.

Cancer of the ovary appears to be more common in highly industrialized nations. However, Japan is highly industrialized, yet the incidence of ovarian cancer was low until just after the end of the Second World War, despite the fact that it had been a highly industrialized nation prior to the Second World War.

Familial and genetic risk factors

Several reports describe families in which women of the same or succeeding generation develop similar neoplasms in the ovary. Most of these neoplasms were serous cystadenocarcinomas, but other types are also observed. Cancers of the breast, colon or other sites were also found in female and male members of two of these families. In families where ovarian cancer has been described in more than one generation, the link between affected individuals has always been through the maternal line.

Unusual susceptibility to neoplasms of the ovaries occurs among females with two rare multisystem syndromes, both of which appear to be inherited as autosomal dominance. Females with the Peutz–Jegher's syndrome are at high risk of developing neoplasms of the ovaries, and females with inherited basal cell naevus syndrome are prone to develop ordinary benign fibromas of the ovary, or less frequently, neoplasms of other cell types.

Osborn and DiGeorge (1963) have reported on ABO blood groups in neoplastic diseases of the ovary, and concluded that ovarian neoplasms which associate with blood group A have a glandular type of epithelium. In contrast, those which do not appear to associate with blood group A are solid rather than cystic. They also noted a four- to sixfold excess of secondary carcinomas of the ovary in women of blood group A compared to women of blood group O.

Reproductive risk factors

Fathalla (1972) has drawn attention to the importance of repeated stimulation of the ovary ovulation in the etiology of malignancy. It would appear that multiple pregnancy (especially more than four children), the use of oral contraceptives, and the suppression of ovulation all protect against ovarian cancer. Nulliparous women appear to have a higher incidence of ovarian cancer, yet there is growing evidence that use of oral contraceptives decreases the risk of ovarian cancer. Moreover, the longer the use of the pill, the lower the risk of ovarian cancer. Reports both from England and the United States support this concept.

Hoover *et al.* (1977) reported a follow-up survey of 908 women who had received Premarin for menopausal symptoms and found eight cases of ovarian cancer. This risk was two to three times greater than expected. The risk increased with the dose of Premarin taken, but not with the duration or use of total dose ingested. The excess risk of ovarian cancer in this group occurred primarily among 21 women who had also used stilbestrol.

Other possible risk factors

Epidemiologic, experimental, and clinical data provide a weak link between asbestos and talc with ovarian cancer. It has been pointed out that direct passage of talc or asbestos-contaminated talc through the female reproductive tract to the ovarian surface may plan an etiologic role. The evidence is suggestive but not conclusive, and further evaluation is needed.

Studies by Speert (1952) and West (1966) showed no relationship between irradiation and ovarian cancer. Speert (1952) followed 958 patients who had received a radio-therapeutic menopause and only one developed cancer of the ovary. He also investigated 343 consecutive patients with ovarian cancer and 247 consecutive patients with cystadenomas of the ovary and of these 590 women only 17 had a record of previous pelvic radiation for benign conditions.

West (1966) in an early study of ovarian cancer utilizing women with benign ovarian conditions as controls, noted that few ovarian cancer patients recalled a prior infection with mumps virus. In a study by Wynder *et al.* (1969) no meaningful differences were noted but it was concluded that because of the relationship of mumps virus to the gonad, this relationship deserves further exploration.

CONCLUSION

The epidemiology and endocrine associations for cancers of the endometrium, ovary, and breast have many factors in common. It suggests that variations in exposure to environmental agents, social practices, and lifestyles are largely responsible for variations in the occurrence of these cancers in different populations.

REFERENCES

Aleem, F. A., Mamdouh, M. A., Hung, H. C., Rommey, S. L. (1976). Plasma estrogen in patients with endometrial hyperplasia and carcinoma. *Cancer*, **38**, 2101.

Beral, V. (1980). *The epidemiology of ovarian cancer* (eds C. E. Newman, H. J. Ford, and J. A. Jordan). Oxford, New York, Toronto, Sydney, Paris, Frankfurt: Pergamon Press.

Dockerty, M. B., Mussey, E. (1951). Malignant lesions of the uterus associated with estrogen-producing ovarian tumors. *American Journal of Obstetrics and Gynecology*, **61**, 147.

Fathalla, M. F. (1972). Factors in the causation and incidence of ovarian cancer. *Obstetrical and Gynecological Survey*, **27**, 751.

Garnet, J. (1958). Constitutional stigma associated with endometrial carcinoma. *American Journal of Obstetrics and Gynecology*, **76**, 11.

Gurpide, E., Tseng, L., and Gusberg, S. B. (1977). Estrogen metabolism and neoplastic endometrium. *American Journal of Obstetrics and Gynecology*, **129**, 809.

Gusberg, S. B. (1947). Precursors of corpus carcinoma: estrogens and adenomatous hyperplasia. *American Journal of Obstetrics and Gynecology*, **54**, 905.

Hammond, C. B., Jelovsek, F. R., Lee, K. L. *et al.* (1979). Effects of long-term estrogen replacement therapy: II Neoplasia. *American Journal of Human Genetics*, **133**, 537.

Hoover, R., Gray, L. A., Sr., and Fraumeni, J. F. (1977). Stilboestrol (diethylstilboestrol) and the risk of ovarian cancer. *Lancet*, **2**, 533.

Horowitz, R. I., and Feinstein, A. R. (1978). Alternative analytical methods for case-control studies of estrogens and endometrial cancer. *New England Journal of Medicine*, **299**, 189.

Lynch, H. T., and Krish, A. J. (1971). Cancer family 'G' revisited 1895–1970. *Cancer*, **27**, 1505.

Mack, T. M., Pike, M. C., Henderson, B. F. *et al.* (1976). Estrogens and endometrial cancer in a retirement community. *New England Journal of Medicine*, **294**, 1262.

Mansell, H., and Hertig, A. T. (1955). Granulosa-theca cell tumors and endometrial carcinoma: a study of their relationship and a survey of 80 cases. *Obstetrics and Gynecology*, **6**, 385.

Osborne, R. H., and DiGeorge, F. V. (1963). The ABO blood groups in the neoplastic disease of the ovary. *American Journal of Obstetrics and Gynecology*, **15**, 380.

Reagan, J. W. (1974). The changing nature of endometrial cancer. *Gynecologic Oncology*, **31**, 702.

Silverberg, B. S. (1980). *Statistical and epidemiological information on gynecologic cancer*. New York City: American Cancer Society Professional Education Publication.

Smith, D. C., Ross, P., Donovan, J. T., and Herrmann, W. L. (1975). Association of exogenous estrogen and endometrial carcinoma. *New England Journal of Medicine*, **293**, 1164.

Smith, G. U. W., Johnson, L. C., and Hertig, A. T. (1942). Relation of ovarian stromal hyperplasia and thecoma of the ovary to endometrial hyperplasia and carcinoma. *New England Journal of Medicine*, **226**, 364.

Speert, H. (1952). The role of ionizing radiation in the causation of ovarian tumor. *Cancer*, **5**, 478.

Way, S. (1951). *Malignant disease of the female genital tract*, Philadelphia: Blakiston Company, p. 165.

West, R. O. (1966). Epidemiologic study of malignancies of the ovaries. *Cancer*, **19**, 1001.

Wynder, E. L., Dodo, H., and Barber, H. R. K. (1969). Epidemiology of cancer of the ovary. *Cancer*, **23**, 352.

Wynder, E. L., Escher, G. C., Mantel, N. (1966). An epidemiological investigation of cancer of the endometrium. *Cancer*, **19**, 489.

Zeil, H. K., and Finkle, W. D. (1975). Increased risk of endometrial carcinoma among users of conjugated esrogens. *New England Journal of Medicine*, **293**, 1167.

Chapter

16 PAUL L. MOOTS and LUCIEN J. RUBINSTEIN

Multiple Neoplasms of the Nervous System

Primary neoplasms of the nervous system are less common than those of most other organ systems and, not surprisingly, multiple primary nervous system neoplasms are distinctly rare. But there is a relatively common disorder, namely neurofibromatosis, in which multiplicity and diversity of neoplasms is the outstanding feature. In this and other hereditary syndromes, genetic predisposition appears to be the best documented factor associated with an increased risk of multiple nervous system neoplasms.

Rather than discuss these neoplasms on the basis of histological classification, we propose to consider them in the context of clinical features that may bear on their multiplicity. First, we will review the multiple tumors that occur as part of well-defined hereditary syndromes; then we will discuss those that are unrelated to these syndromes. Third, we shall comment on tumors that have seemingly arisen in relation to therapy, and finally we will review the association between non-nervous system and nervous system neoplasms.

NEUROFIBROMATOSIS

Three of the four classical phacomatoses (neurofibromatosis, von Hippel–Lindau disease, and tuberous sclerosis) are associated with multiple tumors. The fourth, Sturge–Weber syndrome, is a vascular malformative disorder not associated with neoplasia. In addition to an autosomal dominant pattern of inheritance, common features include a high incidence of sporadic cases, and the occurrence of non-nervous system tumors and of hamartomatous lesions.

Neurofibromatosis is the prototype of neurological syndromes in which tumour multiplicity is the cardinal feature, and a substantial body of data has been gathered on the genetic, biochemical, and clinical features of the disease. The syndrome includes at least two relatively distinct hereditary variants, a peripheral and a central form. Three other types have also been proposed but appear less well defined: a visceral, an autonomic, and a 'fruste' form. While these several variants differ in the predominant localization of the tumors in relation to the peripheral and central nervous systems, and while the central and peripheral variants have been reported to show different biochemical features, they all appear to be bridged by transitional forms.

Peripheral neurofibromatosis

The classical peripheral form of the disease (von Recklinghausen's disease) is a common disorder with an incidence of about 1 in 3000. Autosomal dominant transmission is well established, but in up to half the cases a familial history is not apparent and the sporadic cases are presumed to occur on the basis of spontaneous mutation. Diagnostic features of the disease such as the skin lesions become apparent in childhood. Recent investigations suggest that nerve growth factor (NGF) may be in part responsible for the multiplicity of tumors that occur in these patients. Activity of NGF estimated by biological assay appears to be increased, although NGF concentration as estimated by immunoassay is normal (Fabricant et al., 1979; Fabricant and Todaro, 1981).

The characteristic tumor in this disorder is the neurofibroma. While its cellular origin has long been debated, both Schwann cells and fibroblasts have been shown morphologically to participate in its development (Russell and Rubinstein, 1977). The tumors are most frequently subcutaneous, having originated from the distal portions of the peripheral nerves but, in addition, involvement of major peripheral nerves is frequent. Involvement of one or more segment(s) of the autonomic nervous system, of spinal nerve roots, and, exceptionally, of cranial nerve roots may also occur. Predominant involvement of the sympathetic chain and ganglia, and of visceral nerves, respectively, constitutes the autonomic and visceral subvariants of von Recklinghausen's disease, whereas involvement of spinal and cranial nerve roots is most frequently found in the central form.

Malignant change of a neurofibroma to neurofibrosarcoma may occur, sometimes manifested as a progressive anaplastic change verified by repeated biopsies over a period of years. Estimates of the frequency of sarcomatous change vary considerably, ranging from 2 to 30% (Hope and Mulvihill, 1981) and the variation probably depends on patient case selection and length of patient follow-up. Reports from major cancer centers tend to indicate a 5–10% frequency of malignant change. Sarcomatous change usually does not take place until middle adult life. Reports have recently appeared (see below) suggesting that in some cases, malignant transformation could be radiation-induced (Ducatman and Scheithauer, 1983).

Other peripheral nervous system tumors that may occur in association with von Recklinghausen's disease include pheochromocytomas, which may be bilateral (Glushien *et al.*, 1953). Of 18 pheochromocytomas examined by one of us (LJR), 4 occurred in the context of neurofibromatosis. Single or multiple peripheral ganglioneuromas as well as cases of neuroblastoma have also been described (Russell and Rubinstein, 1977). Multiple Schwannomas may occur, but are more characteristic of the central form of the disease.

A variety of central nervous system neoplasms have been reported in patients with peripheral neurofibromatosis, providing transitional links to the central form of the disease. Optic nerve gliomas are the most frequently encountered in that setting, and may be bilateral and often present in childhood. It has been estimated that neurofibromatosis occurs in at least 10% of patients with optic nerve gliomas, but since the disorder is not always manifest at the time of diagnosis of the optic nerve tumor, the association may be greater than the above figure (Reese, 1956). In the series of 30 optic nerve or chiasmatic astrocytomas reported by Borit and Richardson (1982), neurofibromatosis was present in 25% of the cases or their kin.

Patients with the peripheral form of von Recklinghausen's disease may occasionally develop a solitary glioma, most commonly a pilocytic astrocytoma of the juvenile type situated in the region of the third ventricle (Russell and Rubinstein, 1977). Other types of glioma reported include cerebellar astrocytomas, and diffuse gliomas which may involve the cerebrum or the spinal cord (Russell and Rubinstein, 1977). The incidence of glioblastomas in neurofibromatosis has been reviewed by Manuelidis and Solitaire (1971). When an ependymoma is present, it is most often intraspinal and multiple, and associated with the central form of the disease (see below). Meningiomas too are more often found in the central form, and are then usually multiple.

Non-neural tumors reported in association with neurofibromatosis include carcinoid tumors, thyroid carcinoma, and melanoma. Unlike the association with pheochromocytomas, there is not enough statistical evidence to regard their occurrence as more than coincidental. The same applies to the occasional association of Wilms' tumors, rhabdomyosarcomas, and a number of childhood leukemias, although evidence that the association is significant is stronger in such cases (Hope and Mulvihill, 1981).

Central neurofibromatosis

Central neurofibromatosis is characterized by the presence of multiple tumors originating in the central nervous system and its coverings. These may include multiple meningiomas, cranial and spinal nerve root Schwannomas (especially bilateral acoustic nerve tumors), as well as a variety of primary central neuroepithelial neoplasms, most often spinal ependymomas (Rubinstein, 1963; Rodriguez and Berthrong, 1966; Russell and Rubinstein, 1977). The central form is considerably less frequent than the peripheral form, and while it may be associated with peripheral nerve tumors, the cutaneous lesions of von Recklinghausen's disease are usually inconspicuous or absent (Rubinstein, 1963). However, either peripheral neurofibromas or *café au lait* spots, or both, are said to be present in small numbers in 60% of the cases (Eldridge, 1981).

As in the peripheral form, the inheritance pattern is that of an autosomal dominant trait, but sporadic cases are not infrequent (Rubinstein, 1963). The concentration of NGF as estimated by immunoassay is elevated in the central form, as opposed to its normal concentration in the peripheral form (Fabricant *et al.*, 1979; Fabricant and Todaro, 1981).

There is some confusion in the literature as to what constitutes central neurofibromatosis. Because of its extremely frequent (although not invariable) presence in the disease, the existence of bilateral acoustic Schwannomas associated with minimal lesions elsewhere has been regarded as constituting a distinct subentity (Kanter *et al.*, 1980), but in our view such a concept is much too restrictive. It is true that bilateral acoustic tumors transmitted as a Mendelian autosomal dominant trait with high penetrance and remarkably constant expressivity have been reported in several kindreds (Gardner and Turner, 1940; Moyes, 1968; Alliez *et al.*, 1975; Kanter *et al.*, 1980). The eighth-nerve tumors in these cases are responsible for the majority of initial symptoms (i.e. hearing loss and vestibular dysfunction) which are seldom manifest until the second or third decade.

However, the association of bilateral acoustic Schwannomas with other multiple cranial nerve tumors, with multiple meningiomas and with multiple intra-axial gliomas (especially spinal intramedullary ependymomas) clearly extends the spectrum of the disease. As detailed elsewhere (Rubinstein, 1963; Saran and Winter, 1967), seven out of eight cases with bilateral acoustic Schwannomas examined at autopsy had other lesions of von Recklinghausen's disease, predominantly of the central type. Other multiple cranial nerve tumors were present in six of these cases. Conversely, in all our necropsied cases of neurofibromatosis in which acoustic Schwannomas were present, these were bilateral.

Likewise, multiple meningiomas are classically associated with bilateral acoustic Schwannomas. We have studied six such cases, and further variants of this association have been reported by Delleman *et al.* (1978), in a unique kindred in which the development of multiple familial meningiomas constituted an unusual expression of neurofibromatosis inheritance.

Ependymomas, most often spinal and multiple (Rubinstein, 1963; Rodriguez and Berthrong, 1966; Saran and Winter, 1967; Russell and Rubinstein, 1977) are the most frequent of the central neuroepithelial tumors that are characteristically associated with the combination of bilateral acoustic Schwannomas, multiple cranial and spinal nerve root tumors, and multiple meningiomas. In our autopsy material we noted that ependymoma represented five of the seven central gliomas found to be associated with central neurofibromatosis. In three of the five cases, the ependymomas were multiple, a feature shared by most of the intramedullary examples reported by others (Rodriguez and Berthrong, 1966). An exceptional example of bilateral astrocytic gliomas originating in the optic disks was studied by one of us (LJR) in a 17-year-old girl with the classic multiple lesions of central neurofibromatosis (Saran and Winter, 1967).

In many of the above-quoted examples of central neurofibromatosis, there is a remarkably high incidence of syringomyelia, often closely related to the presence of multiple spinal ependymomas.

It has been stated (Eldridge, 1981) that, in distinction to the peripheral form of neurofibromatosis, neither optic nerve gliomas nor malignant transformation of a neurofibroma into a neurogenic sarcoma have been reported in the central form of neurofibromatosis. The absence of recorded sarcomatous transformation in central neurofibromatosis may, however, partly be due to the fact that central lesions are more likely to affect patients in younger age groups. We noted above that sarcomatous transformation of a neurofibroma usually does not occur until middle or late adult life (the risk being presumably related to the number of neurofibromatous lesions harbored by the patient and to their clinical duration) and, therefore, on statistical ground alone one would expect such a change to be exceptional in central lesions.

Visceral forms of neurofibromatosis

These are rare and predominantly involve the gastrointestinal tract (Lukash *et al.*, 1966; Hochberg *et al.*, 1974). Most commonly involved are the jejunum, stomach, ileum, and duodenum; the colon is only seldom implicated. The tumors are most frequently subserosal and tumor types include neurofibromas, Schwannomas, ganglioneuromas, and occasionally leiomyomas. A characteristic feature of ganglioneuromas is the production of diffuse hyperplasia of Auerbach's plexus.

OTHER HEREDITARY SYNDROMES

Von Hippel–Lindau syndrome

Von Hippel–Lindau syndrome is classically characterized by the presence of one or more capillary hemangioblastomas of the central nervous system (including the retina), accompanied by one or more systemic lesions, some of which are hamartomatous and others true neoplasms. Most of the cases of capillary hemangioblastoma involve the cerebellum and of these cases, 20% have additional manifestations that allow the diagnosis of the syndrome to be made (Melmon and Rosen, 1964). The syndrome is familial in 20% of the cases, the pattern of inheritance being consistent with autosomal dominant transmission (Grossman and Melmon, 1972). The clinical features of the disorder are usually caused by ocular or posterior fossa lesions, with the onset of symptoms occurring typically in middle adult life. Polycythemia is found in 10 to 20% of all cases of cerebellar hemangioblastoma. A tendency for these tumors to recur following resection is an important feature of the syndrome.

The cerebellar capillary hemangioblastoma most commonly presents as a mural nodule enclosed within a cyst and multiple cerebellar tumors occur in 10 to 20% of all patients. Similar neoplasms may also involve the brainstem, especially in the region of the area postrema, and the spinal cord (where they may be multiple) but supratentorial lesions are rare. The retinal neoplasms of von Hippel–Lindau disease are of the same histological type, and bilateral in 35% of cases (Lindau, 1957). Cases with multiple hemangioblastomas in the central nervous system are more likely to have a positive family history than those with solitary tumors (Russell and Rubinstein, 1977).

The systemic lesions which help to define the syndrome are usually benign cysts involving the kidneys or, less frequently, the pancreas. In addition, renal cell carcinoma has been reported in patients with a positive family history (Goodbody and Gamlen, 1974). Pheochromocytomas, which may occasionally be bilateral (Chapman and Diaz-Perez, 1962; Nibbelink *et al.*, 1969), and clinically inapparent islet cell tumors of the pancreas have been reported in some families (Probst *et al.*, 1978; Hull *et al.*, 1979).

The occurrence of central neuroepithelial tumors in the context of von Hippel–Lindau disease would seem to be exceptional. There is a single case report (Pearl *et al.*, 1981), of an intraventricular neuroblastoma in such a patient.

Tuberous sclerosis

Of the three phacomatoses considered in this review, tuberous sclerosis is the least likely to show evidence of central nervous system neoplasia. Like the other phacomatoses, the disorder is inherited as an autosomal dominant trait, while the majority of cases are sporadic. The responsible gene, therefore, may display a high rate of spontaneous mutation. The main clinical features include mental retardation, seizures, and the characteristic hamartomatous skin lesions of adenoma sebaceum, all of which become apparent in childhood.

The proliferative central nervous system lesions include multiple cortical tubers and the subependymal glial nodules described as 'candle gutterings'. These lesions are generally considered to be hamartomatous. In addition, an important CNS component of the disease is the presence of various and widely distributed cytological anomalies involving the morphology, alignment, and intercellular relationships of cortical neurons and glia, often accompanied by abnormalities in cortical lamination.

The cortical tubers usually form relatively well-defined sclerotic superficial cerebral masses that are composed of atypical neuronal and glial elements which expand, disrupt and frequently interrupt the normal cortical lamination. They show on the whole little tendency to enlarge or undergo malignant transformation, although the possibility that they may give rise to gangliogliomas has been suggested in those rare cases in which a massive unilateral ganglioglioma has been interpreted as a 'forme fruste' of the disease (Davis and Nelson, 1961).

By contrast, the subependymal nodules, which may include multiple glial elements but are most frequently almost entirely astrocytic, display a tendency to enlarge and may be the origin of subependymal giant-cell astrocytomas (Russell and Rubinstein, 1977). These tumors, which are relatively benign and circumscribed, cause symptoms by producing ventricular obstruction, typically in the region of the foramen of Monro, the symptoms of hydrocephalus generally appearing late in the first decade (Kapp *et al.*, 1967).

Although neoplasms of the central nervous system are considered to be comparatively rare in tuberous sclerosis (Critchley and Earl, 1932), series have been reported in which their incidence ranges from 5 to 10% (Kapp *et al.*, 1967). In addition to the subependymal giant-cell astrocytomas, which are by far the most frequent tumor type encountered in the disease, other glial tumors have, exceptionally, been reported. These include retinal gliomas, glioblastoma multiforme (Padmalatha *et al.*, 1980), ependymoma and diffuse gliomatosis of the cerebral hemispheres (Russell and Rubinstein, 1977).

Anomalies of visceral organ systems occur as part of the tuberous sclerosis complex. Most frequent are lesions in the kidneys, which occur in 50 to 90% of cases. They are most often of hamartomatous nature and composed of variable amounts of adipose, smooth muscle, and vascular elements. Malignant transformation to sarcoma was said to have been noted in these lesions (Critchley and Earl, 1932; Moolten, 1942) but these were later reclassified as most probably benign angiomyolipomas (Bennington and Beckwith, 1975). Cardiac rhabdomyomas are present in about 25% of cases of tuberous sclerosis and, less frequently, pulmonary cystic hamartomas composed of fibromyomatous elements, or cystic skeletal radiological anomalies in the distal extremities (Donegani *et al.*, 1972).

Other neoplasms with a genetic pattern

Genetic factors may play a role in a few of the nervous system neoplasms that do not form part of the phacomatoses. In most of these examples, familial cases have a greater tendency to multiple neoplasms than non-familial ones, and the best example of these is the retinoblastoma. This neoplasm appears to have a pattern of dominant transmission, although a multiple mutation hypothesis has been proposed (Knudson, 1971, 1975). Of all cases 25 to 30% are bilateral and, not infrequently, more than one tumor is present in the same eye. When familial cases only are considered, 70% of the patients have bilateral tumors and these children also have a high risk of developing additional primary malignancies, especially osteosarcomas (Meadows *et al.*, 1977; François, 1977). Some of these, however, may be related to radiation therapy (see below).

Of particular interest is the recently recorded association of bilateral retinoblastomas with pineoblastoma in children (Bader *et al.*, 1982) and 13 such cases were reported. The suggestion has been made that in these cases which are hereditary, simultaneous or consecutive neoplastic transformation takes place both in the retinoblasts of the retina and in pineal parenchymal cells, which phylogenetically are of photosensory receptor origin. The term 'trilateral retinoblastoma' has been suggested for these patients, with the following hypotheses being put forward to account for tumour multiplicity: (1) a pleiotropic effect of the retinoblastoma gene; (2) different tumor patterns occurring with different alleles of the gene; and (3) interaction between the retinoblastoma gene and environmental factors, either radiation- or virus-mediated, on one or more of the other host genes.

A further variant of the association has been the occurrence of cases which present with a retinoblastoma-like tumor in the suprasellar or parasellar region before the discovery of an intraocular retinoblastoma. Related to this intriguing association is the observation that pineoblastomas occurring in children in the absence of ocular retinoblastomas may exceptionally show, at their primary site of origin, microscopic evidence of photoreceptor differentiation characteristic of retinoblastoma (Rubinstein, 1982).

Neuroblastoma originating in the adrenal medulla or in the sympathetic chain has been reported to be multiple in some familial cases (Knudson, 1975), and examples of congenital bilateral neuroblastomas have been described (Willis, 1967). Other neoplasms that have sometimes been reported as familial and multiple include pheochromocytomas (Tisherman *et al.*, 1962; Cushman, 1962) and some of these cases appear to form part of the multiple endocrine neoplasia syndrome.

The association of solitary nervous system neoplasms with non-nervous system tumors has also been described in other hereditary syndromes. The multiple endocrine neoplasia syndrome (see Chapter 10) may be considered in this group. Glioblastoma and cystic cerebellar astrocytoma have been reported to occur in such a setting (Warner, 1973). Turcot's syndrome consists of familial intestinal polyposis with gliomas, usually glioblastoma multiforme (Turcot *et al.*, 1959; Baughman *et al.*, 1969). Finally, the nevoid basal cell carcinoma syndrome has been associated with cerebellar medullo-blastoma (Neblett *et al.*, 1971).

NON-HEREDITARY MULTIPLE NEOPLASMS

The incidence of multiple primary nervous system neoplasms occurring without evidence of a hereditary predisposition cannot be estimated reliably, but is distinctly uncommon. It has been documented largely through individual case reports but the data on gliomas are exceptional because of the number of series in which multiple tumors of that type have been noted. Some remarks on the nature and merits of the available data are pertinent. Studies from large referral centers (Deen and Laws, 1981; Meadows *et al.*, 1977) and population-based data (Schoenberg *et al.*, 1975) show that multiple neurogenic tumors are distinctly rare.

In reported cases, evidence of multiplicity is based partly on surgical biopsy material and partly on radiological findings, but particularly in the context of multiple gliomas, only careful autopsy examination is acceptable in view of the manifold ways in which these tumors may disseminate throughout the central neuraxis. Many of the data on multiple tumors are derived from case reports. While providing important clinical insights, these reports cannot address in a meaningful way the statistical significance of the reported associations. In the absence of information on the expected frequency of a particular association, biological significance is often implied from the presence of an unusual clinical feature such as the occurrence of a tumor at an unexpected age or in a particular location.

The basis of such an implication may be fragile. Even in those instances in which data on the frequency of different neoplasms are available, the data may be biased by patient referral patterns and variable autopsy rates at reporting institutions, as pertinently analysed by Schoenberg and Myers (1977). Few population-based data are available for either single or multiple tumors. Thus, while many combinations of multiple neoplasms have been reported, the significance of many of these associations remains a matter of speculation.

Multiple gliomas

Autopsy data report a small percentage of multiple gliomas, with a wide range extending from 0.9 to 10% in different series (Batzdorf and Malamud, 1963). These multiple tumors are often regarded as evidence of multifocal neoplastic transformation (multicentric) rather than truly multiple. The majority are malignant astrocytomas or glioblastomas and, in most cases, each of the tumors is of the same histological type and presumed to have arisen at approximately the same time. Moertel *et al.* (1961) found the percentage of multiple gliomas to be three times as high in females but most other studies suggest a slight preponderance in males (Courville, 1936; Batzdorf and Malamud, 1963). The majority of these tumors are diagnosed in the middle decades.

The cerebral hemispheres are most often affected, but a few examples in which one tumor occurred in a cerebral hemisphere and the other in the cerebellum, have been reported (Solomon *et al.*, 1969). In general the principal clinical features of these multicentric gliomas cannot be distinguished from those of their solitary counterparts. However, they may have a relatively shorter duration of symptoms and thus are occasionally referred to as 'acute' brain tumors (Manuelidis and Solitare, 1971).

Other gliomas in which multiplicity has been documented include astrocytomas lacking malignant histological features, but these are exceptional. Courville (1936) found only one example of multiple astrocytomas with benign microscopic features among 21 cases of multiple gliomas. None was found by one of us (LJR) in a series of 173 cerebral gliomas of astrocytic type, in which 4 cases were found to be multiple (3 glioblastomas and 1 anaplastic pilocytic astrocytoma). Solomon *et al.* (1969) cite a single case of multiple oligodendrogliomas.

Multiple ependymomas have been mentioned above in relation to their occurrence in central neurofibromatosis, but are exceptional in the absence of that condition. Multiple subependymomas are occasionally encountered, and have been observed by one of us (LJR) in three instances: in association with a choroid plexus papilloma of the cerebellopontine angle in an 18-year-old girl; in association with a chronic granular ependymitis due to a protracted cryptococcal meningitis of several years' duration in a 59-year-old male; and in association with long-standing hydrocephalus secondary to a diffuse primary leptomeningeal melanomatosis in a 41-year-old male.

Multiple subependymomas have also been reported to occur in association with the presence of heterotopic leptomeningeal glial tissue (Ho, 1983). While these lesions may not infrequently behave as symptom-producing and space-occupying neoplasms (Scheithauer, 1978), their mode of development may be diverse. Some examples may be of hamartomatous nature, a view supported by their occasional occurrence in identical twins (Clarenbach *et al.*, 1979). Others, as in some of the cases examined by one of us in which multiplicity was the dominant feature, may be of reactive origin secondary to long-standing hydrocephalus or chronic ependymitis: microscopically these lesions closely resemble the ependymal granulations that typically accompany chronic low-grade ventricular inflammation.

Multiple papillomas of the choroid plexus have been reported (Ray and Peck, 1956; Laurence, 1974). In some of these cases, the choroid plexus lesions represent examples of diffuse enlargement and villous hypertrophy rather than well-defined neoplasms. Some of these have been reported to be congenital and all have been associated with marked hydrocephalus, attributable to overproduction of cerebrospinal fluid rather than to ventricular obstruction of cerebrospinal fluid flow.

Multiple gliomas of different histological types have been documented in a small number of case reports. Most frequently, concurrent glioblastomas and astrocytomas have been recorded, but multiplicity may involve gliomas of any histological type, either concurrently or consecutively (Manuelidis and Solitare, 1971).

The patterns of growth and spread of gliomas, particularly of their malignant forms, add considerable difficulty in the evaluation of their multiplicity. Diffuse and multifocal spread often involves wide areas of the neural parenchyma and may extensively implicate the ventricular system and craniospinal leptomeninges. Because of this, the distinction between multiple primary neoplasms and multiple metastatic deposits may be established with certainty only after meticulous post-mortem study. Even with these reservations in mind, it is clear from several large series that gliomas which may be either multicentric or truly multiple do occur, and their frequency is in the range of 2 to 4% (Batzdorf and Malamud, 1963; Manuelidis and Solitare, 1971; Russell and Rubinstein, 1977).

Multiple tumors arising from elements covering the neuraxis

These neoplasms include meningiomas, Schwannomas, and their malignant forms. With the exception of meningiomas, multiplicity of these tumor types is extremely rare in the absence of neurofibromatosis. Kepes (1982) reports that 2 to 6% of patients with meningiomas harbor multiple tumors which are usually of the same histological subtype. Occasionally multiplicity is considerable, as detailed elsewhere (Russell and Rubinstein, 1977).

Multiple Schwannomas are exceptional in the absence of other manifestations of neurofibromatosis. One example involving both trigeminal nerves displayed malignant histological features (Liwnicz, 1979). Since sarcomas of the nervous system are rapidly growing tumors that may disseminate widely throughout the subarachnoid space, true multiplicity is difficult to prove.

Nervous system tumors of diverse histologic origin

The combination of neuroepithelial and non-neuroepithelial neoplasms of the nervous system is detailed in a large number of single case reports and in reports embodying a small number of cases. Most commonly it involves the association of meningiomas with various types of glioma (Madonick *et al.*, 1961). In a more recent review of 18 years' experience at the Mayo Clinic, Deen and Laws (1981) found 18 cases of multiple tumors of different histological types. In 15 of these, a combination of meningioma and glioma was observed, and in 9 the two tumors were contiguous. The most frequent glioma was an astrocytoma. In most cases, the meningioma was considered to be an incidental finding.

Meningioma has also been reported in association with glioblastoma (Manuelidis and Solitare, 1971) and with oligodendroglioma (Gass and Van Wagenen, 1950). The two tumors have been reported to occur either simultaneously or consecutively (Fisher, 1968; Deen and Laws, 1981). In a more specific consideration of the ability to diagnose clinically the simultaneous presence of a glioma and of a meningioma, Marra *et al.* (1977) were able to compile only 19 cases from the literature.

There seems little doubt that the relatively infrequent concomitant or consecutive development of these two fairly common types of intracranial tumor is most likely based on chance. However, the ability of one tumor to incite in the adjacent tissues reactive changes that may carry a potential for malignant transformation, is a hypothesis that has often been raised. From the morphological viewpoint, it is contended to be operative only in a different type of neoplastic proliferation occurring within the central nervous system, namely in the mixed gliomas and sarcomas.

Mixed tumors of the central nervous system(gliosarcomas and sarcogliomas)

The possibility of reactive neoplastic transformation must include a consideration of mixed intracranial tumors composed of both glial and mesenchymal elements. The existence of such mixed or composite tumors, partly glioblastoma and partly sarcoma, is well recognized, and their development constitutes the most convincing evidence so far for at least biclonal transformation of cells of different lineage within the central nervous system.

According to Foulds (1940), mixed or combined tumors fall into three types: collision, composite, and dependent. Collision tumors are formed by independent primary tumors apposed to each other and intermingling only at their junction. Composite tumors result from the concurrent participation of both the parenchyma and the stroma in the neoplastic process. In dependent tumors, secondary neoplastic change occurs in the stroma or in the adjacent and included host tissue.

The existence of dependent or consequential tumors in the central nervous system has been brought to light in several studies published by others and ourselves (Feigin *et al.*, 1958; Rubinstein, 1956). Feigin has emphasized the type of mixed glioma and sarcoma (gliosarcoma) in which an exuberant vascular endothelial and fibroblastic proliferation occurs in the stroma of a malignant glioma, proceeding to the formation of a sarcomatous component (Feigin and Gross, 1955; Feigin *et al.*, 1958; Morantz *et al.*, 1976). This development has been estimated to occur in 8% of all glioblastomas. Previous studies (Rubinstein, 1956; Rubinstein, 1964; Lalitha and Rubinstein, 1979), have described the development of mixed sarcoma and glioma (sarcoglioma) in which the gliomatous component is distributed peripherally in relation to a more centrally situated malignant meningioma or intracerebral sarcoma. This type of mixed neoplasm is characterized by the presence of gradual transitions from reactive to frankly neoplastic astrocytes.

Until recently, the mechanisms accounting for this secondary neoplastic development were a matter of speculation, although the respective forms of mixed glioma and sarcoma showed transitional morphological features between vascular endothelial proliferation and angiosarcomatous transformation, or from atypical hyperplastic and hypertrophic reactive astrocytosis to the development of an invasive glioma. The hypothesis of horizontal transmission of malignancy to putatively normal differentiated stromal cells has now gained support from the demonstration in different laboratories, that activation of transforming genes may be induced by the DNA of various human neoplasms and result in the *in vitro* transfer of genetic information coding for malignant transformation in mouse fibroblasts (Pulciani *et al.*, 1982). Induction of mouse sarcoma after transplantation of a human ovarian cystadenocarcinoma in athymic nude mice has also been reported (Goldenberg and Pavia, 1982), thus demonstrating that the phenomenon may occur *in vivo*.

The gliosarcomas and sarcogliomas differ from the intracranial collision tumors in which different neoplastic elements have arisen either independently or conjointly, and either remain separated by a zone of reactive astrocytosis or demonstrate an intermingling that is restricted to a narrow zone of juxtaposition in which no gradual transition is seen from hyperplasia to frank neoplasia (Mayo and Barron, 1966; Whitcomb and Tennant, 1966). A review of these collision tumors by Mayo and Barron (1966) has identified 33 such cases, but no clear distinction is made in that review between the different forms of mixed or combined tumors that may originate in the neural parenchyma.

SECOND NEOPLASMS AS A SEQUEL OF THERAPY

Neoplasia is being recognized with increasing frequency as a possible sequel of chemotherapy or radiation therapy. At present there is no evidence that chemotherapy plays a role in the induction of neoplasms arising from primarily neural tissues but the increased risk of central nervous system lymphomas in iatrogenically immunosuppressed patients is now well recognized (Hoover and Fraumeni, 1973).

Therapeutic radiation given to the central nervous system has been recognized for many years as a potential risk of subsequent new tumor induction. While the number of reported cases is small, the occurrence of unusual tumors within the field of radiation therapy; often following high doses of radiation and a significant latent interval, is a feature that supports the significance of the postulated association (Hutchinson, 1976). A number of cases of intracranial sarcoma are reported following cranial radiation for another type of intracranial tumor, and have usually been classified as fibrosarcomas, although malignant fibrous histiocytomas have also been described (Gonzalez-Vitale *et al.*, 1976).

A number of features common to many of the reported cases serve to define the clinical setting in which these tumors are most apt to arise. The initially treated neoplasm is often a benign tumor of which pituitary adenoma is the most frequent example (Waltz and Brownell, 1966), but other tumors have included ependymoma, glioblastoma, and optic nerve glioma (Noetzli and Malamud, 1962). Soloway (1966), on the other hand, described 25 cases of retinoblastoma in which 3 developed carcinoma and 22 developed sarcoma. Among the latter, the most frequently found were osteogenic sarcomas (nine cases) and fibrosarcomas (six cases). In all these examples of post-radiation sarcoma, the radiation dose tends to be usually well above 3000 rad. The time interval between radiation and the development of the sarcoma has ranged from 2 to 20 years, with the average interval being approximately 11 years (Powell *et al.*, 1977).

Similar observations have been reported on the occurrence of meningiomas following cranial radiation (Waga and Handa, 1976; Watts, 1976). Not surprisingly, some have been malignant (Waga and Handa, 1976). Cases in which meningiomas have developed in young patients have served to strengthen the putative causal relationship to radiation (Watts, 1976).

A recent addition to the list of neurogenic neoplasms that may be induced as a sequel of radiation therapy is neurofibrosarcoma. Ducatman and Scheithauer (1983) reported a series of 12 patients from the Mayo Clinic records in whom a neurofibrosarcoma originated in an area that had been previously radiated, usually for malignant disease. The initially radiated neoplasms included various carcinomas and two examples of optic nerve or chiasmatic glioma. Of the 12 patients 7 were cases of von Recklinghausen's disease, including the two with a glioma of the anterior optic pathways. The mean latency period between radiation and the clinical occurrence of the neurofibrosarcoma was 15.6 years, ranging from 5 to 26 years.

These observations are important in that they not only document the development of a neurogenic sarcoma as a possible post-radiation risk, but present this risk in the clinicopathological context of a hereditary disease characterized by tumor multiplicity, and one in which neoplastic transformation may, therefore, be genetically determined in addition to being the expression of random somatic mutations. Since genetic cell marker studies have shown that the neurofibromas of von Recklinghausen's disease are of multiple-cell origin (the minimal starting number of neoplastic cells in a given neurofibroma has been estimated to be no less than 150, according to Fialkow *et al.*, 1971), the subjection of an individual with a clinically apparent or a family history of neurofibromatosis to prophylactic or therapeutic radiation may, therefore, increase the burden of risk carried by that patient in so far as the development of a malignancy is concerned.

It is only relatively recently that gliomas have been reported as a possible complication of radiation. Experimentally, glioblastomas have appeared in monkeys three to five years after proton radiation (Haymaker *et al.*, 1972). The reported post-radiation gliomas in man have so far been almost all malignant astrocytomas or glioblastomas. Chung *et al.* (1981) collected nine cases from the literature dating back to 1960, with a post-radiation interval ranging from 1 to 26 years. They reported an additional case of a glioblastoma arising in a seven-year-old male who presented five years after prophylactic treatment with radiation and intrathecal methotrexate for acute lymphocytic leukemia. Another report documents the occurrence of a spinal cord glioblastoma following mediastinal radiation for Hodgkin's disease (Clifton *et al.*, 1980).

We have recently examined an example of a malignant astrocytoma of the occipital lobe that arose 25 years after radiation directed to a choroid plexus papilloma of the fourth ventricle. The report, by Kleriga *et al.* (1978), of the development of a malignant cerebellar astrocytoma at the site of a medulloblastoma treated 11 years earlier also raises the suspicion of an astrocytic malignancy induced by radiation, although other hypotheses explaining the development of a second tumor in that case merit consideration without, however, resolving the issue.

The possibility has been raised by Averback (1978) that a mixed sarcoma and glioblastoma might occasionally be a sequel of therapeutic radiation to the head. In view of the relatively short interval reported between the exposure to radiation and the development of a new intracranial tumor (one year), and the discrepancy in one patient between the sites of origin of the first and of the second neoplasm, such a hypothesis rests on a fragile basis.

ASSOCIATION WITH NON-NERVOUS SYSTEM NEOPLASMS

Limited data are available on the association of primary tumors of the nervous system with other primary neoplasms. In a large study reporting the occurrence of second malignant tumors in children, nine histologically unspecified brain tumors were observed as second primaries in a population of 14,610 children with a variety of initial primary neoplasms. In two of these nine patients the initial neoplasm was also in the brain (Miké *et al.*, 1982).

Conversely, patients whose first neoplasm occurred in the brain had a relatively low risk of developing a second neoplasm, except for those with retinoblastoma, where the risk is relatively high (Meadows *et al.*, 1977;

François, 1977; Miké *et al.*, 1982). The second tumors outside the nervous system include mostly sarcomas, most frequently osteogenic sarcomas and rhabdomyosarcomas. Therapeutic maneuvers such as radiation could play a role in the development of these second primary tumors (Li, 1977).

Data on the association of primary nervous system tumors with common neoplasms of adult life have been obtained from the study of a tumor registry. Schoenberg *et al.* (1975) found that meningiomas occurred in association with breast cancer at a frequency in excess of that predicted by chance association but no other significant associations were identified. They suggest that meningiomas, like some breast cancers, may be hormone-sensitive thus accounting for their concurrence and it is noteworthy that estrogen and progesterone receptors have been identified in some meningiomas (Kepes, 1982). The association between the two tumors has been confirmed by others (Mehta *et al.*, 1983), but further information is needed to establish both the statistical and the biological importance of these observations (Smith *et al.*, 1978). There appears to be some statistical evidence, based on the examination of autopsy material, that meningiomas may also be associated with other extraneural malignancies, in particular gastrointestinal tumors (Bellur *et al.*, 1979).

CONCLUSION

Apart from hereditary factors, only radiation exposure is sufficiently well documented to be considered an important risk factor in the iatrogenic development of nervous system tumors. The suspicion that hormonal influence may be important in the development of some meningiomas has been raised and requires further evidence. Finally, the activation of transforming genes is perhaps a useful hypothesis in the case of multicentric neoplasms and of neoplasms composed of histogenetically different cell types.

Some of the ways in which genetic influences are expressed have been discussed in relation to the phacomatoses. Perhaps more intriguing than the type of transmission pattern operative in these genetic syndromes, is the suggestion of a high degree of gene mutability in the light of the high proportion of sporadic cases. The role of tissue growth factors, such as nerve growth factor in neurofibromatosis, may be anticipated to be important in our future understanding of the expression of these genetic traits.

The risk of radiation-induced oncogenesis is discussed. As therapeutic and prophylactic radiation have become the standard treatment for many forms of cancer and the survival of cancer patients continues to improve, radiation-induced neoplasms may be expected to occur with increasing frequency in the years ahead. A similar danger may apply in the case of hormone-dependent neoplasms in view of the increasing use of hormonal preparations in the last two decades. Although some are hormone-sensitive, an increased incidence of meningiomas has not been reported as a long-term complication of the use of these agents (Green, 1977).

REFERENCES

Alliez, J., Masse, J-L., and Alliez, B. (1975). Tumeurs bilatérales de l'acoustique et maladie de Recklinghausen observées daus plusieurs générations. *Revue neurologique*, **131**, 545.

Averback, P. (1978). Mixed intracranial sarcomas: rare forms and a new association with previous radiation therapy. *Annals of Neurology*, **4**, 229.

Bader, J. L., Meadows, A. T., Zimmerman, L. E. *et al.* (1982). Bilateral retinoblastoma with ectopic intracranial retinoblastoma: trilateral retinoblastoma. *Cancer Genetics and Cytogenetics*, **5**, 203.

Batzdorf, U., and Malamud, N. (1963). The problem of multicentric gliomas. *Journal of Neurosurgery*, **20**, 122.

Baughman, F. A., List, C. F., Williams, J. R. *et al.* (1969). The glioma–polyposis syndrome. *New England Journal of Medicine*, **281**, 1345.

Bellur, S. N., Chandra, V., and McDonald, L. W. (1979). Association of meningiomas with extraneural primary malignancy. *Neurology*, **29**, 1165.

Bennington, J. L., and Beckwith, J. B. (1975). *Tumors of the kidney, renal pelvis, and ureter.* (Fascicle 12) *Atlas of tumor pathology*, Second Series. Washington DC: Armed Forces Institute of Pathology.

Borit, A., and Richardson, E. P., Jr. (1982). The biological and clinical behaviour of pilocytic astrocytomas of the optic pathways. *Brain*, **105**, 161.

Chapman, R. C., and Diaz-Perez, R. (1962). Pheochromocytoma associated with cerebellar hemangioblastoma. Familial occurrence. *Journal of the American Medical Association*, **182**, 1014.

Chung, C. K., Stryker, J. A., Cruse, R. *et al.* (1981). Glioblastoma multiforme following prophylactic cranial irradiation and intrathecal methotrexate in a child with acute lymphocytic leukemia. *Cancer*, **47**, 2563.

Clarenbach, P., Kleihues, P., and Metzel, E. (1979). Simultaneous clinical manifestation of subependymoma of the fourth ventricle in identical twins. *Journal of Neurosurgery*, **50**, 655.

Clifton, M. D., Amromin, G. D., Michael, C. P. *et al.* (1980). Spinal cord glioma following irradiation for Hodgkins' disease. *Cancer*, **45**, 2051.

Courville, C. B. (1936). Multiple primary tumors of the brain: review of the literature and report of twenty-one cases. *American Journal of Cancer*, **26**, 703.

Critchley, M., and Earl, C. J. C. (1932). Tuberose sclerosis and allied conditions. *Brain*, **55**, 311.

Cushman, P., Jr. (1962). Familial endocrine tumors. Report of two unrelated kindred affected with pheochromocytomas, one also with multiple thyroid carcinomas. *American Journal of Medicine*, **32**, 352.

Davis, R. L., and Nelson, E. (1961). Unilateral ganglioglioma in a tuberosclerotic brain. *Journal of Neuropathology and Experimental Neurology*, **20**, 571.

Deen, H. G., and Laws, E. R. (1981). Multiple primary brain tumors of different cell types. *Neurosurgery*, **8**, 20.

Delleman, J. W., DeJong, J. G. Y., and Bleeker, G. M. (1978). Meningiomas in five members of a family over two generations, in one member simultaneously with acoustic neurinomas. *Neurology*, **28**, 567.

Donegani, G., Grattarola, F. R., and Wildi, E. (1972). Tuberous sclerosis. Bourneville disease. In *Handbook of clinical neurology* Vol. 14 (eds P. Vinken and G. Bruyn). Amsterdam: North-Holland Publishing Company, p. 340.

Ducatman, B. S., and Scheithauer, B. W. (1983). Post-radiation neurofibrosarcoma. *Cancer*, **51**, 1028.

Eldridge, R. (1981). Central neurofibromatosis with bilateral acoustic neuroma. *Advances in Neurology*, **29**, 57.

Fabricant, R. N., and Todaro, G. J. (1981). Increased serum levels of nerve growth factor in von Recklinghausen's disease. *Archives of Neurology*, **38**, 401.

Fabricant, R. N., Todaro, G. J., and Eldridge, R. (1979). Increased levels of nerve growth factor cross-reacting protein in central neurofibromatosis. *Lancet*, **1**, 4.

Feigin, I. H., and Gross, S. W. (1955). Sarcoma arising in glioblastoma of the brain. *American Journal of Pathology*, **31**, 633.

Feigin, I., Allen, L. B., Lipkin, L., and Gross, S. W. (1958). The endothelial hyperplasia of cerebral blood vessels with brain tumors, and its sarcomatous transformation. *Cancer*, **11**, 264.

Fialkow, P. J., Sagebiel, R. W., Gartler, S. M., and Rimoin, D. L. (1971). Multiple cell origin of hereditary neurofibromas. *New England Journal of Medicine*, **284**, 298.

Fisher, R. G. (1968). Intracranial meningioma followed by a malignant glioma. *Journal of Neurosurgery*, **29**, 83.

Foulds, L. (1940). Histological analysis of tumors. A critical review. *American Journal of Cancer*, **39**, 1.

François, J. (1977). Retinoblastoma and osteogenic sarcoma. *Ophthalmologica*, **175**, 185.

Gardner, W. J., and Turner, O. (1940). Bilateral acoustic neurofibromas. *Archives of Neurology and Psychiatry (Chicago)*, **44**, 76.

Gass, H., and Van Wagenen, W. P. (1950). Meningioma and oligodendroglioma adjacent in the brain. *Journal of Neurosurgery*, **7**, 440.

Glushien, A. S., Mansuy, M. M., and Littman, D. S. (1953). Pheochromocytoma: its relationship to the neurocutaneous syndromes. *American Journal of Medicine*, **14**, 318.

Goldenberg, D. M., and Pavia, R. A. (1982). *In vivo* horizontal oncogenesis by a human tumor in nude mice. *Proceedings of the National Academy of Sciences USA*, **79**, 2389.

Gonzalez-Vitale, J. C., Slavin, R. E., and McQueen, J. D. (1976). Radiation induced intracranial malignant fibrous histiocytoma. *Cancer*, **37**, 2960.

Goodbody, R. A., and Gamlen, R. T. (1974). Cerebellar hemangioblastoma and genito-urinary tumours. *Journal of Neurology, Neurosurgery and Psychiatry*, **37**, 606.

Green, T. H. (1977). *Gynecology: essentials of clinical practice*. Boston: Little, Brown, p. 586.

Grossman, M., and Melmon, K. L. (1972). Von Hippel–Lindau disease. In *Handbook of clinical neurology*, Vol. 14 (eds P. Vinken and G. Bruyn). Amsterdam: North-Holland Publishing Company, p. 241.

Haymaker, W., Rubinstein, L. J., and Miquel, J. (1972). Brain tumors in irradiated monkeys. *Acta Neuropathologica*, **20**, 267.

Ho, K. L. (1983). Concurrence of subependymoma and heterotopic leptomeningeal neuroglial tissue. *Archives of Pathology and Laboratory Medicine*, **107**, 136.

Hochberg, F. H., DaSilva, A. B., Caldabini, J., and Richardson, E. P. Jr. (1974). Gastrointestinal involvement in von Recklinghausen's neurofibromatosis. *Neurology*, **25**, 1144.

Hoover, R., and Fraumeni, J. F. (1973). Risk of cancer in renal transplant patients. *Lancet*, **2**, 55.

Hope, D. G., and Mulvihill, J. F. (1981). Malignancy in neurofibromatosis. *Advances in Neurology*, **29**, 33.

Hull, M. T., Warfield, K. A., Muller, J., and Higgins, J. F. (1979). Familial islet cell tumors in Von Hippel–Lindau's disease. *Cancer*, **44**, 1523.

Hutchinson, G. B. (1976). Late neoplastic changes following medical irradiation. *Cancer*, **37**, 1102.

Kanter, W. R., Eldridge, R., Fabricant, R. *et al.* (1980). Central neurofibromatosis with bilateral acoustic neuroma: genetic, clinical and biochemical distinctions from peripheral neurofibromatosis. *Neurology*, **30**, 851.

Kapp, J. P., Paulson, G. W., and Odom, G. L. (1967). Brain tumors with tuberous sclerosis. *Journal of Neurosurgery*, **26**, 191.

Kepes, J. J. (1982). *Meningiomas: Biology, pathology and differential diagnosis*. New York: Masson Publishing Co., pp. 17–19, 26–28.

Kleriga, E., Sher, J. H., Nallainathan, S. K. *et al.* (1978). Development of cerebellar malignant astrocytoma at site of a medulloblastoma treated 11 years earlier. *Journal of Neurosurgery*, **49**, 445.

Knudson, A. G. (1971). Mutation and cancer: statistical study of retinoblastoma. *Proceedings of the National Academy of Sciences USA*, **68**, 820.

Knudson, A. G. (1975). The genetics of childhood cancer. *Cancer*, **35**, 1022.

Lalitha, V. S., and Rubinstein, L. J. (1979). Reactive glioma in intracranial sarcoma: a form of mixed sarcoma and glioma ('sarcoglioma'). Report of eight cases. *Cancer*, **43**, 246.

Laurence, K. M. (1974). The biology of choroid plexus papillomas and carcinoma of the lateral ventricle. In *Handbook of clinical neurology*, Vol. 17 (eds P. J. Vinken and G. W. Bruyn). Amsterdam: North-Holland Publishing Company, p. 555.

Li, F. P. (1977). Second malignant tumors after cancer in childhood. *Cancer*, **40**, 1899.

Lindau, A. (1957). Capillary angiomatosis of the central nervous system. *Acta Genetica et Statistica Medica*, **7**, 338.

Liwnicz, B. H. (1979). Bilateral trigeminal neurofibrosarcoma. *Journal of Neurosurgery*, **50**, 253.

Lukash, W. M., Morgan, R. I., Sennett, C. P., and Nielson, O. F. (1966). Gastrointestinal neoplasm in von Recklinghausen's disease. *Archives of Surgery*, **92**, 905.

Madonick, M. J., Shapiro, J. H., and Torack, R. M. (1961). Multiple diverse primary brain tumors. *Neurology*, **11**, 430.

Manuelidis, E. E., and Solitare, G. B. (1971). Glioblastoma multiforme. In *Pathology of the nervous system*, Vol. 2. (ed. J. Minckler). New York: McGraw-Hill, p. 2026.

Marra, A., Ramponi, G., and Grimaldi, G. (1977). Simultaneous occurrence of right supratentorial meningioma and glioblastoma multiforme. *Acta Neurochirurgica*, **36**, 83.

Mayo, C. M., and Barron, K. D. (1966). Concurrent glioma and primary intracranial sarcoma. *Neurology*, **16**, 662.

Meadows, A. T., D'Angio, G. J., Miké, V. *et al.* (1977). Patterns of second malignant neoplasms in children. *Cancer*, **40**, 1903.

Mehta, D., Khatib, R., and Patel, S. (1983). Carcinoma of the breast and meningioma. Association and management. *Cancer*, **51**, 1937.

Melmon, K. L., and Rosen, S. W. (1964). Lindau's disease: review of the literature and study of a large kindred. *American Journal of Medicine*, **36**, 595.

Miké, V., Meadows, A. T., and D'Angio, G. J. (1982). Incidence of second malignant neoplasms in children: results of an international study. *Lancet*, **2**, 1326.

Moertel, C. G., Dockerty, M. B., and Baggenstoss, A. H. (1961). Multiple primary malignant neoplasms: III. Tumors of multicentric origin. *Cancer*, **14**, 238.

Moolten, S. E. (1942). Hamartial nature of the tuberous sclerosis complex and its bearing on the tumor problem. *Archives of Internal Medicine*, **69**, 589.

Morantz, R. A., Feigin, I., and Ransohoff, J. (1976). Clinical and pathological study of 24 cases of gliosarcoma. *Journal of Neurosurgery*, **45**, 398.

Moyes, P. D. (1968). Familial bilateral acoustic neuroma affecting 14 members from four generations. *Journal of Neurosurgery*, **29**, 78.

Neblett, C. R., Waltz, T. A., and Anderson, D. E. (1971). Neurological involvement in the nevoid basal cell carcinoma syndrome. *Journal of Neurosurgery*, **35**, 577.

Nibbelink, D. W., Peters, B. H., and McCormick, W. F. (1969). On the association of pheochromocytoma and cerebellar hemangioblastoma. *Neurology*, **19**, 455.

Noetzli, M., and Malamud, N. (1962). Postirradiation fibrosarcoma of the brain. *Cancer*, **15**, 617.

Padmalatha, C., Haruff, R. C., Ganick, D., and Hafez, G-R. (1980). Glioblastoma multiforme with tuberous sclerosis. *Archives of Pathology and Laboratory Medicine*, **104**, 649.

Pearl, G. S., Takei, Y., Stefanis, G. S., and Hoffman, J. C. (1981). Intraventricular neuroblastoma in a patient with von Hippel–Lindau's disease. *Acta Neuropathologica*, **53**, 253.

Powell, H. C., Marshall, L. F., and Ignelzi, R. J. (1977). Post-irradiation pituitary sarcoma. *Acta Neuropathologica*, **39**, 165.

Probst, A., Lotz, M., and Heitz, Ph. (1978). Von Hippel–Lindau's disease, syringo-myelia, and multiple endocrine tumors: a complex neurocristopathy. *Virchows Archiv (Pathologic Anatomy and Histology)*, **378**, 265.

Pulciani, S., Santos, E., Lauver, A. V. *et al.* (1982). Oncogenes in human tumor cells: molecular cloning of a transforming gene from human bladder carcinoma cells. *Proceedings of the National Academy of Sciences USA*, **79**, 2845.

Ray, B. S., and Peck, F. C., Jr. (1956). Papilloma of the choroid plexus of the lateral ventricles causing hydrocephalus in an infant. *Journal of Neurosurgery*, **13**, 405.

Reese, A. B. (1956). *Tumors of the eye and adnexa.* (Fascicle 38) *Atlas of tumor pathology*, Section X. Washington DC: Armed Forces Institute of Pathology.

Rodriguez, H. A., and Berthrong, M. (1966). Multiple primary intracranial tumors in von Recklinghausen's neurofibromatosis. *Archives of Neurology*, **14**, 467.

Rubinstein, L.J. (1956). The development of contiguous sarcomatous and gliomatous tissue in intracranial tumours. *Journal of Pathology and Bacteriology*, **71**, 441.

Rubinstein, L. J. (1963). Tumeurs et hamartomes dans la neurofibromatose centrale. In *Les Phakomatoses cérébrales* (eds L. Michaux and M. Feld). Paris: SPEI Editeurs, p. 427.

Rubinstein, L. J. (1964). Morphological problems of brain tumours with mixed cell population. *Acta Neurochirugica* (Supplement), **10**, 141.

Rubinstein, L. J. (1982). Cytogenesis and differentiation of pineal neoplasms. *Human Pathology*, **12**, 441.

Russell, D. S., and Rubinstein, L. J. (1977). *Pathology of tumours of the nervous system*, 4th edn. London: Edward Arnold.

Saran, N., and Winter, F. C. (1967). Bilateral gliomas of the optic discs associated with neurofibromatosis. *American Journal of Ophthalmology*, **64**, 607.

Scheithauer, B. W. (1978). Symptomatic subependymoma. Report of 21 cases with review of the literature. *Journal of Neurosurgery*, **49**, 689.

Schoenberg, B. S., and Myers, M. H. (1977). Statistical methods for studying multiple primary malignant neoplasms. *Cancer*, **40**, 1892.

Schoenberg, B. S., Christine, B. W., and Whisnant, J. P. (1975). Nervous system neoplasms and primary malignancies of other sites: the unique association between meningiomas and breast cancer. *Neurology*, **25**, 705.

Smith, F. P., Slavik, M., and Macdonald, J. S. (1978). Association of breast cancer with meningioma. *Cancer*, **42**, 1992.

Solomon, A., Perret, G. E., and McCormick, W. F. (1969). Multicentric gliomas of the cerebral and cerebellar hemispheres. *Journal of Neurosurgery*, **31**, 87.

Soloway, H. B. (1966). Radiation-induced neoplasms following curative therapy for retinoblastoma. *Cancer*, **19**, 1984.

Tisherman, S. E., Gregg, F. J., and Danowski, T. S. (1962). Familial pheochromocytoma. *Journal of the American Medical Association*, **182**, 152.

Turcot, J., Despres, J. P., and St. Pierre, F. (1959). Malignant tumors of the central nervous system associated with familial polyposis of the colon: report of two cases. *Diseases of Colon and Rectum*, **2**, 465.

Waga, S., and Handa, H. (1976). Radiation-induced meningioma: with a review of the literature. *Surgical Neurology*, **5**, 215.

Waltz, T. A., and Brownell, B. (1966). Sarcoma: a possible late result of effective radiation therapy for pituitary adenoma. *Journal of Neurosurgery*, **24**, 901.

Warner, T. F. (1973). Rare combination of multiple primary tumours. *Journal of the Irish Medical Association*, **66**, 665.

Watts, C. (1976). Meningioma following irradiation. *Cancer*, **38**, 1939.

Whitcomb, B. B., and Tennant, R. (1966). Brain tumors of diverse germinal origin arising in juxtaposition. Report of three cases. *Journal of Neurosurgery*, **25**, 194.

Willis, R. A. (1967). *Pathology of tumours*, 4th edn. London: Butterworths, p. 856.

Chapter

17 G. W. MILTON and A. SCHEIBNER

Skin Cancers and Multiple Melanoma

The role of sunlight in the development of multiple squamous and basal cell carcinomas of the skin is widely accepted. Although exposure to sunshine is generally regarded as a factor also in the aetiology of cutaneous malignant melanoma, evidence for this in the literature is conflicting. This chapter examines the characteristics of multiple malignant melanoma, and its association with multiple skin cancers in the same group of patients.

INCIDENCE OF MULTIPLE CUTANEOUS LESIONS

Multiple primary cutaneous melanoma is not a common condition, but in any large series of melanoma patients, a number will be found to have had more than one primary lesion. Veronesi *et al.* (1976) calculated that a patient with one melanoma is about 900 times more likely to develop a second primary melanoma, than is an individual in general to develop a melanoma.

The reported incidence of multiple primary melanoma varies from 1.28% (Pack *et al.*, 1952) to 5.3% (Moseley *et al.*, 1979). In our series of 3182 melanoma patients seen at the Melanoma Clinic at Sydney Hospital since 1951, 2.9% had more than one primary melanoma (Scheibner *et al.*, 1982). However, these figures come from special clinics which have a reputation for the treatment of melanoma, and they may not accurately reflect the incidence of multiple lesions among all patients with melanoma.

Queensland has the highest incidence of melanoma in the world and the Queensland Melanoma Project, documenting all the patients in that state, reported the incidence of multiple primary tumours as 3.9% in a series of 1444 melanoma patients (Beardmore and Davis, 1975). It is perhaps surprising that multiple primary melanomas are not more frequent in this series, if sunlight is an important contributing factor in the pathogenesis of the disease as is now becoming apparent from our experiments on human volunteers (Hersey *et al.*, unpublished data).

Basal cell carcinomas (BCC) and squamous cell carcinomas (SCC) of the skin are very frequently multiple, probably as a result of the field damage caused by solar radiation. Supporting evidence is the occurrence of both multiple BCC and SCC in areas of cutaneous solar degeneration, some patients having as many as 20 or more primary tumors, either sequentially or concurrently.

Factors contributing to multiple BCC or SCC formation, other than sun damage to skin, include arsenic administration, radiation skin damage, or immune suppression, e.g. following organ transplantation (Kinlen *et al.*, 1979). On the other hand, the appearance of multiple primary melanoma in immunosuppressed patients is rare, probably because of the high and rapid mortality caused by the original melanoma and/or the original disease process.

Multicentric origin for skin cancers occurs most frequently with BCC and SCC especially on badly sun-damaged skin. Multicentric primary melanoma is difficult to prove if the tumours arise close together, and in our opinion, true multicentric melanoma occurs in only two situations. Firstly, if a giant naevus becomes malignant, then malignant cells may be seen in several parts of the naevus at or about the same time. Secondly, melanoma of the oral mucosa appears in some cases to break out in different parts of the mucosa, with macroscopically benign or normal mucosa between patches of malignancy. These two forms of multiple primary melanoma are rare.

The manifestation of some forms of skin cancer, such as Bowen's disease, has been taken to imply that the patient has an internal malignancy (Graham and Helwig, 1959). There is no evidence to suggest that any form of melanoma (single or multiple primary) is related to the presence of an internal cancer.

However, patients who have a long survival after treatment for melanoma have a higher risk of developing an unrelated malignancy than members of the community at large (Boland *et al.*, 1976). In our series of 90 multiple primary melanoma patients, 7.8% of patients (two men and five women) developed second non-cutaneous, non-melanocytic malignancies (Table 1). All but one of these were diagnosed after removal of the first melanoma.

These findings are consistent with those of Bellet *et al.* (1977) who found that 8.2% of 281 patients with primary cutaneous melanoma had developed primary non-cutaneous, non-melanocytic malignant tumours. Fraser *et al.* (1971) suggest that this association with other neoplasms represents a lower resistance to tumour formation in patients with malignant melanoma.

Table 1 Non-cutaneous, non-melanocytic malignancies in multiple primary melanoma patients

Sex	Number of patients	Type of malignancy
M	1	Brain
M	1	Bladder
F	2	Ovary
F	1	Breast
F	1	Bowel
F	1	Pancreas

SUN EXPOSURE AND MULTIPLE CUTANEOUS LESIONS

Sunlight has long been suspected as an important causative factor in the pathogenesis of melanoma. We found that the skin of patients with multiple melanoma appeared to be more susceptible to sun damage than that of single primary melanoma patients. Although the proportion of men and women with multiple and single primaries who had experienced prolonged sun exposure in the past was almost identical (45% and 10%; 46% and 7% respectively; Table 2), nearly twice as many men with multiple primary lesions as men with single primary lesions had evidence of solar damage in the vicinity of the primary lesions (Table 2).

It is important to note that twice as many men (31%) and about three times as many women (24%) with multiple primary melanoma had had cutaneous squamous or basal cell carcinomas removed than did men and women with single primary lesions at the time of diagnosis of the first primary melanoma (15% and 7% respectively; Table 2). By August 1982, 56% of men and 39% of women with multiple primary lesions had developed cutaneous non-melanocytic malignancies.

The group of patients with multiple primary lesions who had had prolonged sun exposure in the past, had a still higher incidence of basal and squamous cell carcinomas treated prior to the diagnosis of their first melanoma (about 50% of the men and 60% of the women). Their average age was the same as that of the rest of the multiple primary patients (47 years for men and 42 years for women), which was almost identical to that for patients with a single lesion. These patients also had a slightly higher number of multiple primary lesions – an average of 2.40 per patient compared to 2.06 in the rest of the multiple primary lesion patients. Our figures also suggest that even in patients with a skin more prone to sun damage, it takes longer to develop a melanoma than it does a basal or squamous cell carcinoma.

Table 2   Sun exposure and skin lesions. Reproduced by permission of the
Australasian Journal of Dermatology

	Men		Women	
	Multiple lesions	Single lesions	Multiple lesions	Single lesions
Multiple pigmented naevi	42%	10%	42%	10%
Prolonged sun exposure in past	45%	46%	10%	7%
Evidence of solar damage in vicinity of primary lesions	45%	25%	6%	5%
SCC and/or BCC removed	31%	15%	24%	7%

We could not demonstrate any specific racial predisposition to multiple melanomas other than the general susceptibility of fair, blue-eyed people with Celtic ancestors, who reddened and burned easily after sun exposure. As described above, the skin of people who developed multiple primary melanoma appeared to be more susceptible to solar damage as evidenced by the increased number of BCC and SCC seen in these patients.

The male to female ratio in multiple primary patients was slightly higher than 1.0 (1.2 : 1.0), whereas in patients with a single melanoma, the sex incidence is equal. This slight difference could possibly be attributed to the greater number of men with sun-damaged skin who had experienced prolonged sun exposure in the past.

FAMILIAL FACTORS IN MULTIPLE MELANOMA

The tendency for multiple primary melanoma to run in families has been explained by Reimer *et al.* (1978) on the basis of heritable 'dysplastic naevi' which are susceptible to malignant degeneration. The term BK moles, so named after the two original kindreds B and K, is synonymous with familial dysplastic naevi. These naevi can also occur sporadically.

Present evidence suggests that the BK mole syndrome is inherited as an autosomal dominant. Reimer *et al.* (1978) identified this syndrome in 90% of patients with familial melanoma, in 56% of first degree relatives and in 9% of sporadic melanoma cases. As originally described by Clark (1976), these lesions differ from common acquired naevi in the that they are larger (5–15 mm), with an irregular outline, mottled or variegated colour, and a marked variability in appearance from lesion to lesion (Figures 1 and 2).

They are flat or slightly papular and numerous, ranging from less than 10 to more than 100 per person. They are found on both exposed and non-exposed skin, being most common on the trunk (particularly the back) in both men

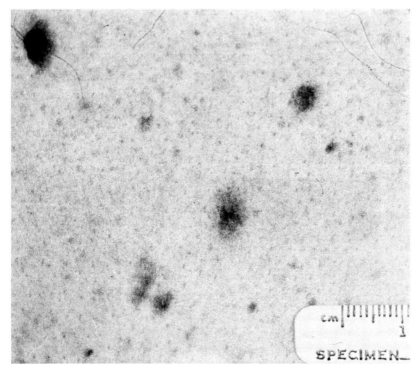

Figure 1   Dysplastic naevi. They are large, irregular in outline and mottled or variegated in colour. There is also variability from lesion to lesion.

and women (Figure 3). However, they can be found almost anywhere including the webs of fingers and feet, buttocks, and scalp. They are absent at birth but begin to appear in early childhood (four to five years) when they increase in number, but remain morphologically normal until adolescence.

In the adult, new dysplastic naevi continue to appear throughout life, even into the sixth and seventh decades. Although most of these naevi do not become malignant, they may experience a number of 'bursts' of activity during which several may become frankly malignant. Histologically, there is focal atypical melanocytic hyperplasia, dense dermal lymphocytic infiltration with fibroplasia, and new blood vessel formation.

Reimer *et al.* (1978) suggest that these sporadic and genetically determined precursors to melanoma may be influenced by ultraviolet light and possibly also by hormonal changes or alterations in host immunity. Patients with these naevi develop their melanomas at a young age, and have a higher frequency of multiple primary tumours than do patients with non-familial melanoma (Anderson, 1971). Reimer *et al.* (1978) found 44% had more than one primary melanoma.

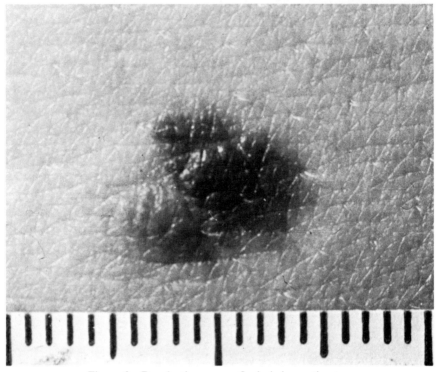

Figure 2   Dysplastic naevus. Scale is in centimetres.

A high proportion (42% of both men and women) of our 90 multiple primary melanoma patients reported 'multiple pigmented' naevi, compared to 10% of both men and women with single primary lesions (Table 2). In August 1982, we contacted 80 of these patients or their relatives and confirmed that these 'multiple pigmented' naevi did in fact fit the description of dysplastic naevi.

At the time of diagnosis of their first primary melanoma, 7.8% of our multiple primary patients reported a family history of melanoma compared to 8% of single primary patients. By August 1982, 16.2% of men and 12.8% of women with multiple primary melanoma had one or more close relatives with the disease, suggesting that the naevi in our series were sporadic rather than of the familial type. Whether sporadic or familial, this syndrome may serve as a cutaneous marker to identify those with a tendency to melanoma formation.

Malignant melanomas share common antigens with other solid tumours, and relatives of patients with certain tumours share common antigens and possibly blocking antibodies. It would follow that in malignant melanoma-prone families, similar and antigenically related tumours and even multiple

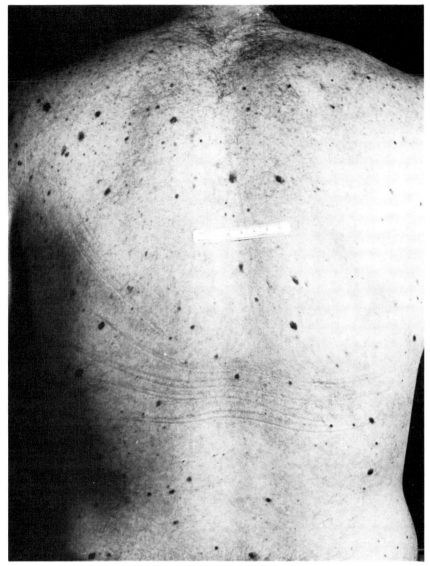

Figure 3   Dysplastic naevi back, in a 36-year-old Anglo-Saxon man.

primary malignant tumours could develop (Lynch *et al.*, 1975). As evidence of this, in our series of 90 multiple primary melanoma patients, we found that 35% of men and 33% of women with multiple primary melanoma had a relative with other primary non-cutaneous, non-melanocytic malignancies. Of this last group, 40% of the men and 20% of the women had a family history of melanoma as well, compared to only 7.8% of all 90 multiple primary melanoma patients.

CLINICAL FEATURES OF MULTIPLE MELANOMA

Although the majority of patients in our series had only two primary melanomas, the maximum noted was five and even larger numbers have been observed by other workers (Wallace *et al.*, 1973). Evidence that the patient has a second primary melanoma and not a metastasis is both clinical and histological. The clinical evidence is the patient's history indicating that the second (or subsequent) lesion was observed to have changed in the same way that the great majority of primary melanomas are observed to change as they evolve, i.e. the lesion grows horizontally at first and later vertically as a nodule.

At the same time as the lesion grows, it usually changes colour and becomes darker, while less frequent symptoms are itching and bleeding (Milton, 1972). The growth and colour changes will have been observed over a period of weeks or months. However, patients who have had one primary melanoma become adept at noticing changes in their 'moles'. As evidence for this, the history of change observed by the patient or his family was about half as long for the second and subsequent melanomas as it was for the first (Scheibner *et al.*, 1982). In addition, patients who have had one melanoma excised, become suspicious of 'moles' even before they can describe definite symptoms. Of second primary lesions 19% were asymptomatic as compared to 6% of the first primary lesions (Scheibner *et al.*, 1982).

The histology of first and second primary lesions tend to be similar (Table 3). In general, the second primary lesions were thinner than the first melanomas in both men and women (Figure 4), not only due to the earlier diagnosis of the second primary lesions but also because of a possible host immune response. This is shown by the increased evidence of regression in the second primary lesions, particularly if these were of the same histological type.

On clinical examination, the lesion resembles a primary melanoma and not a metastasis. The lesion is in the skin, not the subcutaneous tissue, and the benign precursor of either a junctional naevus or a dysplastic naevus (Clark *et al.*, 1978; Reimer *et al.*, 1978) is present at one edge of the melanoma. Events after the excision of the second (or subsequent) primary tumour also imply that it was not a metastasis because the patient may have no evidence of further dissemination.

The histological evidence for each lesion being an independent primary melanoma is that there is continuity between the malignant cells and those of the junctional layer of the adjoining skin or the precursor naevus (Allen and Spitz, 1953; McGovern *et al.*, 1973; Beardmore and Davis, 1975). This relationship between malignant cells and adjacent premalignant or non-malignant cells is usually easily observed unless the melanoma is large and ulcerated, in which case the continuity may be more difficult to demonstrate.

Table 3   Histology of multiple primary lesions. Reproduced by permission of the *Australian Journal of Dermatology*

| | Men | | Women | |
| | Multiple primary lesions | | Multiple primary lesions | |
	First	Second	First	Second
Histology same	67%		83%	
Histology different	33%		17%	
Superficial spreading melanoma	43%	81%	66%	78%
Nodular melanoma	40%	11%	28%	18.5%

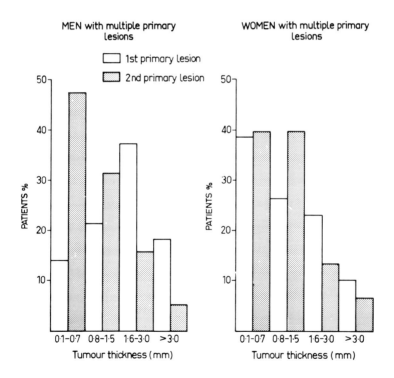

Figure 4   Tumour thickness of first and second primary melanoma lesions in 90 men and women with multiple primary melanoma. Reproduced by permission of *The Australian Journal of Dermatology*.

However, large, ulcerated, primary tumours have not been seen in any of our cases of multiple primary melanoma.

About one-third of the patients had multiple primary melanomas removed concurrently, and about half noted the second lesion within 12–18 months of the diagnosis of the first tumour (Figure 5). Unfortunately, the patient still has some risk of developing a second primary tumour many years after the first is excised. The longest time interval between two tumours in our series was 41 years and this patient eventually died of metastatic melanoma.

The anatomical distribution of multiple melanomas appears to be similar to that of single melanomas (Figure 6). In men, the commonest site was the trunk and in women it was the leg. It appears that the site of the second primary tumour occurs at random, because about half the second primary tumours occurred somewhere in the vicinity of the first lesion, while the remainder developed at distant sites (e.g. one on the leg and one on the back).

TREATMENT AND PROGNOSIS IN MULTIPLE MELANOMA

The treatment of patients with multiple primary melanoma has to be based on the characteristics of each lesion, especially the thickness, the site, and the presence of ulceration (Balch *et al.*, 1979). In addition, the age, general condition, and wishes of the patient have to be taken into account while planning treatment. Thin lesions (i.e. less than 1.0 mm) may be excised with a 2 cm margin and the wound closed. Thicker lesions are, in the present state of knowledge, probably best excised with a wider margin (3–5 cm) and the defect closed with a split skin graft (Milton, 1972).

Elective lymph node dissection in young and otherwise healthy patients with melanoma is still a matter of some debate. Veronesi *et al.* (1982) have evidence to suggest that this operation is not indicated, whereas Balch *et al.* (1979) and Milton *et al.* (1982) have shown that for patients with lesions of intermediate thickness (2–4 mm) there is a better chance of eradicating the disease if elective lymph node dissection is performed at the initial treatment. Fortunately, as stated above, most of the second or subsequent melanomas in any one patient are usually thin, so the question of whether or not to perform elective node dissection does not arise.

In women, the prognosis of those who had a single melanoma and those who had multiple melanomas is similar when taken from the time of diagnosis of the first primary lesion (Figure 7). However, men with more than one melanoma have a significantly better chance of surviving five years than those with a single tumour (Figure 7). We found no significant differences in histology or anatomical distribution of the first lesions, in men with either single or multiple primary lesions, to explain the difference in prognosis.

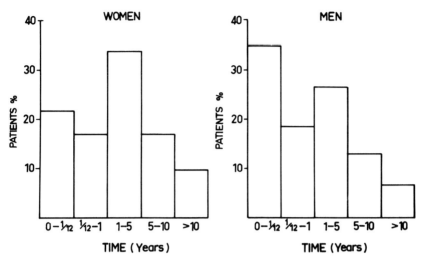

Figure 5   Time between excision of first and second primary melanoma lesions in 90 patients with multiple primary melanoma. Reproduced by permission of *The Australasian Journal of Dermatology.*

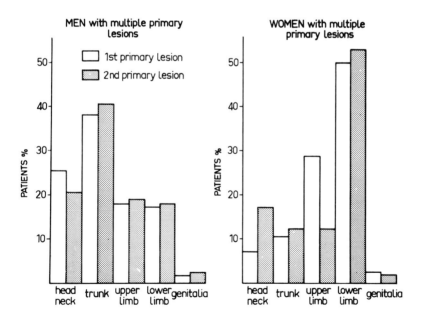

Figure 6   Anatomical distribution of multiple primary melanoma lesions in 90 patients with multiple primary melanoma. Reproduced by permission of *The Australasian Journal of Dermatology.*

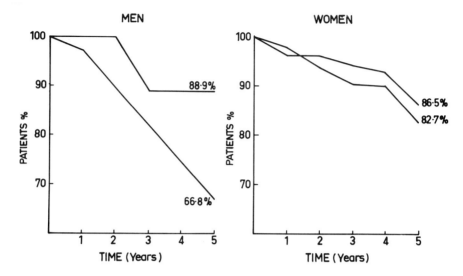

Figure 7   Cumulative survival rate in 49 men and 41 women with multiple primary melanoma (88.9% and 86.5%) taken from the time of diagnosis of the first primary melanoma, compared to survival rate in 372 men and 408 women with single primary melanoma (66.8% and 82.7%) first presenting with clinical Stage I malignant melanoma. Reproduced by permission of *The Australasian Journal of Dermatology.*

In patients with sun-damaged skin and dysplastic naevi, it is unnecessary, if not impossible, to remove all such naevi. Patients should be informed of what features to look for and be followed up every three to six months. Patients with one melanoma should be followed up frequently for the first three years, then annually for the rest of their lives, due to the ever-present risk of developing a second primary lesion.

CONCLUSION

Patients who have had one melanoma run a very much higher risk of developing a second primary melanoma, than does an individual, in general, of developing a melanoma. This risk is greatest in men who have sun-damaged skin and in patients with dysplastic naevi.

Patients suffering from multiple primary melanoma also show a very high incidence of multiple squamous or basal cell carcinoma of the skin. The evidence suggests that in patients with sun-damaged skin, it takes longer to develop a melanoma than it does to develop squamous or basal cell carcinoma.

Acknowledgements

We thank the editor, *Australian Journal of Dermatology*, for permission to reproduce Tables 1, 2, and 3 and Figures 4, 5, 6, and 7 which appear in Scheibner *et al.* (1982).

REFERENCES

Allen, A. C., and Spitz, S. (1953). Malignant melanoma. A clinicopathological analysis of the criteria for diagnosis and prognosis. *Cancer*, **6**, 1.

Anderson, D. E. (1971). Clinical characteristics of the genetic variety of cutaneous melanoma in man. *Cancer*, **28**, 721.

Balch, C. M., Murad, T. M. Soong, S. J. *et al.* (1979). Tumour thickness as a guide to surgical management of clinical stage I melanoma patients. *Cancer*, **43**, 883.

Beardmore, G. L., and Davis, N. C. (1975). Multiple primary cutaneous melanomas. *Archives of Dermatology*, **3**, 603.

Bellet, R. E., Vaisman, I., Mastrangelo, M. J., and Lustbader E. (1977). Multiple primary malignancies in patients with cutaneous melanoma. *Cancer*, **40**, 1974.

Boland, S. L., Shaw, H. M., and Milton, G. W. (1976). Multiple primary cancers in patients with malignant melanoma. *Medical Journal of Australia*, **1**, 517.

Clark, W. H. (1976). The origin of familial melanoma from heritable melanocytic lesions. Read before the American Academy of Dermatology, Chicago.

Clark, W. H. Jr., Reimer, R. R., Greene, M. H. *et al.* (1978). Origin of familial malignant melanomas from heritable melanocytic lesions. *Archives of Dermatology*, **114**, 732.

Fraser, D. G., Bull, J. G. Jr., Dunphy, J. E. (1971). Malignant melanoma and co-existing malignant neoplasms. *American Journal of Surgery* **122**, 169.

Graham, J. H., and Helwig, E. B. (1959). Bowen's disease and its relationship to systemic cancer. *AMA Archives of Dermatology*, **80**, 133.

Hersey, P., Hasic, E., Haran, G. *et al.* (1982). Effects of sunlight exposure on immune function in man. (To be submitted for publication).

Kinlen, L. J., Sheil, A. G. R., Peto, J., and Doll, R. (1979). Collaborative United Kingdom–Australasian study of cancer in patients treated with immunosuppressive drugs. *British Medical Journal*, **2**, 1461.

Lynch, H. T., Frichot, B. C., Lynch, P. *et al.* (1975). Family studies of malignant melanoma and associated cancer. *Surgery, Gynaecology and Obstetrics*, **141**, 517.

McGovern, V. J., Mihm, M. C., Bailly, C. *et al.* (1973). The classification of malignant melanoma and its histologic reporting. *Cancer*, **32**, 1446.

Milton, G. W. (1972). The diagnosis of malignant melanoma. In *Melanoma and skin cancer* (ed W. H. McCarthy). Sydney: Blight, Government Printer, p. 163.

Milton, G. W., Shaw, H. M., McCarthy, W. H. *et al.* (1982). Prophylactic lymph node dissection in clinical stage I cutaneous malignant melanoma: results of surgical treatment in 1319 patients. *British Journal of Surgery*, **69**, 108.

Moseley, H. S., Guiliano, A. E., Storm, F. K. *et al.* (1979). Multiple primary melanoma. *Cancer*, **43**, 939.

Pack, G. T., Scharnagel, I. M., and Hillyer, R. A. (1952). Multiple primary melanoma. A report of sixteen cases. *Cancer*, **5**, 1110.

Reimer, R. R., Clark, W. H. Jr., Greene, M. H. *et al.* (1978). Precursor lesions in familial melanoma. A new genetic preneoplastic syndrome. *Journal of the American Medical Association*, **239**, 744.

Scheibner, A., Milton, G. W., McCarthy, W. H. *et al.* (1982). Multiple primary melanoma – a review of 90 cases. *Australasian Journal of Dermatology*, **23,** 1.

Veronesi, U., Adamus, J., Bandiera, D. C. *et al.* (1982). Delayed regional lymph node dissection in stage I melanoma of the skin of the lower extremities. *Cancer*, **49,** 2420.

Veronesi, U., Cascinelli, N., Bufalino, R. (1976). Evaluation of the risk of multiple primaries in malignant cutaneous melanoma. *Tumori*, **62,** 127.

Wallace, D. C., Beardmore, G. L., and Exton, L. A. (1973). Familial malignant melanoma. *Annals of Surgery*, **177,** 15.

Risk Factors and Multiple Cancer
Edited by B.A. Stoll
© 1984 John Wiley and Sons Ltd.

Chapter

18 R. J. HEALD

Multiple Primary Cancers of the Bowel

INTRODUCTION

Bowel cancer provides a clue to the understanding of multiple primary cancers because of the evidence that it may arise in a pre-existing benign adenomatous polyp. Progression from polyp to cancer, and from localized cancer to infiltrating and then to metastasizing tumour, appears to be relatively slow and orderly.

It was thought in the first half of the century (Lockhart-Mummery and Dukes, 1939) that the presence of one bowel cancer had an inhibitory effect upon the development of another, but it later became clear that the incidence of multicentric colorectal primaries is higher than would be expected by chance (Warren and Gates, 1932; Slaughter, 1944). Wide variations in the incidence are quoted in the literature, from 1.8% (Muller, 1930) to 9.8% (Brindley and Rico, 1952) of cases. At the Mayo Clinic, Moertel et al. (1958, 1961) reported the incidence of multicentric large bowel cancers to be 4.3% compared to the incidence of 5.1% for multiple primary cancer at all sites.

In recent years, an association of bowel cancer with primary cancer at other sites has also been recognized. In a series of 524 rectal cancers and 809 colon cancers (Adelstein et al., 1979), 5% colorectal double primaries (rather than the 1.3% expected by chance) occurred within the large intestine while 39 of the second cancers occurred at other sites (rather than the expected 22). Most significantly increased was the association between cancers of the colon and breast, between cancer of the rectum and gynaecological cancer and between rectal and prostatic cancers.

INCIDENCE OF MULTIPLE TUMOURS

The author has previously reviewed the records of St Mark's Hospital, London, for synchronous cancer of the bowel (Heald and Bussey, 1973), and for metachronous cancer of the bowel (Heald and Lockhart-Mummery, 1972). Of 4884 survivors from operations from cancers of the large bowel (apart from those associated with major polyposis or colitis), 83 of the operations (1.6%) were for second, i.e. metachronous growths. A second but synchronous growth was found at or within a month of operation in 157 patients (3%) – nearly double the incidence of metachronous cancer in the same series. However, the true incidence is probably even greater, since 18 of those classified as metachronous were certainly present at the time of the original operation. They were really 'missed synchronous' growths.

The true incidence of synchronous cancer was, therefore, about 3.5% (which accords with many other published series) and this is almost exactly the same figure as the cumulative long-term risk in our series of developing metachronous cancer. Thus, when we diagnose colonic or rectal cancer, there is a 3.5% risk that a second cancer is present at the same time, and if we cure the patient, there is a further 3.5% risk that another cancer will develop over the years.

Triple carcinoma was observed in less than 0.25% of all operations at St Mark's Hospital. The Mayo Clinic series (Agrez *et al.*, 1982) had a slightly higher incidence of third tumours in that 11% of those patients having surgery for metachronous tumours subsequently required operation for a third cancer.

Only the second of Bilroth's (1889) postulates is necessary for stating that two primary tumours coexist in the bowel (i.e. they can be clearly identified macro- and microscopically as arising in different locations). Histologically, most large bowel tumours have many similarities, although variations in the degree of differentiation are common within and between tumours. Similarly, metastases from one lesion are unlikely to be recognizably different from those of another. Distinguishing a second primary growth from local recurrence of a previously excised cancer is not usually difficult. The second primary arises on the mucosal surface of the bowel and invades outwards, i.e. it has a characteristic appearance both macro- and microscopically. Conversely even a small 'suture-line recurrence' usually appears to arise outside the bowel and only secondarily invades towards the lumen.

Timing, site, and stage

In the St Mark's series, the average interval between the first and second operations was just over 11 years. In the Mayo Clinic series (Agrez *et al.*, 1982) 50% of the patients had their second operations with 5.5 years of the first. The low incidence in the first five years probably reflects the selection of patients with a 'clean colon' by the first operation and by the exclusion of the 'missed synchronous' cancers. The subsequent rise in the incidence may simply be the result of increasing age of the survivors.

The site of second or subsequent cancers in the St Mark's series showed approximately the same pattern of distribution as did single cancers. However, in the Mayo Clinic series, the proportion of carcinomas in the right colon rose from 21% of first cancers to 48% of second lesions. It is clear that review of residual colonic mucosa must be *complete* to be of value.

It has been reported that the histopathological grade of the first growth in the St Mark's metachronous cancer series tended to be unusually favourable (Bussey *et al.*, 1971). This is probably because there are more long-term survivors from less malignant and less advanced growths, but does not necessarily imply an intrinsic tendency for multiple growths to be more benign. However, there is a suggestion that second growths appear somewhat more favourable in stage than would be expected in 'first-time' cancers. The higher proportion of 'A' tumours probably reflects the value of the clinic in detecting such lesions, as second tumours discovered presymptomatically tend to be more favourable than those with symptoms.

HIGH RISK FACTORS

Familial and genetic

In patients with minor polyposis or cancer occurring without polyps, only a minimal familial tendency can be demonstrated but a so-called 'cancer family syndrome' was studied extensively by Lynch *et al.* (1973). They showed an increased incidence of adenocarcinoma in certain families, usually manifest as colonic and endometrial cancers but sometimes as gastric and breast tumours. It is inherited as an autosomal dominant, and this rare syndrome is now well established as an example of genetically determined bowel cancer. In addition, close relatives of 'ordinary' bowel cancer patients are found to have a higher incidence of similar tumours than a control population. The figures vary from 3 to 10% and these high figures are not found in spouses. Thus, a genetic factor is probably present in most patients with a positive family history (see Chapter 9).

Patients affected by multiple cancers do not differ in age or sex distribution from those with single cancers. The average age in the St Mark's group was 65 years with a male : female preponderance of 4 : 3. This seems to argue against an increased genetic determination of multiple as against single cancer. On the other hand, when hundreds or thousands of adenomas occur in a teenager, conferring a high cancer risk before the age of 40, the condition is based on familial adenomatosis. This disease is passed on as an autosomal dominant to 50% of offspring of either sex and a genetic causation is readily apparent.

A further example of genetic causation is Gardner's syndrome, in which familial adenomatosis is associated with predisposition to mesenchymal tumours. These include osteomas of the jaw, epidermoid cysts, and a tendency to form desmoid tumours in the abdominal wall of retroperitoneum. There are also recorded examples of associated ampullary duodenal cancer and small bowel adenomas and carcinoids. The condition is rare but important because it illustrates a genetically determined predisposition to tumour formation both in colonic epithelium and in other epithelia and soft tissues. The approximately equal sex incidence implies an environmental cause, and the observed geographical incidence and dietary association suggest that faecal carcinogens may play a major part in causation.

The most obvious dietary difference between low incidence and high incidence bowel cancer populations is a reduction in dietary fibre and a consequent increase in transit times. Correlation of cancer incidence with transit times is, however, poor so that other factors presumably contribute. Search for the actual carcinogen points to the possibility of a bacterial degradation product of bile acids and a possible relationship with dietary fat or meat (see Chapter 6). The association of bowel cancer with breast cancer (Isa *et al.*, 1981) may have a genetic basis, although high fat consumption could provide an alternative explanation for this connection.

Association with benign disease

The association between adenomas and bowel cancer is well documented, and adenomatous polyps increase the risk of developing cancer by five times (Rider *et al.*, 1964). True adenomas are classified by the WHO as tubular, tubulovillous or villous, and range from the pedunculated 'raspberry on a stalk' (tubular) through a spectrum of intermediate types to the mass of 'seaweed' of the typical sessile villous papilloma. The epithelial cells of these neoplasms are tall and their nuclei larger and hyperchromatic. Dysplasia is said to be marked when nuclear pleomorphism, hyperchromatism and mitotic activity increase, and the cells become dissimilar to normal mucosa and less regularly arranged.

The criterion of change to carcinoma in an adenoma is that invasion of the muscularis mucosae by dysplastic cells is seen to have occurred, and in about 1 in 10 adenomas such malignant transformation can be demonstrated. This is very much size-related, ranging from a 1% chance for a tubular adenoma of less than 1 cm, to over 50% for a villous lesion of more than 2 cm.

All series of multiple cancers show a high incidence of associated benign tumours. Metaplastic polyps must be specifically excluded and rigid criteria applied to define an 'adenoma'. Villous lesions and 'intermediate' forms such as papillary adenoma are less prone to cause confusion since they are all clearly benign epithelial neoplasms of bowel mucosa. The terms 'polyp' and 'adenoma', on the other hand, continue to cause virtual chaos in the world literature.

In the St Mark's series, two-thirds of all multiple cancers showed evidence of associated benign lesions at a time which largely antedated the colonoscope. The true figures might, therefore, be even higher. More than one-half had adenomas and about one-tenth had villous lesions. This incidence is three times that found in resection specimens for single cancers, and more than ten times that in the population as a whole. In approximately one-quarter of these the malignancy was actually identified as arising within a pre-existing benign tumour.

The Mayo Clinic series (Agrez *et al.*, 1982) shows a similar trend but a lower figure (40%) for associated benign lesions. Furthermore, if adenomas are identified on an operation specimen in association with a cancer, Bussey *et al.* (1967) showed that the risk of developing a subsequent cancer was doubled. All this evidence links colorectal multiple malignancy with benign tumours of large bowel epithelium, and reinforces the observations of Morson (1974) that the adenoma–cancer sequence is important in the genesis of large bowel malignancy.

Association of colonic cancer with ulcerative colitis is well documented and has probably received more attention in the literature than is merited by its miniscule contribution to the problem of bowel cancer. It constitutes a negligible risk in the first 10 years of the disease but reaches 25–30% after 25 years (Lennard-Jones *et al.*, 1977). Endoscopic recognition of epithelial atypia (which may be focal or widespread) is important in the difficult decision of whether to perform prophylactic proctocolectomy.

According to Thompson and Pearlman (1982) one or more of the following risk factors are recognized in only 12–15% of patients with colorectal cancers: familial polyposis; previous polyps; inflammatory bowel disease; cancer family syndrome; family history of colonic cancers; previous colonic cancer; previous cancer of kidney, bladder or breast (? also prostatic or gynaecological cancer).

Thompson and Pearlman (1982) screened this high risk group for colorectal cancer while leaving the remainder of the population as controls. The percentage of A and B lesions in the high risk group was found to be 66% compared with 43% in the controls, and the percentage of inoperable cases 7% compared with 23% in the controls. However, the average age of onset was little different (60 years and 63 years respectively) despite the screening, and over 90% in the screened group had symptoms at the time of diagnosis. These figures are comparable with the St Mark's experience and support the idea that both screening and follow-up are valuable. Both series argue against the assertion that cancer in high risk groups is in any way more virulent than in low risk groups.

The basic problem remains that 85% of patients do not belong to a recognizable high risk group. There is some preliminary evidence that intestinal resections might predispose to colonic malignancy, and this provides a further group that might usefully be screened. Cholecystectomy patients also are alleged to have a higher risk, and if confirmed, would provide a sizable group for screening. There is no evidence that a procedure such as cholecystectomy is in itself a risk factor, but it is possible that the aetiological factors which cause gallstones may also be relevant in large bowel carcinogenesis (probably through the mechanism of fat metabolism).

MANAGEMENT OF MULTIPLE TUMOURS

For practical purposes the management of polyps is by endoscopic excision and that of cancer is by excision of the relevant segment of bowel with its mesentery. The extent of the operation when two growths have been discovered will be a matter for individual choice. St Mark's surgeons have elected to use a conservative approach, each growth being resected in a radical fashion but normal colon being retained where possible. Thus, right hemicolectomy and an anterior resection might be combined in a patient.

More extensive colonic resections have many advocates in the United States, since the cumulative risk that survivors will develop a metachronous growth rises from about 3.5% after resection of a single cancer to more than 8% after removal of two growths. But the time interval is around 13 years, and there is a strong argument for conservative surgery backed by careful follow-up. The increased morbidity (and perhaps mortality) or total colectomy must be weighed against the risk of developing a subsequent cancer which will have a very good chance of cure provided it is detected early.

Familial adenomatosis

This disease provides a perfect model for preventive cancer surgery and careful family tracing and screening. Adenomas are always found in the rectum so that the screening tool can be the sigmoidoscope. Barium enema and colonoscopy are both unnecessarily deterrent to younger brothers and sisters. Similarly, screening should not start until the mid-teens since the cancer risk is small before 25 though very high by 40.

The choice of operation also needs to take account of other family members' reaction to their elders undergoing permanent ileostomy. For this reason, the St Mark's policy has been to perform total colectomy and ileo-rectal anastomosis, and to fulgurate and continue careful observation of the rectum for life. Thomson (1983) has recently reported on the success of this policy of ileo-rectal anastomosis supplemented by stringent follow-up. Careful three to six month surveillance was carried out between 1948 and 1981, and 105 out of the 157 patients required a total of over 500 fulguration sessions. Only 10 have required abdomino-perineal resection and only 2 have so far died of carcinomatosis due to rectal carcinoma.

Compared with the cumulative cancer risk of 100% in untreated adenomatosis, the 25-year risk was approximately 10% in this series, although it may rise above this when the follow-up extends to 30–40 years. The timing of the operation should take regard of family circumstances and marriage plans, but should seldom be deferred beyond 30 years. Ileal pouches have made ileo-anal anastomosis a more acceptable operation, and some believe it is now the surgical procedure of choice for polyposis.

Follow-up and metachronous cancer

Detection of metachronous cancer is probably the most valuable aspect of a follow-up clinic and the colonoscope has revolutionized the routine examination. First class double contrast radiology can produce comparable pick-up rates for the larger lesions but the tiny adenoma is easily missed. Furthermore, the colonoscope is able to deal with the lesions as they are found. The examination is considerably facilitated by the removal of the sigmoid loop with straightening of the left colon which occurs after left colon or rectal excision.

The haemoccult slide test is of some value in detecting presymptomatic tumours, and most patients who have had major bowel surgery will comply with such examination annually. Colonoscopy probably does not need to be more frequent than once in two to three years since Morson (1971) showed that the polyp–cancer sequence is usually spread over many years. A good view of the whole colonic mucosa can lead to the assumption that the patient is 'safe' for a considerable time, but a *good* view is crucial. Again, a normal barium enema report is almost valueless unless the examination is a high grade double contrast examination.

Occasionally, colorectal tumours with rapid growth rates will appear which no practicable prevention routine is likely to detect, but it is reasonable to practise the following routine: annual consultation, physical examination and haemoccult test, plus colonoscopy or double contrast enema every two to three years.

The reverse argument was, however, propounded by Wangensteen (1943) and recently reiterated by Fagler and Welner (1980) and the extirpative approach finds wide acceptance by surgeons in the United States. They point to the ever-rising incidence of multiple lesions if they are searched for with the colonoscope, which they now regard as a mandatory pre-operative investigation. They would not hesitate to perform subtotal colectomy in every case of multiple malignancy, and imply that we should be moving towards subtotal colectomy for *every* colorectal cancer.

Few British surgeons accept these arguments as the long-term morbidity of ileo-anal anastomosis is unacceptably high. Ileal pouch operations to reduce stool frequency are gaining ground on both sides of the Atlantic, but they are formidable surgical undertakings and their widespread introduction outside centres of special interest would undoubtedly lead to fatalities. Furthermore, the stool frequency is an unacceptably high price to pay for the avoidance of stringent follow-up.

If the rectum, which can be readily visualized by the sigmoidoscope, can be left *in situ*, the argument for sacrificing the whole colon with two colon cancers is rather stronger. Even here British surgeons would argue that a functional price must be paid by the patient, while the colonoscope permits all the remaining mucosa at risk to be readily inspected. We remain conservative: each cancer should be managed as if it were a single lesion, and multiplicity constitutes an indication for rigorous follow-up.

Prognosis after treatment

For *synchronous* multiple cancers the operability rate of 82% for radical resections was higher than the St Mark's figure of 68% quoted for single rectal cancers over the same period though lower than current operability figures. The corrected five-year survival rate for radical resection was 66%. Thus, one can say that four of five patients were operable, and that two out of three of these were cured of both growths by the operation. These figures are certainly no worse than those in most comparable series of single cancers, and even suggest that a patient with two colorectal cancers fares slightly better than a patient with one.

Examination of the five-year survivals by stage demonstrates the expected distribution of cures, and patients with two Dukes' B or C growths do not show the adverse effect that might be expected if the malignant potentials of the two were to summate.

Similarly favourable information about the excised second tumours was obtained from the histopathological data in the St Mark's *metachronous* group. The actual five-year cumulative survival probability in the Mayo Clinic metachronous group was 50% for C tumours and 75% for B tumours while only 7 of the series of 62 had distant spread at the time of the second operation. These figures do not differ significantly from those expected for first cancers at the Mayo Clinic. The lower incidence of more advanced lesions at St Mark's may reflect follow-up activity which is geographically more difficult in the Mayo Clinic situation.

The nine cases of triple synchronous carcinoma in this series showed the same favourable trend. Four of the eight survivors lived for more than ten years, and the average survival time for all resections, including one classified as palliative, was seven years and eight months, which is almost exactly the average for single cancers.

TUMOURS OTHER THAN ADENOCARCINOMA

Since Lubarsch's account in 1888, the multicentricity of carcinoids of the small and large intestine has been widely recognized and its frequency varies between 20 and 40% of all cases of carcinoid tumour. Kothari and Mangla (1981) recently reviewed the associated tumours in a series of 96 gastrointestinal carcinoids and found 23 malignant neoplasms in 17 of the patients. They observed that appendiceal carcinoids have a very high tendency to be associated with malignant tumours elsewhere, and five appendiceal carcinoids were associated with no less than three endometrial cancers, two colonic cancers, and one gastric cancer. At the other end of the scale, the rectal carcinoid had no tendency to association with other cancers while the ileal lesions occupied an intermediate position with an incidence of 36%. In four patients death occurred as a result of metastasis of the other tumour before the carcinoid had spread.

Careful search must, therefore, be made for other tumours, particularly in the colon but also in other possible sites, in every case where a carcinoid tumour is detected other than in the rectum. Conversely the small intestine, which is not readily assessed pre-operatively should always be carefully examined at laparotomy prior to colorectal cancer surgery. There is one case on record of a carcinoid tumour occurring in association with Gardner's syndrome.

Other multiple tumours of the small intestine are rare although lymphomatous small bowel polyposis provides an occasional example of multiple small bowel tumours.

CONCLUSION

This review suggests that the prognostic significance of second and third lesions is no worse for the patient than a single bowel cancer, and that the main purpose of follow-up is to detect missed synchronous or metachronous lesions at an early stage. The observation that multiple synchronous lesions do not appear to summate in their malignant potential needs to be explained on a biological basis.

REFERENCES

Adelstein, P., Baldwin, J. A., and Fedrich, J. (1979). Cancers of the large bowel: associated disorders in individuals. *Cancer*, **43**, 2553.

Agrez, M. V., Ready, R., Ilstrup, D., and Beart, R. W. (1982). Metachronous colorectal malignancies. *Diseases of the Colon and Rectum*, **25**, 569.

Bilroth, H. (1889). *Die allgemeine chirurgische, Pathologie und Therapie*, Berlin: R. Reimer, p. 908.

Brindley, G. V., and Rice, J. S. (1952). Multiple primary malignancies of the large intestine. *Surgical Clinics of North America*, **32**, 1499.

Bussey, H. J. R., Wallace, M. H., and Morson, B. C.)1971). *Proceedings of the Royal Society of Medicine*, **60**, 208.

Fagler, R., and Weiner, E. (1980). Multiple foci of colorectal carcinoma: argument for subtotal colectomy. *New York State Journal of Medicine*, **80**, 428.

Heald, R. J., and Bussey, H. J. R. (1973). Clinical experience of St Mark's Hospital with multiple synchronous cancers of the colon and rectum. *Diseases of the Colon and Rectum*, **18**, 6.

Heald, R. J., and Lockhart-Mummery, H. E. (1972). The lesson of the second cancer of the large bowel. *British Journal of Surgery*, **59**, 16.

Isa, S. S., Attiyeh, F. F., and Quan, S. H. (1981). Double primary carcinoma of large bowel and breast. *Clinical Bulletin*, **11**, 22.

Kothari, T., and Mangla, J. C. (1981). Malignant tumours associated with carcinoid tumours of the gastrointestinal tract. *Journal of Clinical Gastroenterology*, **3** (Suppl. 1), 43.

Lennard-Jones, J. E., Morson, B. C., Ritchie, J. K. *et al.* (1977). Cancer in colitis: assessment of individual risks by clinical and histological criteria. *Gastroenterology*, **73**, 1280.

Lockhart-Mummery, H. E., and Fukes, C. E. (1939). Familial adenomatosis of the colon and rectum: relationships to cancer. *Lancet*, **2**, 586.

Lubarsch, O. (1888). Über den primaren krebs des ileum nebst bemerkungen uber das gleichzeitige vorkommen von krebs und tuberculose. *Virchows Archiv (Pathologic Anatomy and Histology)*, **111**, 280.

Lynch, H. T., Krush, A. J., Guirgis, H. (1973). Genetic factors in families with combined gastrointestinal and breast cancer. *American Journal of Gastroenterology*, **59**, 31.

Moertel, C. G., Bargen, J. A., and Dockerty, M. B. (1958). Multiple carcinomas of large intestine; review of literature and study of 261 cases. *Gastroenterology*, **34**, 85.

Moertel, C. G., Dockerty, M. B., and Baggenstoss, A. H. (1961). Multiple primary malignant neoplasms. *Cancer*, **14**, 221.

Morson, B. C. (1971). *Cancer of the bowel. Proceedings of the Royal Society of Medicine*, **64**, 959.

Morson, B. C. (1974). The polyp–cancer sequence in the large bowel. *Proceedings of the Royal Society of Medicine*, **67**, 451.

Muller, R. F. (1930). Über multiple nichtsystematisierte primare carcinome und ihre hanfigker. *Zeitschrift Krebsforsch*, **31**, 339.

Rider, J. A., Kirsner, J. B., Moeller, H. C., and Palmer, W. L. (1964). Polyps of the colon and rectum. *American Journal of Medicine*, **16**, 555.

Slaughter, D. P. (1944). Multiplicity of origin of malignant tumours; collective review. *International Abstract of Surgery*, **79**, 89.

Thomson, J. P. S. (1983). Paper read at the Section of Proctology, Royal Society of Medicine, London.

Thompson, J. S., and Pearlman, M. D. (1982). Cancer of the colon and rectum in high-risk patients. *Diseases of the Colon and Rectum*, **25**, 461.

Wangensteen, O. H. (1943). Primary resection of the colon – accompanying excision of carcinoma of the rectal ampulla. *Surgery*, **14**, 403.

Warren, S., and Gates, O. (1932). Multiple primary malignant tumours. *American Journal of Cancer*, **16**, 1358.

Risk Factors and Multiple Cancer
Edited by B.A. Stoll
© 1984 John Wiley and Sons Ltd.

Chapter

19 FRED ROSNER and HANS W. GRÜNWALD

Multiple Hemolymphatic Cancers

The association of two hemolymphatic neoplasms in the same patient is not rare and, although it may occur as a result of chance, evidence is increasing that both cancer treatment and host susceptibility may play a role. This chapter examines the appearance of second neoplasms (predominantly acute myelocytic leukemia or one of its variants) in patients being treated for multiple myeloma, Hodgkin's disease, non-Hodgkin's lymphoma, acute lymphoblastic and chronic lymphocytic leukemia, or myeloproliferative disorders. The frequency of second neoplasms, the factors that may be involved, and possible preventive measures are discussed.

MULTIPLE MYELOMA AND ACUTE LEUKEMIA

We have reviewed 145 reported cases of multiple myeloma associated with acute leukemia (Rosner and Grünwald, 1980a). The two diseases were either diagnosed simultaneously or within several months of each other in 19 cases and these are excluded from the analysis, as is also one patient whose diagnosis of leukemia could not be established with certainty. There remain 125 patients with multiple myeloma whose disease terminated in acute leukemia (72 men, 44 women, 9 of unspecified sex). The mean age at the time of diagnosis of multiple myeloma was 59 years, with a range of 26 to 81 years.

Treatment given for multiple myeloma is summarized as follows: 51 patients received melphalan therapy only for periods varying from 10 to 102 months (mean 40 months), and developed acute leukemia between 15 and 180 months (mean 51 months) after initiation of therapy. Thirty-six patients who were treated with melphalan for 14 to 100 months (mean 45 months) also received radiation therapy, 1400 to 6800 r, during the course of their multiple myeloma and developed acute leukemia 17 to 120 months (mean 54 months) from the beginning of treatment. Sixteen patients who were treated with other chemotherapy, mostly cyclophosphamide, procarbazine, and/or nitrosoureas, also received melphalan for 20 to 96 months (mean 51 months), and leukemia developed after 27 to 180 months (mean 65 months). In at least two patients, the development of acute leukemia appears to be associated with long-term cyclophosphamide therapy, while in 51 patients, the acute leukemia is clearly associated with or related to the melphalan therapy, since no other cytotoxic drug was given, nor was irradiation administered.

The morphologic type of acute leukemia is variously described as myeloblastic in 56 cases; monomyelocytic, monomyeloblastic, or myelomonocytic in 42 cases; erythroleukemia in 14 cases; monoblastic or monocytic in 4 cases; promyelocytic in 2 cases; erythromyelomonocytic in 1 case; lymphoblastic in 1 case; stem cell in 1 case; poorly differentiated in 1 case; undifferentiated in 1 case; megakaryocytic in 1 case; and reticulosarcoma cell leukemia in 1 case. Serum and/or urinary lysozyme was increased in at least 10 patients and normal in at least 4 patients. The immunoglobulin types of the multiple myeloma showed a distribution similar to that observed in large series of patients with multiple myeloma.

At least 40 patients had a pancytopenic preleukemic phase, and at least 19 patients had sideroblastic anemia, weeks or months before the development of frank acute leukemia. In some patients, various dyserythropoietic changes are described even in the absence of sideroblasts. This pancytopenic or sideroblastic preleukemic phase has only recently become recognized, and was rarely described prior to 1974 in patients with multiple myeloma terminating in acute leukemia. In some patients, specific mention is made of the absence of sideroblasts.

The outcome of the acute leukemia is nearly invariably fatal within days to weeks, or at most several months. Only two complete remissions of the leukemia have been described, and in many instances antileukemic therapy was considered futile and not administered. In those patients on whom autopsies were performed, acute leukemia was found in 37 instances and in 17 of these patients, residual myeloma was also observed. In two patients, amyloidosis was found at autopsy. Several of the patients had additional neoplasms found clinically or detected at autopsy.

Karyotypic analysis of peripheral blood and/or bone marrow cells at the time of acute leukemia was reported in 28 patients. In three patients showing simultaneous multiple myeloma and acute leukemia, the chromosomes showed normal findings. Of the 25 patients whose myeloma terminated in acute leukemia, 22 had abnormal karyotypes, mostly hypodiploidy but also hyperdiploidy with the not-infrequent occurrence of a marker chromosome.

The frequency of acute leukemia reported following treatment of multiple myeloma and related paraproteinemias has been variously reported as 0.6% (Marcovic *et al.*, 1974), 1.3% (Gonzalez *et al.*, 1977), 2.0% (Dubovsky and

Jacobs, 1974), 3.8% (Bergsagel *et al.*, 1979), and 7.0% (Law and Blom, 1977). Recently, Kyle (1982) described 17 cases of multiple myeloma terminating in acute myelocytic leukemia from the Mayo Clinic, and calcu lated the actuarial risk of developing acute leukemia at 5 and 10 years respectively, as 2.8% and 10.1%.

OTHER PARAPROTEINEMIAS AND ACUTE LEUKEMIA

There are 18 reported cases of Waldenström's macroglobulinemia associated with acute leukemia (Rosner and Grünwald, 1980a; Bergsagel, 1982). In six of these patients, both diseases occurred simultaneously or within a few months of each other, another patient developed hairy cell leukemia, and yet another received no cytotoxic therapy. Of the remaining 10 patients (3 myeloblastic, 4 myelomonocytic, 1 undifferentiated and 2 erythroleukemias), 7 are men, 2 are women and the sex is not noted in 1 patient. Their mean age at primary diagnosis ranged from 42 to 81 years (mean 65 years).

All received alkylating agents (4 melphalan, 4 chlorambucil, 1 cyclophos-phamide, and 1 melphalan, chlorambucil and cyclophosphamide), and de-veloped acute leukemia 8 to 168 months (mean 54 months) after initiation of therapy. In two patients, the leukemia was preceded by a period of pancy-topenia, with sideroblastic anemia in one. Serum and/or urinary lysozyme concentrations were increased in at least three patients. Two patients achieved brief partial, and another patient a complete, remission of the leukemia after specific antileukemic chemotherapy. The presence of acute leukemia was confirmed at autopsy in seven patients.

At least three cases of amyloidosis, two cases of scleromyxedema, two cases of monoclonal paraproteinemia, and one case of cold agglutinin disease treated with alkylating agents and terminating in acute myeloblastic leukemia, or one of its variants have been reported (Rosner and Grünwald, 1980a). One of the patients with monoclonal paraproteinemia had a pancytopenic period of one year with increased serum and urinary lysozyme levels prior to the development of acute myelomonocytic leukemia.

MULTIPLE MYELOMA AND OTHER HEMATOPOIETIC NEOPLASMS

Multiple myeloma and chronic lymphocytic leukemia in the same patient have been reported in at least 17 patients (Bergsagel, 1982). Hairy cell leukemia has also been described in association with multiple myeloma (Catovsky *et al.*, 1981) and macroglobulinemia (Golde *et al.*, 1977). In the latter case, hairy cells were shown by immunofluorescence to be producing monoclonal IgM, thereby substantiating the B lymphocyte derivation of the neoplastic cells.

Most authors emphasize the wide clinical and biologic spectrum of B-cell neoplasms, and consider the association of the two diseases in the same patient to be a clinical manifestation of closely related disorders arising from divergent differentiation from a common B-cell precursor, rather than a chance association. Recently, plasma cell myeloma in a patient with a cutaneous T-cell lymphoma was reported (Bryant *et al.*, 1982).

HODGKIN'S DISEASE AND ACUTE LEUKEMIA

The number of patients with Hodgkin's disease and acute leukemia reported in the literature up to July 1980 exceeds 300 (Grünwald and Rosner, 1982). We have examined various characteristics of these patients, including the stage and histopathology of the Hodgkin's disease and the type of treatment given. Our goals were to quantify the risk of acute leukemia developing after cure of Hodgkin's disease, and to attempt to find predictive parameters that might identify patients for whom the risk of leukemia developing is particularly high.

Approximately 90% of these patients had one of the varieties of myeloid (or 'non-lymphocytic') leukemia, that is to say types M_1 through M_6 of the FAB classification of acute leukemias (Bennett *et al.*, 1976). The relatively few patients with lymphoblastic, undifferentiated, or other types of acute leukemia (half of which were described as coincidental, initial, or autopsy findings) are excluded from the subsequent analyses. Also excluded are 4 patients in whom the diagnosis of Hodgkin's disease cannot be established with certainty, 3 patients in whom the diagnosis of acute leukemia is questionable, 11 patients with the simultaneous occurrence (within three months) of Hodgkin's disease and acute leukemia, and 50 patients where the case reports provide insufficient data for analysis.

There remain 216 individual patients with Hodgkin's disease whose disease terminated in acute myeloid leukemia: 116 are men, 96 are women, and the sex is not indicated in 4. The mean age at the time of diagnosis of Hodgkin's disease was 35.5 years (range 4–74 years). The mean interval from diagnosis of Hodgkin's disease to the development of acute leukemia was 73.4 months (range 9–222 months).

The histologic types of Hodgkin's disease are comparable with the expected frequencies in patients with this disease. The stage of the disease at the time of diagnosis of Hodgkin's disease is also fairly evenly distributed. Of the 216 patients 75% received both radiotherapy and chemotherapy. The mean duration from first exposure to radiation until the development of acute leukemia was slightly less than six years. The mean time from first exposure to drugs until the appearance of acute leukemia was only 4.6 years, probably reflecting the fact that chemotherapy is usually employed as the second modality of treatment, either immediately following radiation therapy or when relapse of the Hodgkin's disease occurs.

The type and frequency of radiation therapy administered suggest that amount, extent, and frequency of radiation play a significant role in the ultimate development of acute leukemia. Less than one-third of the irradiated patients received a single course of regional or extended field therapy, while two-thirds of the patients in whom acute leukemia developed were treated with multiple courses of therapy or total nodal irradiation.

The type, duration, and intensity of chemotherapy also seem to play a major role in the development of acute leukemia. Only one-fifth of the patients had less than eight months' drug exposure, either single or in combination. The great majority of patients received either prolonged maintenance treatment with one or more drugs or multiple courses of combination chemotherapy. With regard to the specific drugs used, the overwhelming majority of patients had received a MOPP-type combination of drugs with or without additional drugs. Only seven (4%) of the patients had not been exposed to alkylating agents and only 37 (21%) of the patients had not received procarbazine during their treatment.

When acute leukemia developed, there was no evidence of residual Hodgkin's disease in over two-thirds of the patients. In at least 73 patients (one-third of the total 216), a period of pancytopenia (and in some patients, bone marrow sideroblastosis) ranging from 1 to 35 months (mean 8.2 months) preceded the full clinical and hematologic expression of the acute leukemia. Among 49 patients in whom chromosomal analysis was reported at the time of acute leukemia, only 6 had normal karyotypes. More than half the patients received specific antileukemic chemotherapy and, in these, complete or partial remission was achieved in 25%. Several complete remissions lasting more than two years have been reported. Similar findings have recently been published by the Cancer and Leukemia Group B (Glicksman *et al.*, 1982), the Southwest Oncology Group (Coltman and Dixon, 1982), and the Danish Lymphoma Study (Pedersen-Bjergaard and Larsen, 1982).

Other types of acute leukemia may also rarely occur as terminal events following treatment of Hodgkin's disease. These include acute lymphoblastic leukemia (Saleem and Johnston, 1980), acute B-cell leukemia (Arkin *et al.*, 1981), atypical T-cell leukemia (Boucheix *et al.*, 1979), and Burkitt cell leukemia (Nassar *et al.*, 1982). Also reported is the occurrence of Hodgkin's disease during the course of acute lymphoblastic leukemia in remission (Woodruff *et al.*, 1977; Garwicz *et al.*, 1978; Wingen *et al.*, 1979).

Acute myeloid leukemia or one of its variants appears as a late complication of Hodgkin's disease or its treatment in up to 4.65% of cases (Borum, 1980; Brody and Schottenfeld, 1980) but in several large series, the figures are only 0.9% (Neufeld *et al.*, 1978), 1.0% (Jouet *et al.*, 1979), 1.1% (Svahn-Tapper *et al.*, 1976), 1.3% Kuse and Hausmann, 1977; Wolf *et al.*, 1979),

1.4% (Glicksman *et al.*, 1982), 1.5% (Larsen and Brincker, 1977), 1.7% (Toland *et al.*, 1978), and 2.0% (Cavallin-Stahl *et al.*, 1977). The experience at the Stanford University Medical Center (Coleman *et al.*, 1977, indicates that the actuarial risk of leukemia at five and seven years is 1.5% and 2.0%, respectively, following the diagnosis of Hodgkin's disease. The figure at seven years for patients receiving both irradiation and chemotherapy is 3.9%.

The proportion of patients developing leukemia is greater for series reported after 1970 than for those reported before that date (Brody and Schottenfeld, 1980). Crosby (1959) calculated the risk of leukemia developing in patients with Hodgkin's disease to be 10 times greater than that for normal individuals while Larsen and Brincker (1977) cited the risk to be 75 times greater than the expected one, based on Danish Cancer Registry Data. The Southwest Oncology Group experience (Toland *et al.*, 1978; Coltman and Dixon, 1982) shows the actuarial risk of developing leukemia at seven years to be 6.2% for patients receiving chemotherapy alone, 6.4% for combined modalities, and 7.7% for patients treated with salvage chemotherapy.

At the National Cancer Institute, DeVita *et al.* (1970) reported a 29-fold increased risk of leukemia in Hodgkin's disease patients treated with both intensive radiotherapy and intensive chemotherapy, over that calculated for a comparable normal population. The Cancer and Leukemia Group B reported (Glicksman *et al.*, 1982) a relative risk ratio of 133 and life-table estimate of 5.6%. The Finsen Institute in Copenhagen (Pedersen-Bjergaard and Larsen, 1982) cited an actuarial risk of acute leukemia of 3.9% at 5 years, and of 15.3% at 15 years, among 391 non-selected patients with Hodgkin's disease.

HODGKIN'S DISEASE AND OTHER HEMATOPOIETIC NEOPLASMS

There are at least 20 reported cases of non-Hodgkin's lymphoma developing after treatment for Hodgkin's disease (Rosner and Grünwald, 1983). Although there is a strong suspicion that non-Hodgkin's lymphoma following Hodgkin's disease occurs as a second neoplasm with greater frequency than would be expected by chance alone, it is premature to draw such a conclusion as there are too few reported cases. Hodgkin's disease has also been reported in association with chronic myelocytic leukemia (Swain *et al.*, 1971).

NON-HODGKIN'S LYMPHOMA AND ACUTE LEUKEMIA

In 1979, we reported 12 cases of non-Hodgkin's lymphoma associated with acute myeloblastic leukemia or one of its variants, and an additional 33 cases from the literature (Zarrabi *et al.*, 1979). The mean interval between the diagnosis of lymphoma and acute leukemia was 5.2 years. In five patients the two diseases occurred simultaneously or within six months of each other. All but 10 of the 45 patients received radiation therapy for their lymphoma, and 9 patients had either total nodal or total body irradiation or both. Eight patients received chemotherapy alone. No patient was untreated. Survival after the diagnosis of acute leukemia ranged from 3 days to 14 months, with a median of 3 months. Four patients achieved complete hematological remission following antileukemic therapy.

Since then, there have been reports of at least eight additional cases of non-Hodgkin's lymphoma terminating in acute myeloblastic leukemia or erythroleukemia (Carobell *et al.*, 1979; Dumont *et al.*, 1980; Herrmann *et al.*, 1980; Kauer *et al.*, 1981) and an additional patient with the simultaneous occurrence of both diseases. Another patient developed acute myelofibrosis three years after successful multimodality therapy of non-Hodgkin's lymphoma, and subsequently showed a gradual evolution into acute myeloblastic leukemia (Puckett and Cooper, 1981).

A unique case was reported of chronic myelocytic leukemia developing in a patient with non-Hodgkin's lymphoma treated with alkylating agents (Erskine *et al.*, 1977). These two diseases can also coexist unrelated to therapy (Wilson and Van Slyck, 1966). The leukemic phase of non-Hodgkin's lymphoma is part of the spectrum of the disease and does not represent transformation of the lymphoma into a new leukemia. This leukemic phase should not be confused with treatment-related acute myeloblastic leukemia discussed above.

ACUTE LYMPHOBLASTIC LEUKEMIA AND OTHER HEMATOPOIETIC NEOPLASMS

We recently reviewed the occurrence of second neoplasms in patients with acute lymphoblastic leukemia (Zarrabi *et al.*, 1983) and found 17 patients who developed acute myeloblastic leukemia or one of its variants. At least four of the patients were adults. In three instances, the acute myeloblastic leukemia was noted within six months of the diagnosis of acute lymphoblastic leukemia and the two leukemias are, therefore, considered coincidental or simultaneous occurrences. In the other 14 cases, the new leukemia developed 7 to 180 months (mean 38 months) after the initial leukemia. The new acute leukemia was myeloblastic in most cases but myelomonocytic in two cases and promyelocytic in one case. The new acute leukemia was confirmed morphologically and histochemically in nearly all instances.

All patients had received extensive chemotherapy. At least seven patients were also given cranial or craniospinal irradiation and two patients received organ (spleen, liver, and kidney) or mediastinal radiation, respectively. In six of seven cases where chromosome analysis was performed at the onset of the new leukemia, the karyotype was abnormal. Survival from diagnosis of the second leukemia ranged between four weeks and nine months. In the four cases where an autopsy was reported, there was no evidence of residual lymphoblastic leukemia. One other case of acute myelomonocytic leukemia developing in a patient with acute lymphocytic leukemia has been reported (Madoff et al., 1981).

There are 12 reported cases of acute lymphoblastic leukemia followed by chronic myelocytic leukemia (Zarrabi et al., 1983) and half of the patients were adults. All 12 patients received intensive chemotherapy for their acute leukemia and five also had cranial or craniospinal irradiation. The chronic leukemia developed after an interval of 2 to 60 months and was Philadelphia-chromosome-positive in seven cases. In one patient, the Ph[1] chromosome was present at the time acute leukemia was initially diagnosed but the patient did not develop typical clinical and hematological features of chronic myelocytic leukemia until three years later. Two patients, both Ph[1] negative, had juvenile chronic myelocytic leukemia.

In one patient, acute lymphoblastic leukemia recurred four months after the chronic leukemia was diagnosed and the patient died within a week. In two patients, the clinical, hematological, and cytogenetic features of chronic myelocytic leukemia occurred within a few months of the initial diagnosis of acute lymphoblastic leukemia, so that the authors suggest their patients may have originally presented as an unrecognized lymphoblastic crisis of chronic myelocytic leukemia.

Nineteen patients with acute lymphoblastic leukemia followed by lymphoma have been reported (Zarrabi et al., 1983). All eight patients (three adults and five children) who developed Hodgkin's disease achieved a complete remission of their acute leukemia. At least seven of the eight patients received cranial or craniospinal irradiation and combination chemotherapy, and developed Hodgkin's disease 10 to 29 months later. All eight patients also achieved a complete remission of their Hodgkin's disease following appropriate chemotherapy or radiotherapy. In one patient the acute leukemia recurred three years later and, at autopsy, there was evidence of acute leukemia but none of Hodgkin's disease.

Two patients developed non-Hodgkin's lymphoma. One was a child who died in complete remission 12 months after acute leukemia was diagnosed but in whom an intracerebral reticulum cell sarcoma was found unexpectedly at autopsy. The second was a four-year-old girl who had a 15-month remission from acute leukemia but then developed anaplastic histiocytic lymphoma. The lymphoma cells did not form rosettes with sheep erythrocytes nor did they show surface immunoglobulin. A complete response was achieved following nitrogen mustard, vincristine, procarbazine, and prednisone (MOPP) chemotherapy.

There are nine reported cases of acute lymphoblastic leukemia in association with histiocytic medullary reticulosis (Zarrabi et al., 1983). They ranged in age from 2 to 24 years (median 13.3 years). All were treated for their acute leukemia with combination chemotherapy and at least six of the nine also received cranial or craniospinal irradiation. The diagnosis of histiocytic medullary reticulosis was made at autopsy in three patients. All nine patients responded promptly to chemotherapy for their acute leukemia but within 3 to 8 months (median 4.8 months) developed rapidly-progressive histiocytic medullary reticulosis terminating in fever, sepsis, and death. In four patients, the acute leukemic lymphoblasts had T-cell surface markers and, in another patient, some of the leukemic cells had convoluted nuclear membranes, an observation interpreted to be characteristic of T-cell acute lymphoblastic leukemia.

CHRONIC LYMPHOCYTIC LEUKEMIA AND ACUTE LEUKEMIA

In 1977, we reviewed 31 proven cases of chronic lymphocytic leukemia terminating in acute leukemia (Zarrabi *et al.*, 1977). Not included were 10 additional reported cases where the two diseases were diagnosed simultaneously or within four months of each other, 10 cases where the diagnosis of chronic lymphocytic leukemia could not be substantiated due to lack of lymphocytosis in peripheral blood and bone marrow, and 6 cases that probably represent duplication of previously reported ones. Of the cases reviewed, 9 are men, 9 are women, and the sex is not indicated in the remaining 13 cases. At the time of diagnosis of chronic lymphocytic leukemia, the patients ranged in age from 38 to 89 years, with a mean of 64.6 years. The mean interval between the initial diagnosis and the occurrence of acute leukemia is 5.6 years.

The acute leukemia was variously described as lymphoblastic (10 cases), myeloblastic (4 cases), myelomonocytic (2 cases), 'acute' or 'acute terminal phase' (11 cases), and 1 case each of 'stem cell', 'acute plasma cell', 'undifferentiated', and 'erythroleukemia'. Twelve patients had received radioactive phosphorus therapy and eight patients received local or total body radiation. One additional patient had been exposed to numerous diagnostic X-rays. Chemotherapy used in these patients included chlorambucil (12 cases), prednisone (8 cases), and 1 case each of cyclophosphamide, vincristine, uracil mustard, and L-phenylalanine mustard.

Six patients received chemotherapy only and developed acute leukemia 1 to 8½ years later (mean 4.2 years). In addition, two patients received no therapy at all but developed acute leukemia 15 and 20 years after the original diagnosis. Since our 1977 report, additional cases of acute myeloblastic leukemia have been described in both treated (Sebahoun *et al.*, 1980; Stern *et al.*, 1981) and untreated (Hamilton, 1976; Lawlor *et al.*, 1979) patients with chronic lymphocytic leukemia. The incidence of acute leukemia occurring in patients with chronic lymphocytic leukemia varies from 0 to 6.9% in 11 large series, with an overall incidence of 1.7%.

CHRONIC LYMPHOCYTIC LEUKEMIA AND OTHER HEMATOPOIETIC NEOPLASMS

The association of chronic lymphocytic leukemia and multiple myeloma in 17 patients (Bergsagel, 1982) has already been mentioned above. The transformation of chronic lymphocytic leukemia to non-Hodgkin's lymphoma, the so-called Richter syndrome, is well known (Sebahoun *et al.*, 1980). The overlap between chronic lymphocytic leukemia and well-differentiated lymphoma wil not be discussed here since there is a wide clinical and biologic spectrum of B-cell neoplasms and two such neoplasms in the same patient may, in fact, be part of the spectrum of one B-cell precursor disorder.

It is outside the scope of this chapter to discuss the well-recognized increased incidence of second primary non-hematopoietic tumors (particularly of the lung, stomach, colon, and skin) in patients with chronic lymphocytic leukemia.

MYELOPROLIFERATIVE DISORDERS AND ACUTE LEUKEMIA

The term 'myeloproliferative disorders' was introduced (Dameshek, 1951) to describe a group of disorders characterized by varying degrees of overgrowth or abnormal growth of one or more cell lines of the bone marrow elements. There are well-known interrelationships of these disorders, such as the termination of polycythemia vera in myelofibrosis, the blastic transformation of chronic myelocytic leukemia, and the conversion of sideroblastic anemia or idiopathic myelofibrosis to acute myelocytic leukemia. Rarer interrelationships have been reported, such as idiopathic sideroblastic anemia terminating in acute myelofibrosis (Yeung and Trowbridge, 1977) and idiopathic myelofibrosis followed by acute lymphoblastic leukemia (Marino *et al.*, 1979).

These conversions and transformations are traditionally thought to be part of the natural history of these disorders. Recently, however, it has been suggested that the chemotherapy given for the initial myeloproliferative disorder may be responsible (at least in part) for the conversion to acute leukemia (Rosenthal and Moloney, 1977) or other myelodysplasia (Sultan *et al.*, 1981). Thus, chlorambucil-induced acute leukemia in polycythemia vera (Berk *et al.*, 1981) has been well documented. The substitution of busulfan for the chemotherapy of polycythemia has been suggested (Brodsky, 1982) although an erythroleukemia-like syndrome due to busulfan toxicity in polycythemia has been observed (Pezzinenti *et al.*, 1976).

FACTORS INVOLVED IN DEVELOPMENT OF SECOND NEOPLASMS

There is disagreement as to the mechanism of leukemogenesis or carcinogenesis involving drugs such as alkylating agents, nitrosoureas, and procarbazine. While Penn (1974, 1976, 1978) and Arsenau *et al.* (1977) believe that the immunosuppressive activities of cytotoxic drugs are primarily responsible for their carcinogenic effects, Schmähl (1977) suggests that chemical carcinogenesis is not related to the immune status of the host (see Chapter 4).

Patients with primary immunodeficiency disorders have a sharply increased incidence of malignant neoplasms (Walpole, 1958), an incidence as high as 10,000 times that of the general age-matched population (Gatti and Good, 1971). The most common types of such neoplasms are lymphoreticular (Louie *et al.*, 1980) and epithelial tumors and leukemias (Kersey *et al.*, 1973). Iatrogenic suppression of immunity in the course of management of patients with organ homografts is also associated with an increased frequency of malignant neoplasms (Penn, 1977).

Although it is highly likely that the therapy administered to patients with malignant neoplasms is directly related to the subsequent development of acute leukemia or other second neoplasm such as lymphoma, sarcoma or bladder cancer, it is by no means certain. One can argue that the natural history of the primary neoplasm is such that a small number of patients will terminate in acute leukemia. No one questions the correctness of such an assertion in the myeloproliferative syndromes where polycythemia vera, agnogenic myeloid metaplasia and thrombocythemia may all occasionally terminate as acute leukemia. In chronic myelogenous leukemia, the vast majority of patients die of acute leukemic transformation and a similar change may occur in multiple myeloma, Hodgkin's disease and non-Hodgkin's lymphoma.

One might postulate that acute leukemia as a late manifestation of these neoplasms was rare until a few years ago because patients with these neoplasms did not live long enough to develop leukemia as part of the natural history of their disease. Since the introduction of melphalan for the treatment of multiple myeloma (Waldenström, 1964) and the four drug combination known as MOPP for the treatment of advanced Hodgkin's disease (DeVita *et al.*, 1970), survival has improved somewhat in the former disease and considerably in the latter. Nevertheless, the increasingly large number of patients developing acute leukemia following treatment with these drugs seems to implicate strongly the drugs as a direct or indirect cause of the leukemia.

The mechanisms whereby antineoplastic drugs produce acute leukemia and perhaps other second neoplasms are discussed in Chapter 4. Is the induction of chromosomal abnormalities by alkylating agents (Sieber and Adamson, 1975) directly or indirectly responsible for the leukemia? Do the drugs activate a latent leukemogenic virus? Is the development of leukemia a reparative response to the marrow hypoplasia or aplasia induced by the chemotherapy (Potolsky and Creger, 1973)? How do drugs potentiate the effects of radiation and vice versa? Why is radiation followed by chemotherapy more leukemogenic than the reverse? Do the drugs mediate their leukemogenicity by immunosuppression of the host? Do patients with multiple myeloma, Hodgkin's disease, and other neoplasms suffer from immunoincompetence even prior to any therapy? These questions require investigation.

The syndrome of acute leukemia as a second neoplasm has certain characteristic features. The syndrome is often preceded by a period of pancytopenia and/or dyserythropoiesis with or without the presence of ringed sideroblasts in the bone marrow. These changes may be related to previous chemotherapy. Also typical of this syndrome is the occurrence of chromosomal aberrations, mostly hypodiploidy with loss of a number 5 or 7 chromosome, but also hyperdiploidy (Rowley *et al.*, 1977). The hypodiploid chromosome number and karyotypic pattern support the notion that the leukemic cells arise independently of the Hodgkin's disease.

The syndrome of acute leukemia following treatment for a primary cancer is often associated with a refractoriness to antileukemic chemotherapy and a very short survival. However, although only 25% of such patients achieve complete or partial remission following specific antileukemic therapy, several complete remissions lasting more than two years have been reported (Beltran and Stuckey, 1978; Clément, 1979). Such treatment is, therefore, worth administering.

CAN WE REDUCE THE FREQUENCY OF SECOND NEOPLASMS?

What approaches are possible to reduce the risk of leukemia in these patients? Sultan (1976) has suggested that serial bone marrow cultures may help. Incipient marrow damage results in a reduced colony-forming capacity, and withdrawal of alkylating therapy may allow the marrow to recover. Another approach might be to substitute antimetabolites for alkylating agents wherever the choice is equal, since their carcinogenicity (if any) is certainly of a lesser degree. It may also be possible to obtain good therapeutic results with somewhat less aggressive multi-drug chemotherapy.

Unnecessary or unproved programs of combined radiation therapy and chemotherapy should be avoided. For patients with Hodgkin's disease Stages I, II, and IIIA, radiotherapy alone is probably sufficient, and chemotherapy might be reserved for the 10 to 40% of patients who have recurrence of their disease, and of whom more than half can be salvaged by chemotherapy (Hoppe *et al.*, 1980). Combination chemotherapy with six cycles of the MOPP program can be used for patients with Stages IIIB and IV disease and those who fail the initial radiation treatment. Perhaps six courses of MOPP are as effective as 9 or 12 courses, with significantly less immediate and late toxicity, including leukemia. Randomized clinical trials are needed to answer these questions.

For patients with acute leukemia achieving complete remission following intensive induction combination chemotherapy, the concept of maintenance therapy may have validity. However, for patients with lymphomas or other neoplasms who achieve complete remission from the neoplasm such maintenance chemotherapy may be not only unnecessary but, in fact, detrimental. Patients with Hodgkin's disease in remission who receive daily oral chlorambucil maintenance chemotherapy have a higher frequency of acute leukemia than comparable patients who were given no maintenance therapy (Glicksman *et al.*, 1982). In disseminated testicular cancer, maintenance chemotherapy following remission induction has been shown in a prospective study (Einhorn *et al.*, 1981) to be unnecessary. The duration of adjuvant chemotherapy for breast cancer (Bonadonna *et al.*, 1976) and other neoplasms is presently being evaluated.

The CMF regimen (cyclophosphamide, methotrexate and 5-fluorouracil) recommended by Bonadonna *et al.* (1976) contains at least one leukemogenic and carcinogenic agent. Perhaps another non-leukemogenic cytotoxic drug can substitute for cyclophosphamide in the CMF program without losing any of the therapeutic efficacy in the new combination. Perhaps the substitution of non-leukemogenic drugs for nitrogen mustard and/or procarbazine in the MOPP regimen for advanced Hodgkin's disease can provide equal therapeutic benefit but lesser incidence of leukemia or other second neoplasm. The ABVD regimen (adriamycin, bleomycin, vinblastine, and DTIC) is said to be associated with a lower incidence of acute leukemia as a late complication (Valagussa *et al.*, 1980) than is the MOPP combination.

Of even greater concern than the cancer patients terminating in acute leukemia are the patients with non-neoplastic diseases such as rheumatoid arthritis and renal disease who are treated with cytotoxic immunosuppressive chemotherapy and who develop acute leukemia (Grünwald and Rosner, 1979). We have described (Rosner and Grünwald, 1980b) 93 patients with non-neoplastic diseases treated with cytotoxic immunosuppressive drugs who developed acute leukemia. Eighty-four of the patients received single or multiple alkylating agent therapy. The increasing use of these drugs in the past decade is at least partly responsible for the sharp increase in incidence of leukemia in patients so treated.

In a recent review of 1884 recipients of renal transplants receiving immunosuppressive drugs (Sheil, 1977), 24% of patients surviving beyond five years with successful transplants had developed a malignant neoplasm. The necessity for continuous use of such immunosuppressive therapy has been seriously questioned (Sheriff *et al.*, 1978). Another review of 2006 patients receiving cyclophosphamide for the treatment of rheumatoid arthritis revealed the development of acute myeloid leukemia in 19 patients (Kahn *et al.*, 1979). Unless a patient has a life-threatening disorder, one should hesitate before using immunosuppressive cytotoxic drugs for indolent non-neoplastic diseases.

CONCLUSION

Acute myeloid leukemia or one of its variants is being reported with increasing frequency as a second neoplasm in patients being treated for multiple myeloma, Hodgkin's disease, non-Hodgkin's lymphoma, and a variety of other primary neoplasms. Although many of these patients were treated with both chemotherapy and radiotherapy, many received no radiotherapy at all. Drugs most frequently implicated in the causation of acute leukemia and other second neoplasms are the alkylating agents, procarbazine and the nitrosoureas.

Suggestions for reducing the frequency of second neoplasms include the possible substitution of non-leukemogenic antimetabolites for alkylating agents, the possible use of somewhat less aggressive multi-drug chemotherapy, and the elimination of adjuvant or 'maintenance' chemotherapy where such therapy has not been shown to be efficacious.

There could develop a reluctance to use cytotoxic agents to treat malignant neoplasms for fear of inducing acute leukemia. Although one has to consider this potential complication, one should certainly not withhold these drugs from a patient with a neoplasm (or other potentially fatal disease) for whom such therapy is the treatment of choice. We seem to be faced with the paradox that patients benefiting most from chemotherapy may be at highest risk to its undesirable consequences.

Meanwhile, the incidence of leukemia in patients treated either for cancer or non-neoplastic diseases with chemotherapy, or combined chemotherapy and radiotherapy, is still quite small and the number of patients benefited by such therapy is large. Although the risk of leukemogenesis or carcinogenesis in man may be small, these drugs should be used with caution in patients with indolent non-neoplastic diseases such as rheumatoid arthritis.

REFERENCES

Arkin, C. F., Kurtz, S. R., and Sparks, J. T. (1981). Acute B-cell leukemia occurring with Hodgkin's disease. *American Journal of Clinical Pathology*, **75**, 406–410.

Arsenau, J. C., Canellos, G. P., Johnson, R., and DeVita, V. T. (1977). Risk of new cancers in patients with Hodgkin's disease. *Cancer*, **40**, 1912–1916.

Beltran, G., and Stuckey, W. J. (1978). Successful therapy for acute myelogenous leukemia in patients with malignant lymphomas. *Blood*, **52**, 239 (Supplement) (Abstract 493).

Bennett, J. M., Catovsky, D., Daniel M. T. *et al.* (1976). Proposals for the classification of the acute leukemias. French-American-British (FAB) Cooperative Group. *British Journal of Haematology*, **33**, 451–458.

Bergsagel, D. E. (1982). Plasma cell neoplasms and acute leukemia. *Clinics in Haematology*, **11**, 221–234.

Bergsagel, D. E., Bailey, A. J., Langley, G. R. *et al.* (1979). The chemotherapy of plasma–cell myeloma and the incidence of acute leukemia. *New England Journal of Medicine*, **301**, 743–748.

Berk, P. D., Goldberg, J. D., Silverstein, M. N. *et al.* (1981). Increased incidence of acute leukemia in polycythemia vera associated with chlorambucil therapy. *New England Journal of Medicine*, **304**, 441–447.

Bonadonna, G., Brusamolino, E., Valagussa, P. *et al.* (1976). Combination chemotherapy as an adjuvant treatment in operable breast cancer. *New England Journal of Medicine*, **294**, 405–410.

Borum, K. (1980). Increasing frequency of acute myeloid leukemia complicating Hodgkin's disease. A review. *Cancer*, **46**, 1247–1252.

Boucheix, C., Zittoun, R., Reynes, M. *et al.* (1979). Atypical T-cell leukemia terminating Hodgkin's disease. *Cancer*, **44**, 1403–1407.

Brodsky, I. (1982). Busulfan treatment of polycythemia vera. *British Journal of Haematology*, **52**, 1–6.

Brody, R. S., and Schottenfeld, D. (1980). Multiple primary cancers in Hodgkin's disease. *Seminars in Oncology*, **7**, 187–201.

Bryant, E., Ronan, S. G., and Iossifides, I. A. (1982). Plasma cell myeloma in a patient with cutaneous T-cell lymphoma. *Cancer*, **50**, 2122–2125.

Carobell, S. C., Chaffey, J. T., Rosenthal, D. S. *et al.* (1979). Results of total body irradiation in the treatment of advanced non-Hodgkin's lymphoma. *Cancer*, **43**, 994–1000.

Catovsky, D., Costello, C. Loukopoulos, D. *et al.* (1981). Hairy cell leukemia and myelomatosis: chance association or clinical manifestations of the same B-cell disease spectrum. *Blood*, **57**, 758–763.

Cavallin-Stahl, E., Landberg, T., Ottow, Z., and Mittelman, F. (1977). Hodgkin's disease and acute leukemia. A clinical and cytogenetic study. *Scandinavian Journal of Haematology*, **19**, 273–280.

Clément, F. (1979). Les hémopathies malignes induites. Six nouvelles observations dont l'une avec survie de 45 ans. *Schweizerische Medizinische Wochenschrift*, **109**, 544–551.

Coleman, C. N., Williams C. J., Flint, A. *et al.* (1977). Hematologic neoplasia in patients treated for Hodgkin's disease. *New England Journal of Medicine*, **297**, 1249–1252.

Coltman, C. A. Jr., and Dixon, D. O. (1982). Second malignancies complicating Hodgkin's disease: a Southwest oncology group 10 year follow-up. *Cancer Treatment Reports*, **66**, 1023–1033.

Crosby, W. H. (1969). Acute granulocytic leukemia, a complication of therapy in Hodgkin's disease? *Clinical Research*, **17**, 463.

Dameshek, W. (1951). Some speculations on the myeloproliferative syndromes. *Blood*, **6**, 372–375.

DeVita, V. T., Serpick, A., and Carbone, P. P. (1970). Combination chemotherapy in the treatment of advanced Hodgkin's disease. *Annals of Internal Medicine*, **73**, 881–895.

Dubovsky, D., and Jacobs, P. (1974). Acute leukemia and myeloma. *Lancet*, **1**, 1113–1114.

Dumont, J., Thiery, J. P., Mazabraud, A. *et al.* (1980). Acute myeloid leukemia following non-Hodgkin's lymphoma: danger of prolonged use of chlorambucil as maintenance therapy. *Nouvelle Revue Française D'Hématologie*, **22**, 391–404.

Einhorn, L. H., Williams, S. D., Troner, M. *et al.* (1981). The role of maintenance therapy in disseminated testicular cancer. *New England Journal of Medicine*, **305**, 727–731.

Erskine, J.G., Wang, I., and Hutton M.M. (1977). Chronic granulocytic leukaemia developing upon a follicular lymphoma. *British Medical Journal*, **4**, 1329.

Garwicz, S., Aronson, S., Andréasson, B. *et al.* (1978). Hodgkin's disease during acute leukemia in remission. *Lancet*, **1**, 269.

Gatti, R. A., and Good, R. A. (1971). Occurrence of malignancy in immunodeficiency diseases. *Cancer*, **28**, 89–98.

Glicksman, A. S., Pajak, T. F., Gottlieb, A. *et al.* (1982). Second malignant neoplasms in patients successfully treated for Hodgkin's disease: a Cancer and Leukemia Group B study. *Cancer Treatment Reports*, **66**, 1035–1044.

Golde, D. W., Saxon, A., and Stevens, R. H. (1977). Macroglobulinemia and hairy cell leukemia. *New England Journal of Medicine*, **296**, 92–93.

Gonzalez, F., Trujillo, J. M., and Alexanian, R. (1977). Acute leukemia in multiple myeloma. *Annals of Internal Medicine*, **86**, 440–443.

Grünwald, H. W., and Rosner, F. (1979). Acute leukemia and immunosuppressive drug use. A review of patients undergoing immunosuppressive therapy for non-neoplastic diseases. *Archives of Internal Medicine*, **139**, 461–466.

Grünwald, H. W., and Rosner, F. (1982). Acute myeloid leukemia following treatment of Hodgkin's disease: a review. *Cancer*, **50**, 676–683.

Hamilton, P. J. (1976). Concomitant myeloblastic and lymphocytic leukemia. *Lancet*, **1**, 373.

Herrmann, R., Han, T., Barcos, M. P. *et al.* (1980). Malignant lymphoma of pre-T-cell type terminating in acute myelocytic leukemia. *Cancer*, **46**, 1383–1388.

Hoppe, R. T., Rosenberg, S. A., Kaplan, H. S., and Cox, R. S. (1980). Prognostic factors in pathological stage III-A Hodgkin's disease. *Cancer*, **46**, 1240–1246.

Jouet, J. P., Huart, J. J., Bauters, F., and Goudemand, M. (1979). Leucémies aigües compliquant la maladie de Hodgkin. Cinq nouvelles observations. *Nouvelle Presse Médicale*, **8**, 613–614.

Kahn, M. F., Arlet, J., Bloch-Michel, H. *et al.* (1979). Leucémies aigües après traitement par agents cytotoxique en rhumatologie. 19 observations chex 2006 patients. *Nouvelle Presse Médicale*, **8**, 1393–1397.

Kaur, P., Miller, D. R., Andreeff, M. *et al.* (1981). Acute myeloblastic leukemia following non-Hodgkin lymphoma in an adolescent. A report of a case with preleukemic syndrome and review of the literature. *Medical and Pediatric Oncology*, **9**, 69–80.

Kersey, J. H., Spector, B. D., and Good, R. A. (1973). Primary immunodeficiency diseases and cancer: the immunodeficiency-cancer registry. *International Journal of Cancer*, **12**, 333–347.

Kuse, R., and Hausmann, K. (1977). Akute myeloische leukämie im krankeits verlauf des morbus Hodgkin. *Deutsche Medizinische Wochenschrift*, **102**, 1824.

Kyle, R. A. (1982). Second malignancies associated with chemotherapeutic agents. *Seminars in Oncology*, **9**, 131–142.

Larsen, J., and Brincker, H. (1977). The incidence and characteristics of acute myeloid leukaemia arising in Hodgkin's disease. *Scandinavian Journal of Haematology*, **18**, 197–206.

Law, I. P., and Blom, J. (1977). Second malignancies in patients with multiple myeloma. *Oncology*, **34**, 20–24.

Lawlor, E., McCann, S. R., Whelan, A. *et al.* (1979). Acute myeloid leukaemia occurring in untreated chronic lymphatic leukaemia. *British Journal of Haematology*, **43**, 369–373.

Lerner, H. (1977). Second malignancies diagnosed in breast cancer patients while receiving adjuvant chemotherapy at the Pennsylvania hospital. *Proceedings of the American Association for Cancer Research*, **18**, 340 (Abstract #C-295).

Louie, S., Daost, P. R., and Schwartz, R. S. (1980). Immunodeficiency and the pathogenesis of non-Hodgkin's lymphoma. *Seminars in Oncology*, **7**, 267–284.

Madoff, L., Davey, F. R., Gordon, G. B. *et al.* (1981). The development of acute myelomonocytic leukemia in a patient with acute lymphocytic leukemia. *Cancer*, **48**, 1157–1163.

Marcovic, N., Hansson, G. B., and Hallen, J. (1974). Myelomatosis and acute monocytic leukemia. *Scandinavian Journal of Haematology*, **12**, 32–36.

Marino, R., Altshuler, G., and Humphrey, G. B. (1979). Idiopathic myelofibrosis followed by acute lymphoblastic leukemia. *American Journal of Diseases of Children*, **133**, 1194–1195.

Nassar, V. H., Jacobs, J., Mirra, S. S. *et al.* (1982). Burkitt cell leukemia following therapy for Hodgkin disease. *American Journal of Hematology*, **12**, 73–76.

Neufeld, H., Weinerman, B. H., and Kemel, S. (1978). Secondary malignant neoplasms in patients with Hodgkin's disease. *Journal of the American Medical Association*, **239**, 2470–2471.

Pedersen-Bjergaard, J., and Larsen, S. O. (1982). Incidence of acute non-lymphocytic leukemia, preleukemia, and acute myeloproliferative syndrome up to 10 years after treatment of Hodgkin's disease. *New England Journal of Medicine*, **307**, 965–971.

Penn, I. (1974). Chemical immunosuppression and human cancer. *Cancer*, **34**, 1474–1480.

Penn, I. (1976). Second malignant neoplasms associated with immunosuppressive medications. *Cancer*, **37**, 1024–1032.

Penn, I. (1977). Development of cancer as a complication of clinical transplantation. *Transplantation Proceedings*, **9**, 1121–1127.

Penn, I. (1978). Malignancies associated with immunosuppressive or cytotoxic therapy. *Surgery*, **83**, 492–502.

Pezzinenti, J. F., Kim, H. C., and Lindenbaum, J. (1976). Erythroleukemia-like syndrome due to busulfan toxicity in polycythemia vera. *Cancer*, **38**, 2242–2246.

Potolsky, A., and Creger, W. P. (1973). Radiation and drug therapies, and leukemia. *Annual Review of Medicine*, **24**, 75–82.

Puckett, J. B., and Cooper, M. R. (1981). Acute myelofibrosis evolving into acute myeloblastic leukemia. *Annals of Internal Medicine*, **94**, 545–546.

Rosenthal, D. S., and Moloney, W. C. (1977). Occurrence of acute leukaemia in myeloproliferative disorders. *British Journal of Haematology*, **36**, 373–382.

Rosner, F., and Grünwald, H. W. (1980a). Multiple myeloma and Waldenström's macroglobulinemia terminating in acute leukemia. Review with emphasis on karyotypic and ultrastructural abnormalities. *New York State Journal of Medicine*, **80**, 558–570.

Rosner, F., and Grünwald, H. W. (1980b). Cytotoxic drugs and leukaemogenesis. *Clinics in Haematology*, **9**, 663–681.

Rosner, F., and Grünwald, H. W. (1983). Hodgkin's disease terminating in non-Hodgkin's lymphoma: a review (in preparation).

Rowley, J. D., Golomb, M. H., and Vardiman, J. (1977). Nonrandom chromosomal abnormalities in acute nonlymphocytic leukemia in patients treated for Hodgkin's disease and non-Hodgkin's lymphomas. *Blood*, **50**, 759–770.

Saleem, A., and Johnston, R. L. (1980). Acute lymphoblastic leukemia following Hodgkin's disease. *Annals of Clinical and Laboratory Science*, **10**, 100–104.

Schmähl, D. (1977). Carcinogenic action of anticancer drugs with special reference to immunosuppression. *Cancer*, **40**, 1927–1929.

Sebahoun, G., Blanc, A. P., Sainty, D. *et al.* (1980). Syndrome de Richter et transformation aigue: deux complications hematologiques terminales de la leucémie lymphoide chronique. *Semaine Hôpital de Paris,* **56,** 414–417.

Sheil, A. G. R. (1977). Cancer in renal allograft recipients in Australia and New Zealand. *Transplantation Proceedings,* **9,** 1135–1136.

Sheriff, M.H.R., Yayha, T., and Lee, H.A. (1978). Is azathioprine necessary in renal transplantation? *Lancet,* **1,** 118–120.

Sieber, S. M., and Adamson, R. H. (1975). Toxicity of antineoplastic agents in man: chromosomal aberrations, antifertility effects, congenital malformations and carcinogenic potential. *Advances in Cancer Research,* **22,** 57–155.

Stern, N., Shemesh, J., and Ramot, B. (1981). Chronic lymphatic leukemia terminating in acute myeloid leukemia: review of the literature. *Cancer,* **47,** 1849–1851.

Sultan, C. in discussion following: Tchernia, G., Mielot, F., Subtil E., and Parmentier, C. (1976). Acute myeloblastic leukemia after immunodepressive therapy for primary nonmalignant disease. *Blood Cells,* **2,** 78.

Sultan, C., Sigaux, F., Imbert, M., and Reyes, F. (1981). Acute myelodysplasia with myelofibrosis: a report of eight cases. *British Journal of Haematology,* **49,** 11–16.

Svahn-Tapper, G., Baldetorp, L., and Landberg, T. (1976). Mantle treatment of Hodgkin's disease. Results and side effects. *Acta Radiologica (Therapy Physics Biology),* **15,** 369–386.

Swain, W. R., Windschitt, H. E., Doscherhoimen, A. *et al.* (1971). Chronic myelogenous leukemia in Hodgkin's disease: immunofluorescence of cells. *Cancer,* **27,** 569–573.

Toland, D. M., Coltman, C. A. Jr., and Moon, T. E. (1978). Second malignancies complicating Hodgkin's disease: the Southwest Oncology Group experience. *Cancer Clinical Trials,* **1,** 27–33.

Valagussa, P., Santoro, A., Kenda, R. *et al.* (1980). Second malignancies in Hodgkin's disease: a complication of certain forms of treatment. *British Medical Journal,* **280,** 216–219

Waldenström, J. (1964). Melphalan therapy in myelomatosis. *British Medical Journal,* **1,** 859–865.

Walpole, A. L. (1958). Carcinogenic action of alkylating agents. *Annals of the New York Academy of Sciences,* **68,** 750–761.

Wilson, B. D., and Van Slyck, E. J. (1966). Coexistent lymphosarcoma and chronic granulocytic leukemia. *Cancer,* **19,** 809–816.

Wingen, A. M., Olischläger, A., and Kleihauer, E. (1979). Morbus Hodgkin als zweiterkrankung bei akuter lymphatischer leukämie. *Klinische Pädiatrie,* **191,** 1–7.

Wolf, M. M., Cooper, I. A., and Ding, J. C. (1979). Hodgkin's disease terminating in acute leukemia: report of seven cases. *Australia, New Zealand Journal of Medicine,* **9,** 398–402.

Woodruff, R. K., Lister, T. A., Brearley, R. L. *et al.* (1977). Hodgkin's disease occurring during acute leukemia in remission. *Lancet,* **2,** 900–903.

Yeung, K. Y., and Trowbridge, A. A. (1977). Idiopathic acquired sideroblastic anemia terminating in acute myelofibrosis. *Cancer,* **39,** 359–365.

Zarrabi, M. H., Grünwald, H. W., and Rosner, F. (1977). Chronic lymphocytic leukemia terminating in acute leukemia. *Archives of Internal Medicine,* **137,** 1059–1064.

Zarrabi, M. H., Rosner, F., and Bennett, J. M. (1979). Non-Hodgkin's lymphoma and acute myeloblastic leukemia. A report of 12 cases and review of the literature. *Cancer,* **44,** 1070–1080.

Zarrabi, M. H., Rosner, F., and Grünwald, H. W. (1983). Second neoplasms in acute lymphoblastic leukemia. *Cancer,* **52,** 1712–1719.

Index